Student Learning Guide

Medical-Surgical Nursing

Concepts & Practice

Susan C. deWit, MSN, RN, CNS, PHN
Formerly, Instructor of Nursing
El Centro College
Dallas, Texas

Candice K. Kumagai, MSN, RN
Clinical Instructor
Dallas County Community College District
Dallas, Texas

SAUNDERS
ELSEVIER

SAUNDERS
ELSEVIER

11830 Westline Industrial Drive
St. Louis, Missouri 63146

STUDENT LEARNING GUIDE FOR *MEDICAL-SURGICAL NURSING: CONCEPTS & PRACTICE*

ISBN 13: 978-1-4160-5011-7
ISBN 10: 1-4160-5011-6

ISBN 13: 978-1-4160-5011-7
ISBN 10: 1-4160-5011-6

Executive Publisher: Tom Wilhelm
Managing Editor: Robin Levin Richman
Developmental Editor: Mayoor Jaiswal
Publishing Services Manager: Jeffrey Patterson
Senior Production Manager: Mary G. Stueck

Printed in the United States of America

Last digit is the print number: 9 8 7 6 5 4 3

To the Student

The *Student Learning Guide* has been constructed to assist you in achieving the objectives of each textbook chapter and establishing a solid base of knowledge in medical-surgical nursing. Completing the exercises in this guide will help to reinforce the material studied in the textbook and learned in class. Additional exercises and activities are provided on the Evolve web site for this textbook. Many exercises will assist you to develop solid critical thinking and priority setting skills. Some exercises require you to call upon previously learned information and to synthesize to reach an answer. Completing the exercises will help you be successful on the NCLEX-PN® Exam.

In an effort to assist Limited English Proficient (LEP) students in mastering communication in English, a section has been included in each chapter called *Steps Toward Better Communication*. The exercises in this section are aimed at improving communication while reinforcing the content of the chapter. The exercises have been constructed so that they will be helpful to other students as well.

STUDY HINTS FOR ALL STUDENTS

Ask Questions!

There are no stupid questions. If you do not know something or are not sure, you need to find out. Other people may be wondering the same thing but may be too shy to ask. The answer could mean life or death to your patient! That is certainly more important than feeling embarrassed about asking a question.

Chapter Objectives

At the beginning of each chapter in the textbook are objectives that you should have mastered when you finish studying that chapter. Write these objectives in your notebook, leaving a blank space after each. Fill in the answers as you find them while reading the chapter. Review to make sure your answers are correct and complete. Use these answers when you study for tests. This should also be done for separate course objectives that your instructor has listed in your class syllabus.

Reading Hints

When reading each chapter in the textbook, look at the subject headings to learn what each section is about. Read first for the general meaning. Then reread parts you did not understand. It may help to read those parts aloud. Carefully read the information given in each table and study each figure and its caption.

Concepts

While studying, put difficult concepts into your own words to see if you understand them. Check this understanding with another student or the instructor. Write these in your notebook.

Key Points

Use the Key Points at the end of each chapter in the textbook to help you recall topic information. Try to elaborate about the topic of each key point from what you have learned.

Class Notes

When taking lecture notes in class, leave a large margin on the left side of each notebook page and write only on right-hand pages, leaving all left-hand pages blank. Look over your lecture notes soon after each class, while your memory is fresh. Fill in missing words, complete sentences and ideas, and underline key phases, definitions, and concepts. At the top of each page, write the topic of that page. In the left margin, write the key word for that part of your notes. On the opposite left-hand page, write a summary or outline that combines material from both the textbook and the lecture. These can be your study notes for review.

Study Groups

Form a study group with some other students so you can help one another. Practice speaking and reading aloud. Ask questions about material you are not sure about. Work together to find answers. Attempt to answer the textbook and syllabus objectives in your own words.

References for Improving Study Skills

Good study skills are essential for achieving your goals in nursing. Time management, efficient use of study time, and a consistent approach to studying are all beneficial. There are various study methods for reading a textbook and for taking class notes. Some methods that have proven helpful can be found in *Saunders Student Planner*. This book contains helpful information on test taking and preparing for clinical experiences. It includes an example of a "time map" for planning study time and a blank form that you can use to formulate a personal time map. Another good study reference is Palau and Meltzer's *Learning Strategies for Allied Health Students* (Saunders, 2007).

ADDITIONAL STUDY HINTS FOR ESL/LEP STUDENTS

First-Language Buddy

LEP/ESL students should find a first-language buddy—another student who is a native speaker of English and who is willing to answer questions about word meanings, pronunciations, and culture. You might schedule some study time together. Maybe your buddy would like to learn about your language and culture too. This could help in his or her nursing experience as well.

Vocabulary Notebook

Keep a small alphabetized notebook or address book in your pocket or purse. Write down new non-technical words you read or hear along with their meanings and pronunciations. Write each word under its initial letter (A, B, etc.) so you can find it easily, as in a dictionary. For words you do not know or for words that have a different meaning in nursing, write down how they are used and sound. Look up their meanings in a dictionary or ask your instructor or first-language buddy. Then write the different meanings or usages that you have found in your book, including the nursing meaning. Continue to add new words as you discover them. For example:

Primary
- the most important; main: the primary problem or disease
- the first one; elementary: primary school

Secondary
- less important; resulting from another problem or disease: a secondary symptom
- the second one; secondary school (in the United States, high school)

Vocabulary

If you find a non-technical word you do not know (e.g., *drowsy*), try to guess its meaning from the sentence (e.g., *With electrolyte imbalance, the patient may feel fatigued and drowsy*). If you are not sure of the meaning, or if it seems especially important, look it up in the dictionary. Many of these words are included in the Vocabulary Building Glossary in each chapter of the *Student Learning Guide*. It is useful to look at this glossary before reading the chapter. (If you guessed that drowsy means something like sleepy, you were correct!)

If there is a technical word you do not understand or remember, look for it in the Vocabulary Building Glossary in this guide, in the index at the back of the textbook, or in your medical dictionary. Write it in your notebook. Keep an alphabetical list of words you have difficulty remembering so you can look them up easily and review them before a test.

Pronunciation Notes

The pronunciation of words in the Vocabulary Building Glossary in each chapter in this guide is shown by a simple respelling. It follows the pronunciation guide in Miller-Keane *Encyclopedia and Dictionary of Medicine, Nursing, and Allied Health, 7th edition* (Saunders, 2006):

Long Vowels: "Long" vowels (a, e, i, o, u, y) are pronounced with the sound of the name of the letter.

1. An unmarked vowel ending a syllable is long *(ba' be=baby).*
2. A long vowel in a syllable ending with a consonant is marked with a long symbol or macron (¯) *(be hāv'yer).*

Short Vowels: "Short" vowels have varying pronunciations.

3. An unmarked vowel in a syllable ending with a consonant is short *(ab dukt'=abduct).*
4. A short vowel at the end of a syllable is marked with a short mark or breve (˘) *(lip ĭ do' sis).* Sometimes, the vowel is followed by a silent *h* instead of using the breve *(lip ih do' sis).*
5. Some sounds are represented by two letters:
   - ah': In stressed syllables, *ah* represents the "a" sound heard in father *(fah' ther).*
   - ah: In unstressed syllables, *ah* represents the "a" sound heard in sofa *(so'fah).* (It often sounds like uh. This sound, called a *schwa,* is represented in many dictionaries by an upside-down *e.* Many people pronounce any unaccented vowel as a schwa.)
   - aw: The *aw* in paw.
   - oi: The *oi* in oil.
   - oo: The *oo* in food.
   - ou: The *ou* in out.
6. A stressed syllable is indicated by an accent mark (') at the end of the syllable.

Good Luck!

Susan C. deWit, Candice Kumagai, and Gail Boehme, ESL Consultant

To the Instructor

The *Student Learning Guide for Medical-Surgical Nursing: Concepts & Practice* is designed to provide reinforcement for the terms and concepts presented in the text. It will assist students to set priorities, apply the nursing process, practice critical thinking, make good judgments and decisions, increase ability to communicate therapeutically, and meet chapter objectives.

ORGANIZATION OF THE TEXT

Included are a wide variety of exercises, questions, and activities. Most chapters include Terminology, Short Answer, NCLEX-PN® Exam Review, Critical Thinking Activities, and a special section called *Steps Toward Better Communication* written by a specialist in English as a second language. Other sections that appear where appropriate are Completion, Identification, Review of Structure and Function, Priority Setting, and Application of Nursing Process. Additional activities and exercises, including Meeting Clinical Objectives, are provided on the Evolve web site for the textbook.

Description of Exercises

The exercises are as follows:

- **Terminology** – matching or fill-in-the-blank questions to reinforce correct use of words from the chapter terms list.
- **Short Answer** – list of brief answers to reinforce knowledge and assist students to meet the chapter objectives.
- **NCLEX-PN® Exam Review** – questions in NCLEX-PN® format (both multiple choice and new alternate item formats), based on real-life situations and requiring knowledge, synthesis, analysis, evaluation, and application.
- **Critical Thinking Activities** – brief scenarios and questions to foster problem-solving skills in nursing care which may be practiced individually or in study groups.
- **Completion** – this exercise reinforces the chapter content with fill-in-the-blank questions.
- **Identification** – the student names appropriate steps in a process or procedure or verifies normal or abnormal laboratory values.
- **Review of Structure and Function** – this is re-examination of the anatomy and physiology of the body system pertinent to the text chapter.
- **Priority Setting** – students analyze information and make decisions to set priorities within tasks or clinical situations.
- **Application of the Nursing Process** – critical thinking skills are used and the steps of the nursing process are applied to real-life patient care.
- **Meeting Clinical Objectives** (Evolve) – suggestions for practicing learned skills and obtaining experience in the clinical area. These exercises help students meet the clinical practice objectives and encourage focusing on the school's clinical objectives. These exercises are found on the Evolve web site for the textbook.

All answers to the exercises are included in the TEACH Instructor Resources on Evolve web site for *Medical-Surgical Nursing: Concepts & Practice*. The answers can be printed out and put on reserve in the library or posted so that students can check them should the instructor choose not to use the *Student Learning Guide* for class credit activities.

Students with Limited English Proficiency

Because so many students from other countries, whose primary language is not English, are entering nursing programs in the United States and Canada, we have enlisted the aid of a specialist in English as a Second Language who has worked with many health care occupation students. She helped construct the exercises in the *Steps Toward Better Communication* within each chapter. Her letter to you follows. I hope you find this section helpful to your students with limited English proficiency.

Susan C. deWit, MSN, RN, CNS, PHN

STEPS TOWARD BETTER COMMUNICATION

Imagine yourself back in nursing school – trying to read the texts and understand the lectures in Spanish or German. Students studying in a language that is not their native language face not only the challenge of learning the medical and physiological lessons that are required of all nursing students, but they must also decipher and use a language whose nuances and grammar are unfamiliar to them. In order to ease some of that burden, we've attempted to simplify and regularize the language of *Medical-Surgical Nursing: Concepts & Practice* and the student learning guide, and to explain some of the colloquial uses of English that occur.

A major part of the nursing process could be described as "knowing your patient inside and out," and one key to that knowledge is being able to accurately and sensitively communicate with the patient and colleagues. To this end, after the regular exercises, we added a section for the ESL student titled *Steps Toward Better Communication*, which offers help in pronunciation, vocabulary building, and use of grammatical issues such as verb tense, and encourages asking for help and clarification. In addition, a section on understanding cultural nuances and mannerisms helps student face real-life situations and clarify feelings. Another section offers facility in appropriately asking questions and carrying on conversations.

A note about pronunciation: we assume that the important medical terms will be used and modeled correctly by the instructor. In terms of conversation, intelligibility rather than native-like accuracy should be the goal. Correct stress is the major determining factor in how easily a person can be understood. Therefore, we chose to indicate stressed syllables in words and phrases, rather than giving phonetic pronunciations that students often find difficult to understand.

Description of Exercises

The following exercises appear in the *Steps Toward Better Communication* section as appropriate.

- **Vocabulary Building Glossary** – explains and defines idiomatic or unusual use of non-medical terms used in the chapter and indicates the stressed syllables for capitalizing them.
- **Completion Sentences** – offer opportunities to use the words presented in the Glossary, often in different context than they are used in the text, thereby offering yet another way to increase vocabulary.
- **Vocabulary Exercises** – use words from the chapter in various ways to increase ease of understanding.
- **Word Attack Skills** – deal with word segments, suffixes, prefixes, and types of words to help the student learn to decode new words and their usage.
- **Pronunciation Skills** – offer practice in pronouncing difficult terms as well as phrases and sentences, with emphasis on stress and intonation.
- **Grammar Points** – are made occasionally, especially when there is a recurring point raised by the chapter, such as the use of the past tense in taking case histories.
- **Communication Exercises** – encourage communicative interchange, writing, and dialogues that might actually be used by a practicing nurse. The value of this section is enhanced if students can be paired in first- and second-language speaker combinations, giving each the opportunity to experience the other's accent and offering the possibility for cross-cultural exchange. Answers to the Communication Exercises are provided in the TEACH Instructor Resources on Evolve web site for the text, and could be printed out for student use.

- **Cultural Point(s)** – present explanations and questions about issues and customs that may differ across the cultures represented in the class, and in the prospective patient community. They can explain the normative culture in which the individual will be working, while at the same time, acknowledge and validate an individual's cultural difference.

In preparing these materials, I have drawn on my teaching experience of practicing and aspiring health care personnel. I have found them to be dedicated and eager to improve their own lives while helping others. I have learned much from them about hard work, perseverance, humor, and what they need in order to do a better job. My colleagues in teaching English, and nurses with whom I have worked have been helpful with ideas for teaching projects, indicating language areas needing to be addressed, and offering suggestions and solutions for problems. However, any omissions and errors are my own.

I have been impressed with the similarity between learning language skills and nursing skills. Both require access to academic knowledge, but mastery occurs with hands-on practice and experience. The exercises are geared to provide this opportunity. Encourage your students to interact as often as possible. Look at each lesson with the question, "How can I structure this lesson so the students will have to generate their own language to complete the exercise?" Offer real-life challenges and tasks for speaking and communicative interaction with other students, colleagues, and patients whenever possible. An encouraging, open, and interactive classroom is the best setting for language learning and improvement. I wish you well in working with this special group of people.

Gail G. Boehme, BA
ESL Teaching Certification
University of California at Santa Barbara

Illustration Credits

Chapter 17

Ignatavicius, D.D., & Workman, M.L. (2006). *Medical-Surgical Nursing: Critical Thinking for Collaborative Care* (5th ed.). Philadelphia: Saunders.

Chapter 19

Aehlert, B. (2002). *EKGs Made Easy* (2nd ed.). St. Louis: Mosby.

Chapter 29

deWit, S.C. (2005). *Fundamental Concepts and Skills for Nursing* (2nd ed.). Philadelphia: Saunders.

Chapter 33

Lewis, S.M., Heitkemper, M.M., & Dirksen, S.R. (2007). *Medical- Surgical Nursing: Assessment and Management of Clinical Problems* (7th ed.). St. Louis: Mosby.

Chapter 34

Ignatavicius, D. D., & Workman, M. L. (2006). *Medical–Surgical Nursing: Critical Thinking for Collaborative Care* (5th ed.). Philadelphia: W.B. Saunders.

Chapter 42

Lewis, S.M., Heitkemper, M.M., Dirksen, S.R., et al. (2007). *Medical-Surgical Nursing: Assessment and Management of Clinical Problems* (7th ed.). St. Louis: Mosby.

Contents

CHAPTER 1

Caring for Medical-Surgical Patients

evolve Go to http://evolve.elsevier.com/deWit for additional activities and exercises.

SHORT ANSWER

Health Care System

Directions: Provide the answers to the following questions.

1. List three factors that contribute to the rising cost of health care. *(7)*

   a. ______________________________

   b. ______________________________

   c. ______________________________

2. List at least six indicators that reflect the major health concerns according to the U.S. *Healthy People 2010* agenda. *(7)*

   a. ______________________________

   b. ______________________________

   c. ______________________________

   d. ______________________________

   e. ______________________________

   f. ______________________________

Nursing Functions and Responsibilities

Directions: Provide the answers to the following questions.

1. List the four functions of the LPN/LVN. *(2, 3)*

   a. ______________________________

   b. ______________________________

   c. ______________________________

   d. ______________________________

2. What are the five rights of delegation according to The National Council of State Boards of Nursing's position paper, *Delegation: Concepts and Decision-Making Process (NCSBN:1996)*? ***(4)***

   a. ______________________________

   b. ______________________________

   c. ______________________________

   d. ______________________________

   e. ______________________________

3. Describe three ways in which you as a nurse can actively participate in health promotion and disease prevention. ***(2)***

   a. ______________________________

   b. ______________________________

   c. ______________________________

4. List at least five examples of patient teaching activities performed by the LPN/LVN. ***(2)***

   a. ______________________________

   b. ______________________________

   c. ______________________________

   d. ______________________________

   e. ______________________________

COMPLETION

Directions: Fill in the blanks to complete the statements.

1. Delegation is ____________________ to competent unlicensed assistive personnel (UAP) the authority to perform a selected nursing task/activity in a selected patient situation that is within the job description of the LPN/LVN. ***(3)***
2. The traditional method of financing health care services, ______________________________ involves direct reimbursement by an insurance company to a provider. ***(5)***
3. In all clinical situations, the LPN/LVN has the opportunity to identify ____________________ and ____________________ routines in the work setting; correction of these problems contributes to cost containment. ***(7)***
4. Delegation is a ______________________________ function. ***(3)***
5. You must provide unlicensed assistive personnel with the necessary ________________, ____________________, ________________________, and ____________________ to safely carry out the delegated task/activity. ***(4)***

SHORT ANSWER

Dealing with Different Patient Behaviors

Directions: Read the clinical scenario and answer the questions that follow.

Scenario A: Mrs. Gay, age 78, has been hospitalized for a broken hip. She is very quiet, does not seem to want to be touched, and responds with "I'm just fine" when asked if she is worried about anything.

1. Mrs. Gay's behavior is typical of anxiety or fear and is an expression of a need for ____. *(10)*

2. Write four appropriate nursing interventions to help meet Mrs. Gay's needs and modify her withdrawn behavior. *(11)*

   a. ______________________________

   b. ______________________________

   c. ______________________________

   d. ______________________________

Scenario B: Mr. Tong has had one arm amputated as a result of injuries suffered in an automobile accident. He has supported his wife and three small children by working as a carpenter. During his hospitalization, Mr. Tong has become increasingly abusive and critical and has threatened to report his nurse on several occasions. *(10)*

1. Mr. Tong's behavior probably indicates feelings of ______________ and ______________.

2. His hostile behavior is an expression of a need to ____.

3. Write three appropriate nursing interventions to satisfy Mr. Tong's need and modify his behavior.

   a. ______________________________

   b. ______________________________

   c. ______________________________

Scenario C: Mrs. Barton has become manipulative with the nursing staff. She is demanding and attempts to bargain to get out of what she is supposed to do for rehabilitation after her myocardial infarction. She insists that she get something other than the broiled chicken breast for dinner, stating that she wants steak, mashed potatoes, and gravy. She announces that she will not walk in the halls anymore until she gets something "decent" to eat.

1. List four nursing interventions and approaches that might help in dealing with Mrs. Barton's behavior. *(11)*

   a. ______________________________

   b. ______________________________

   c. ______________________________

   d. ______________________________

PRIORITY SETTING

Directions: Read the scenario and prioritize as appropriate. (11)

Scenario: You are caring for five patients. They have various behavioral issues that you must address. Prioritize the order in which you will assist these patients with their needs.

_____ a. Mrs. Bora is calling for assistance to the bathroom. She is capable of managing this for herself, but she routinely calls for assistance for many tasks that she can do for herself.

_____ b. Mr. Foegelle has locked himself in the bathroom. The nursing assistant is speaking to him through the door, but he "wants some time to himself."

_____ c. Mr. Ahrens is yelling at his wife. You can hear him say, "These nurses are so stupid. You should have never brought me here! You are stupid too!"

_____ d. Ms. Schott wants you to immediately call her doctor. "Call him right this second, or I will make sure you get fired for incompetence!"

_____ e. Mr. McGinnis refuses to get out of bed. The nursing assistant has tried to encourage him, but he just gazes off and then starts crying.

NCLEX-PN® EXAM REVIEW

Directions: Choose the best answer(s) for the following questions.

1. The LPN/LVN assigns the certified nursing assistant to give a patient a tap water enema. During the procedure, the patient is burned because the nursing assistant uses water that is too hot. Who is held accountable for this incident? *(3)*
   1. RN
   2. Nursing assistant
   3. Hospital
   4. LPV/LVN

2. The doctor asks the LPN/LVN student to hang a unit of blood on a patient who has suddenly become very critical. The best action would be to: *(2)*
   1. follow the doctor's orders because of the emergency situation.
   2. refuse to do it and explain that it is outside the scope of practice.
   3. immediately get an RN to assist the physician.
   4. obtain the equipment for the doctor, but tell him that he will have to hang the blood himself.

3. The nurse must be instrumental in helping contain the cost of health care. This can be accomplished by doing which of the following? *(Select all that apply.) (7)*
   1. Follow policies for charging for supplies used in patient care.
   2. Document patient care for reimbursement.
   3. Reuse and recycle supplies whenever possible.
   4. Organize patient care for effective and efficient use of time.
   5. Decrease patient length of stay by recommending patients leave.

4. The nurse is caring for a patient who is depressed about his health condition and he is concerned about how it will affect his ability to care for his family. He tells the nurse, "I just don't know how my wife is going to cope if I die." What is the best response? ***(10)***
   1. "You are not going to die. For goodness sakes, cheer up! Don't be so pessimistic."
   2. "What makes you think you are going to die? Your prognosis is actually quite good."
   3. "Your wife is coming to see you today and you wouldn't want her to worry about this or about you."
   4. "It sounds like you are really worried about several issues. What have you been thinking about?"

5. The patient is constantly using the call bell and the entire nursing staff is quite frustrated with and tired of this behavior. A team approach to help the patient gain independence would be to: ***(11)***
   1. assign a different nurse every day to prevent the patient's dependency on one person.
   2. tell the patient that someone will check on him every 30 minutes if he does not use the call bell.
   3. refuse to answer the call bell if the patient uses it too much.
   4. tell the patient to do things for himself and then follow through by refusing to help him.

6. The doctor has just told the patient that she has a terminal illness. She is softly crying and the doctor instructs you to "take care of her." What would be the best intervention to meet the immediate spiritual needs of this patient? ***(13)***
   1. Offer to sit with her.
   2. Offer to call the hospital clergy.
   3. Offer to call family or friends.
   4. Offer to pray for her.

CRITICAL THINKING ACTIVITIES

Scenario: You are caring for Mr. Huang, a young man who recently emigrated from a Southeast Asian country. You notice a strange bruising pattern on his back. When you question him about it, he appears to be embarrassed and just shakes his head. When you report the finding to the RN, she tells you that it may be from a culturally based home remedy known as "coin rubbing."

1. What might his nonverbal behavior mean? ***(12)*** ______________________________

   ____

   ____

2. List three interventions that would help Mr. Huang to feel more relaxed and open in giving information for the data collection. ***(10)***

   a. ______________________________

   b. ______________________________

   c. ______________________________

3. How can you increase your "cultural competence" to prepare yourself in working with coworkers and patients from a variety of different cultural backgrounds? *(12)*

____

____

STEPS TOWARD BETTER COMMUNICATION

VOCABULARY BUILDING GLOSSARY

Term	**Definition**
signif'icant others	important people in the life of the patient; may include family, loved ones, and close friends
collab'orative (co lab' ah ra tive)	working together
pre'mium (pree' mee um)	rate amount paid for insurance
fee'-for-service	amount paid to the doctor depending on the service given
em'pathy	understanding of another's feelings
feed'back	return information about actions or an idea
self-esteem'	feelings of worth
eye contact	looking into a person's eyes while talking to him or her
compass'ion	caring
com'petence	knowing what to do
interact'ing	acting on each other; communicating
el'derly	polite term for people who are over age 65 years

COMPLETION

Directions: Fill in the blanks with the appropriate words from the Vocabulary Building Glossary to complete the statements.

1. The LPN/LVN, the RN, the physician, and the respiratory therapist form a ____________________ team that provides the best and most efficient care for the patient.
2. The patient's insurance was not valid, because he forgot to pay the monthly ______________________.
3. The patient needed an explanation of ______________________________ in order to understand that the insurance company would directly pay the doctor.
4. When a patient is an adult and not married, you should inquire about ____________________________ ____________________ who are part of the patient's support system.
5. When evaluating your patient teaching, it is important to obtain ____________________________ from the patient.
6. Being able to feel _____________________________ helps you to understand the patient and to provide compassionate care.

VOCABULARY EXERCISE

1. The word **site** means "place." In this chapter, the places talked about are work sites, or places LVNs might work. On the job, you might talk about the **site** of the wound, or the **site** of the infection. Make two sentences using the word in the two different ways.

____

____

Two other words with the same pronunciation are **sight**: to see (verb), or something to see (noun) and **cite**: to quote or make reference to.

2. Complete the sentences using the correct word above: **Site/sight/cite**
   a. It was quite a _______________ to see Mr. Benson tangled in his oxygen tubes.
   b. This is the _______________ for the new clinic.
   c. When you write your paper, be sure to _______________ your sources.
   d. The original _______________ of the infection is not known.

3. If medical personnel were *demeaning* and *aloof* would that be good for the patient? Why or why not?

____

____

SPECIAL VOCABULARY MEANINGS

Directions: Explain in your own words the meaning of the words in the quotation marks.

1. What does "bending the rules" mean? ____

____

2. Why is "skyrocketing" a good description for the cost of health care? _______________________

____

____

3. What is meant by "unraveling… and stitched back together" with reference to the health care systems?

____

____

4. Why would expensive and specialized medical care be called "boutique medicine"?

____

____

CLINICAL SCENARIOS

Directions: Study the following scenarios.

1. Mrs. Bazan was admitted with weight loss, abdominal pain, and a diagnosis of "rule out cancer of the colon." She underwent a colonoscopy and a bone scan. A member of her church group has come to visit and stops you in the hall to ask if Mrs. Bazan's tests show that she has cancer. You know that they did and that Mrs. Bazan has been told her diagnosis. To protect your patient's privacy and confidentiality, which of the following is the *best* response? ***(8)***
   a. "You will have to speak to Mrs. Bazan's doctor about that."
   b. "I really have no idea what the tests showed."
   c. "I cannot reveal the results of a patient's tests."
   d. "What did Mrs. Bazan tell you?"

2. *Communication example:* Jane is talking with a nursing assistant. "Barry, I would like you to assist Mr. Januz with his range of motion exercises now. Put each joint of his affected arm through the range of motion five times. If he has discomfort, stop and let me know. I will be in room 212."

   Later, Jane checks with Barry about the task delegated. "Barry, how did the range of motion exercises go for Mr. Januz? Did he have any discomfort? Did you encounter any problems? How many times was each joint exercised?"

3. Write out how you would delegate the following task and then describe how you would verify that the task was completed.

   Mrs. Paul needs to be dangled and then ambulated twice on your shift. Ann, the nursing assistant working with you, is capable of performing this task.

CHAPTER 2

Critical Thinking and Nursing Process

evolve Go to http://evolve.elsevier.com/deWit for additional activities and exercises.

IDENTIFICATION

Phases of the Nursing Process

There are five major phases or components of the nursing process: assessment, nursing diagnosis, planning, implementation, and evaluation. Four of these apply to the LPN/LVN assessment (data collection), planning, implementation, and evaluation. ***(26-30)***

Directions: For each nursing action on the right, identify the name of the phase in which the action occurs.

1. ______________________	Noting whether the application of heat has relieved muscle pain.
2. ______________________	Referring patient and family to a community support group.
3. ______________________	Setting a goal for prevention of damage to the skin from prolonged pressure.
4. ______________________	Assisting a patient to turn, cough, and breathe deeply every 2 hours after surgery.
5. ______________________	Changing the types of nourishing fluids offered to a patient to ones that he prefers.
6. ______________________	Asking how often the patient normally has a bowel movement.
7. ______________________	Writing on a patient's care plan a request that she be allowed to have her bedtime snack at 8:30 because she likes to go to sleep early.
8. ______________________	Looking at the laboratory report on a patient's chart to determine the results of a urinalysis.
9. ______________________	Teaching a patient to administer his own insulin.
10. ______________________	Reaching the conclusion that a patient has a fluid volume deficit.

COMPLETION

Directions: Fill in the blanks to complete the statements.

1. The nursing process is a rational way of helping nurses perform their tasks more ______________________ ______________________. ***(18)***

2. Graduates of practical nursing programs are expected to ______________________ to the development of nursing care plans. *(19)*

3. The focus of nursing should be on ________________ patient needs, ________________ nursing care, and ________________________ the plan. *(17)*

4. Ongoing ________________________ is a necessary and important part of the nursing process. *(30)*

5. Formulating the nursing care plan and writing outcome criteria are joint processes between the nurse and the ________________________________. *(28)*

Assessment (Data Collection)

Directions: Answer the following questions about the process of data gathering, which occurs during the assessment phase of the nursing process.

1. A nursing history is obtained from what three sources? *(19)*

   a. ____

   b. ____

   c. ____

2. An interview should be conducted in a ____________________________ and should take no longer than 20–30 minutes. *(21)*

3. When interviewing an elderly patient, the nurse should ______________________________ because the person probably has more health history information to relate and may speak slowly if ill. *(19)*

4. Three important aspects of the psychosocial data collection process are determining with whom the patient ____________________________, financial ____________________________, and other concerns or problems she might have other than her state of health. *(21)*

5. Cultural values that may affect a patient's care or health practices are best assessed by asking about ____. *(19)*

6. Part of a psychological assessment is determining how a patient reacts to ________________ and then determining present ____________________ abilities. *(8)*

7. One way to begin a spiritual assessment is to ask if ______________________ is important to the patient. *(8)*

8. Your patient weighs 155 pounds. Convert the patient's weight to kilograms: ____________ kg

9. Your patient is an infant. She weighs 11 pounds, 4 ounces. Convert the patient's weight to kilograms: ____________ kg

SHORT ANSWER

LPN/LVN's Role and Use of Nursing Process

Directions: Write a short essay answer for each question.

1. During the evaluation, you find that an intervention is not effective and the patient is not meeting the goal. What is the next step? ***(30)***

____

____

2. Explain why documentation of nursing care is important. (Include at least three reasons.) ***(30)***

____

____

____

____

____

APPLICATION OF THE NURSING PROCESS

Directions: Provide the answers to the following questions.

Scenario A: The nursing diagnosis on the nursing care plan states "Pain related to surgical incision." Nursing interventions include the following: "Monitor PCA morphine effectiveness; reposition every 2 hours; provide quiet environment and rest periods; offer distraction to minimize pain." The expected outcomes state "morphine will control pain effectively; patient says pain is not interfering with rest." What would be appropriate evaluation data to determine that these expected outcomes are being met? ***(27)***

____

____

____

____

Scenario B: Your diabetic home care patient is experiencing a flare-up of rheumatoid arthritis and has considerable pain in her knees and fingers. The nursing care plan has a nursing diagnosis of "Self-care deficit related to joint pain." Write two expected outcomes for this nursing diagnosis relevant to this patient. ***(28)***

a. ____

b. ____

PRIORITY SETTING

Directions: Read each scenario and prioritize the needs for these patients.

Scenario A

1. Your patient has a complex health condition and as you are assessing the patient you discover several problems. You realize that priorities of care are determined by a hierarchy of needs. Which of the following problems has the highest level of need? *(28)*
   a. Patient is vomiting and cannot retain meals.
   b. Blood pressure is elevated to 160/100.
   c. Respiratory rate is 32 breaths per minute.
   d. Patient has not had a bowel movement in 3 days.

Scenario B

1. Your patient is hospitalized with pneumonia. There are several important tasks that must be accomplished in the early part of the shift. It is 8:30 AM. What should be done first? *(28)*
   a. Administer the 9:00 AM medication for hypertension.
   b. Have the patient turn, cough, and deep breathe with the incentive spirometer as scheduled.
   c. Get the patient up to the chair as ordered and make the bed.
   d. Obtain the medication ordered for constipation that the patient has requested.

NCLEX-PN® EXAM REVIEW

Directions: Choose the best answer(s) for the following questions.

1. The LPN/LVN contributes to the nursing care plan by: *(26)*
   1. devising the nursing diagnoses.
   2. collaborating with the RN on the nursing diagnoses.
   3. independently choosing nursing diagnoses from a list.
   4. collaborating with the patient concerning the nursing diagnoses.

2. The focus of the planning step of the nursing process is: *(28)*
   1. implementing nursing interventions.
   2. collecting data to determine appropriate nursing diagnoses.
   3. determining goals and identifying expected outcomes.
   4. revising interventions according to outcomes

3. The most important part of writing expected outcomes for nursing diagnoses is to: *(28)*
   1. state the outcome so that it is measurable.
   2. include health promotion and resource management.
   3. make the outcome "short-term."
   4. base it on objective patient data.

4. Which of the following are considered to be objective data? *(Select all that apply.)* *(19)*
   1. Nausea and dizziness when rising too quickly
   2. A fecal odor on the patient's breath
   3. Skin color appears pale and is cool to touch
   4. Blood pressure is 150/90 and pulse is 112
   5. Relief 1 hour after pain medication.

5. The nurse is performing the morning assessment on a patient. There is a sweet, fruity odor of acetone noted on the patient's breath. This odor is most likely to associated with which of the following conditions? *(20)*
   1. Hepatic coma
   2. Diabetic ketoacidosis
   3. Poor hygiene
   4. Chronic sinusitis

6. In order to correctly palpate the abdomen, the nurse uses which of the following techniques? *(21)*
   1. Depresses gently with the fingertips and thumb.
   2. Uses a sweeping motion with the back of the hand.
   3. Gently feels with the flat palmar surface of the hand.
   4. Warms the stethoscope bell before listening to four areas.

7. The nurse is looking at the patient's chart and other documentation to determine when the patient received the last dose of blood pressure medication. Where would be the best place to locate this information? *(24)*
   1. Physician's orders
   2. Medication reconciliation form
   3. Nurse's narrative notes
   4. Medication administration record

8. An increased number of WBCs is most likely to be associated with which of the following? *(25)*
   1. Dehydration
   2. An improper diet
   3. An iron deficiency
   4. An infection

9. The nurse knows that current vital signs are an important indication of what is happening at a given moment. In addition, vital signs should be correlated with which of the following patient data? *(19)*
   1. Trends of the past readings
   2. Standardized normal readings
   3. The patient's ideal body weight
   4. Accuracy of the equipment

CRITICAL THINKING ACTIVITIES

1. You are caring for a patient with a nursing diagnosis of Constipation related to medication side effects. Identify which of the following interventions you would select for this diagnosis and briefly explain why you selected each intervention. Also, for interventions that you rejected, give your rationale in the space provided on the next page.
   a. Encourage a healthy diet that includes lean meat and low-fat dairy.
   b. Encourage fluids (if not contraindicated).
   c. Monitor vital signs at least once per shift.
   d. Encourage ambulation at least three times per shift.
   e. Teach about high-fiber foods.
   f. Give positive feedback for selecting fruit (i.e., whole apple) for lunch.
   g. Keep the patient clean and dry.
   h. Discontinue any medications that are causing constipation.

STEPS TOWARD BETTER COMMUNICATION

VOCABULARY BUILDING GLOSSARY

Term	Definition
base'line data	data for reference; measure later information against it
cor'relate	make to match, compare points of several things
clue	added information or hints
da'tabase (da' tah bas)	basic information collected about the patient
dis'count	disregard, not pay attention to
enhance'	improve, make better, add to
entail'	includes or involves as a necessary inclusion
evalua'tion	process of judging
hi'erarchy (hi' er ark ee)	in order according to importance
in'put	information from someone about facts, feelings, or attitudes
implementa'tion	the carrying out of actions
men'tate	patient's capacity to think
on'going	in progress; continuing
pru'dent	wise or careful

COMPLETION

Directions: Fill in the blanks with the appropriate words from the Vocabulary Building Glossary above to complete the statements.

1. The patient and family should have ______________ on the goals of care and the treatment plan in order to increase compliance and success.
2. You should ______________________________ with the respiratory therapist about how the patient is to perform her respiratory exercises and how to work them into her schedule of other treatments.
3. A _____________________________ is a person with whom the patient shares closeness, intimacy, and trust in a long-term relationship.
4. When items or concepts are placed in order according to their priority, they are in a __________________ ________________________.
5. If you have a cold or cough, it is not ____________________________ to work with patients with low resistance.
6. Don't _______________________ the statements the patient makes because it will give you some _______________________ as to how he is feeling.
7. Think of some ways you can ____________________ your patient's stay in the hospital.
8. Try to _____________________ the lab reports with what you observe with the patient.
9. Taking a good history ___________________ getting adequate information from the patient.

CLINICAL ACTIVITIES

Asking for Assistance

Directions: Seek assistance when something is unclear or not understood.

1. If you feel awkward auscultating the heart and lungs, ask the instructor to demonstrate the skill on your patient by saying, "Would you please show me how to auscultate my patient's lungs (or heart) properly?"
2. If you are having difficulty hearing a patient's blood pressure accurately, ask for help by saying, "I'm not certain I'm getting my patient's blood pressure accurately. Could you help me?"

SHORT ANSWER

To assist patients with spiritual concerns, rather than saying, "Do you want . . .?", the patient might be more receptive if you would use a more polite form of question, such as "Would you like . . .?". Other polite phrases include "Might I . . .?", "May I . . .?", and "I would like to . . . if that is all right with you."

Directions: In the spaces below, write polite phrases for asking a patient about reading to her, praying with her, sitting with her, calling a spiritual advisor, and calling friends. Example: "Would you like me to bring you something to read?"

1. ______________________________

2. ______________________________

3. ______________________________

4. ______________________________

5. ______________________________

Writing Expected Outcomes

Directions: Write two expected outcomes for each of the following nursing diagnoses. Example: Patient will use PCA pump before pain becomes severe for 48 hours after surgery. ***(8)***

1. Pain related to surgical incision.

   a. ______________________________

   b. ______________________________

2. Self-care deficit related to paralysis of left side.

   a. ______________________________

   b. ______________________________

3. Constipation related to side effects of medications.

   a. ______________________________

   b. ______________________________

GRAMMAR POINTS

When taking a history, you need to be sure that you and the patient are talking about the same time period.

- When you are asking about past medical history, you need to ask "Have you had...*breathing problems*...?" (chronic conditions) or "Have you **ever** had...*a stroke*...?" (a one-time happening).
- If you are asking about current symptoms, you will need to ask "Do you have...*vision or hearing problems*...?" (now).

If you do not pronounce the words carefully, or are dealing with an older person with a hearing loss or with someone who is distracted, or is a native speaker of another language, you may not receive the correct information.

CHAPTER 3

Fluids, Electrolytes, Acid-Base Balance, and Intravenous Therapy

evolve Go to http://evolve.elsevier.com/deWit for additional activities and exercises.

MATCHING

Directions: Select the principle on the right that most accurately completes the statement on the left.

1. Maintaining normal composition and distribution of body fluids is essential to health because __________. ***(35)***
2. The composition of the internal environment remains fairly stable because __________. ***(35)***
3. Intravascular fluid normally moves throughout the body because ______________. ***(35)***
4. The substances in the body fluids can move in and out of capillaries and cell bodies because ______________. ***(36)***
5. A deficit of water in the extracellular compartment leads to cellular dehydration because ______________. ***(36)***

a. The heart acts as a pump to distribute blood.

b. All the life processes of every cell of every organ take place in a fluid medium.

c. When a semipermeable membrane separates fluids of unequal concentration, molecules of water move from the less concentrated to the more concentrated solution.

d. Virtually every organ in the body is involved in maintaining homeostasis.

e. Diffusion provides a spontaneous mixing of molecules.

COMPLETION

Directions: Fill in the blanks to complete these statements about fluid and electrolyte balance.

1. Whenever sodium is retained by the body and not excreted by the kidneys, ________________ is also retained. ***(48)***
2. Normal transmission of nerve impulses and normal muscular activity, including that of the heart, require the presence of __________________________. ***(49)***
3. A potassium deficit can cause cardiac ____________________________________. ***(48)***
4. When a patient becomes dehydrated from insufficient fluid intake, serum sodium levels ________________. ***(48)***
5. Signs of dehydration include ______________________________________, ________________ ____________________________, and ____. ***(39)***

6. Four conditions that can lead to hypokalemia are improper use of ____________________, as well as ____________________, ____________________, and continuous ____________________. *(46)*

7. Examples of three foods high in potassium are ____________________, ____________________, and ____________________. *(48)*

8. Symptoms of hypokalemia include general weakness, ____________________, and ____________________. *(46)*

9. Magnesium is important in reactions related to ____________________ metabolism. *(50)*

10. Good sources of magnesium include ____________________ ____________________. *(47)*

11. ____________________ is essential for the formation of bone. *(50)*

12. ____________________ is also important as a ____________________ to promote acid-base balance. *(51)*

SHORT ANSWER

Fluids and Electrolytes

Directions: Fill in the blank or supply a short answer to complete the following statements about fluid balance and intake.

1. The average intake of liquids during a 24-hour period is ______________ mL. *(35)*

2. A urinary output of less than ______________ mL per hour indicates fluid deficit. *(40)*

3. List three treatments or nursing measures that can lead to water intoxication. *(43)*

   a. ____________________

   b. ____________________

   c. ____________________

4. Name three nursing actions that can help relieve nausea and vomiting. *(41)*

   a. ____________________

   b. ____________________

   c. ____________________

5. When a patient vomits, he loses water and which electrolytes? *(41)* ____________________

____

6. To help in the assessment of fluid volume deficit related to diarrhea, list three observations the nurse should note and record. ***(42, 43)***

   a. ______________________________

   b. ______________________________

   c. ______________________________

7. Name four nursing measures useful for treating fluid volume deficit related to diarrhea. ***(41, 42)***

   a. ______________________________

   b. ______________________________

   c. ______________________________

   d. ______________________________

8. Name two practices that can lead to a fluid volume deficit in a patient with gastric suction. ***(38)***

   a. ______________________________

   b. ______________________________

9. List three nursing actions that should be included in the care plan of a patient with generalized edema. ***(44)***

   a. ______________________________

   b. ______________________________

   c. ______________________________

10. List three common nursing diagnoses for patients with problems of vomiting, diarrhea, or draining wounds. ***(40)***

    a. ______________________________

    b. ______________________________

    c. ______________________________

TABLE ACTIVITY

Fluid Deficits

Directions: Complete the following table which compares the three major conditions related to fluid deficits. ***(38-43)***

	Vomiting	Diarrhea	Draining Wounds
Clinical manifestations to be documented			
Possible causes			
Nursing interventions			
Medical management			

IDENTIFICATION

Intravenous Therapies

Directions: For each type of intravenous therapy on the left, identify and list all interventions on the right that apply.

1. ______ Total parenteral nutrition (TPN) ***(62-63)***
2. ______ Intravenous therapy ***(55-56)***
3. ______ Blood transfusion ***(55, 393-394)***

a. Two nurses must check and verify the bag label with the patient's ID band and information.
b. Started at no more than 60–80 mL per hour.
c. Take baseline vital signs including temperature before starting.
d. Monitor the site, flow rate, and how patient is tolerating the infusion hourly.
e. Monitor blood sugar frequently during the first week.
f. Monitor the elderly patient carefully for signs of fluid overload.
g. Stop the infusion if the patient becomes short of breath.
h. Always use an IV infusion pump to administer it.
i. Slowly decrease the rate of infusion before stopping it.
j. Take vital signs every hour while administering it.

CALCULATIONS

Directions: Calculate the correct flow rates for the following orders and situations. ***(58)***

1. Ordered: 1000 mL D_5RL over 8 hours
   Administration set delivers 15 gtts/mL
   How many drops per minute should be administered? __________

2. Ordered: 500 mL D_4MRL over 10 hours
   Administration set delivers 60 gtts/mL
   How many drops per minute should be administered? __________

3. Ordered: 500 mL $D_{10}W$ at 150 mL/hour
   Administration set delivers 15 gtts/mL
   How many drops per minute should be administered? __________

4. Your patient had an IV count of 525 mL at the beginning of your shift. You infused two piggybacks during the shift; the first was 125 mL and the second was 100 mL. You hung a new 1000 mL bag of fluid at 1:00 PM. The IV count at the end of your shift was 800 mL.
   What was the total IV intake for the shift? __________

PRIORITY SETTING

You are assigned to care for the following patients:

a. Ms. Toms, age 76, who has nausea, vomiting, and dehydration.
b. Mr. Wilson, age 68, who had surgery and is receiving a transfusion of packed red cells.
c. Mr. Whitts, age 36, who has pancreatitis and is receiving TPN.

1. After you receive report, which patient would you visit and check first? __________

You have a nursing assistant assigned to help you with your patients. You need vital signs on all three patients at 8:00 AM.

2. Which patient would you assign to the nursing assistant for measuring vital signs? __________

3. You need to do an initial shift assessment on each of the three patients. Which one would you assess first?
____

IDENTIFICATION

Blood Gas Analysis

Directions: Under each laboratory value given below, add ↓ if the value is below normal, ◊ if normal, and ↑ if above normal. Then decide whether the data set indicates metabolic acidosis, respiratory acidosis, metabolic alkalosis, or respiratory alkalosis. ***(52)***

	pH	pCO_2	HCO_3
Example:	*7.32*	*44 mm Hg*	*21 mEq/L*
	↓	◊	↓

Indicates metabolic acidosis

	pH	pCO_2	HCO_3
1.	7.33	50 mm Hg	26 mEq/L

Indicates ______________________________

	pH	pCO_2	HCO_3
2.	7.48	32 mm Hg	25 mEq/L

Indicates ______________________________

	pH	pCO_2	HCO_3
3.	7.50	45 mm Hg	28 mEq/L

Indicates ______________________________

	pH	pCO_2	HCO_3
4.	7.30	45 mm Hg	20 mEq/L

Indicates ______________________________

NCLEX-PN® EXAM REVIEW

Directions: Choose the best answer(s) for the following questions.

1. Assessment data indicative of hypokalemia include: *(Select all that apply.)* ***(46)***
   1. hyperactive bowel sounds.
   2. a potassium level of 2.8 mEq.
   3. brisk reflexes.
   4. poor skin turgor.
   5. weakness.
   6. urinary retention.

2. A nursing intervention appropriate for the patient with hyponatremia is: ***(46)***
   1. encourage intake of milk.
   2. restrict fluid intake.
   3. administer ordered diuretic.
   4. give foods high in potassium.

3. Safe administration of intravenous fluids includes: ***(57)***
   1. shaking the bag to mix the solution thoroughly.
   2. checking the infusion rate every 30–60 minutes.
   3. weighing the patient daily.
   4. checking electrolyte levels before hanging a new bag of IV solution.

4. The *best* data indicating effectiveness of interventions for an elderly patient with a fluid volume deficit is: ***(39)***
   1. weight gain of 3 pounds.
   2. successful infusion of 3000 mL of normal saline.
   3. patient can answer questions without confusion.
   4. moist mucous membranes in the mouth.

5. Nursing actions for a patient receiving intravenous fluids should include: *(Select all that apply.)* ***(58)***
   1. re-dress the IV insertion site each shift.
   2. stabilize the cannula in the vein to prevent trauma to the surrounding tissues.
   3. set the intravenous fluid to run at the prescribed rate of flow.
   4. speed up the flow rate of intravenous fluids when necessary to catch up on fluids that have not been administered at the prescribed rate.
   5. observe and record the patient's response to the administration of fluids.
   6. maintain strict asepsis when changing the intravenous tubing and bag.

6. When a patient shows signs of a transfusion reaction, the nurse must: ***(55, 394-395)***
   1. increase the rate of flow of the saline via the "Y" tubing.
   2. take the vital signs and wait 15 minutes, then take them again.
   3. slow down the rate of flow and notify the physician.
   4. stop the transfusion, notify the physician, and keep the intravenous line open with normal saline.

7. Calculation: Find the correct number of drops per minute for the following order: 500 mL D5½NS IV q 8 hr. Available: Microdrip tubing. ____________________ ***(58)***

8. Place an "X" on the diagram below where a central line would most likely be inserted for the administration of TPN. *(62)*

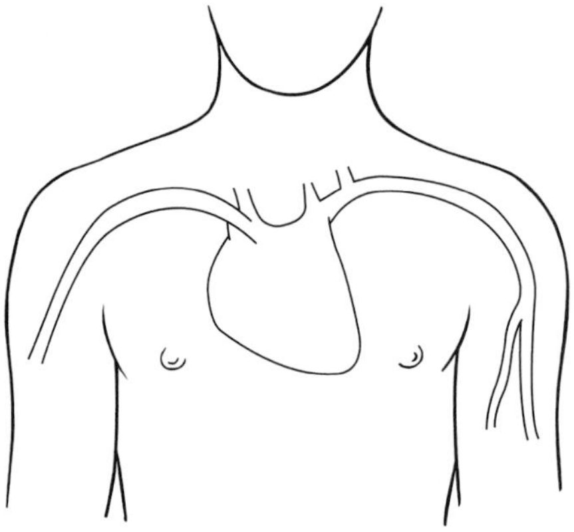

9. Metabolic acidosis is more likely to occur in a person who: *(53)*
   1. is unable to metabolize carbohydrates normally or who ingests few or no carbohydrates.
   2. is unable to metabolize fats normally.
   3. suffers from kidney failure with excessive reabsorption of bicarbonate from the urine.
   4. has diarrhea with excessive loss of bicarbonates in the feces.

10. Hypoventilation results in: *(52, 53)*
    1. blowing off too much carbon dioxide, resulting in respiratory acidosis.
    2. retention of oxygen in the lungs and resulting respiratory acidosis.
    3. inadequate release of carbon dioxide through the lungs, resulting in formation of carbonic acid and respiratory acidosis.
    4. excessive loss of oxygen and accumulation of carbonic acid in the blood.

CRITICAL THINKING ACTIVITIES

Scenario: Intestinal Surgery

Your patient is a 68-year-old female who had intestinal surgery 4 days ago. She is NPO, has a nasogastric tube set to intermittent suction, an intravenous line with D5½NS at 125 mL/hr. Physical assessment data includes: Alert and oriented but groggy, diaphoretic, fine crackles in the lower lobes of both lungs, moving all extremities, and complaining of abdominal pain and a dry mouth. Bowel sounds are hypoactive, no BM since surgery, and is voiding dark amber urine without difficulty. Urine sp. gr. is 1.030. NG output in last 2 hours is 200 mL of dark green secretions. Vital signs: T 101.2° F, P 92, BP 128/78. Intake last 24 hours: 2480 mL/, output was 2010 mL. Laboratory values: K^+ 3.1 mEq/L, Na^+ 140 mEq/L, Cl^- 91 mEq/L.

1. What other assessment data should you acquire related to her fluid status? *(39)*

2. Do the assessment findings indicate a fluid deficit or fluid excess problem? Explain using the assessment data. *(39)*

3. What is her electrolyte status? Does she have any electrolyte abnormalities? If so, which one(s)? Give your rationale for your answers. ***(46)***

STEPS TOWARD BETTER COMMUNICATION

VOCABULARY BUILDING GLOSSARY

Term	**Definition**
syno'via (sin o' vee ah)	secreting membrane found in joints
a'queous (a' kwee us) hu'mor	transparent fluid between the lens of the eye and the cornea
paren'teral (pah ren' ter al)	by subcutaneous, intramuscular, intravenous, or method other than by the gastrointestinal tract
cru'cial (kru'shul)	of extreme importance
diaphore'sis (di ah for ee'sis)	excessive perspiration
clam'my	cool and damp
sprue	disorder causing lack of absorption from the intestine
per'meable (per'mee a bul)	permitting passage of a substance
vis'cous (vis' kus)	thick, like honey (a property of fluids)

VOCABULARY EXERCISE

Table of Prefixes to Remember:

Prefix	Meaning	Examples
extra-	outside	extracellular
hyper-	more	hypertonic hyperglycemic
hypo-	less	hypotonic hypoglycemic
inter-	between among	internal interstitial intervention
intra-	within	intracellular intravascular intravenous
iso-	same, equal	isotonic isometric
trans-	through	transcellular transfusion transport

COMPLETION

Directions: Fill in the blanks with the correct terms from the glossary list.

1. ____________________ fluid is located in the joints and acts as a lubricant for the joints.

2. Fluid balance is __________________ to the well-being of an elderly person.
3. The patient with a high fever often experiences ______________________________.
4. Normal saline intravenous solution is ___________________________.
5. A 10% dextrose intravenous solution is ___________________________.
6. An intravenous infusion places fluid in the ______________________________ space.
7. The patient who is experiencing shock has skin that feels ______________________.
8. Enteral feeding solutions are more ___________________ than intravenous solutions.
9. Patients who have _____________________ often experience considerable diarrhea.
10. A membrane must be ______________________ for diffusion to take place across it.

COMMUNICATION EXERCISE

Patient Teaching

A. *Directions: A nurse is instructing a patient about input and output. Note their interaction.*

Nurse: "Mrs. T., the doctor wants us to measure everything you drink. This sheet will be here for you to write down the amount each time you drink something."

Mrs. T.: "How will I know how much I drank?"

Nurse: "See how this cup is marked with lines indicating the amount of fluid?"

Mrs. T.: "Oh, yes, I do see that now."

Nurse: "Now tell me what you will do."

Mrs. T.: "I need to look to see how much fluid is in the cup and then how much is left when I have had a drink. Do I subtract to determine the exact amount I drank?"

Nurse: "Yes, that's correct. If you have trouble, just call me and I'll help you. Let's try it now. The cup has 120 mL in it. Take a drink. Good. Now it has 60 mL left. So if we subtract 60 from 120, we find that you drank 60 mL. Let's write that down."

Mrs. T.: "It doesn't seem too complicated. Leave the paper and pencil next to the cup to remind me to write the amount down each time I drink, please."

Nurse: "Of course, Mrs. T. Also, I need to measure your urine output. So whenever you use the toilet, be certain that the little white "hat" is sitting in it. Call me when you have finished and I will measure and record it. Try to drop any toilet paper into the toilet behind the hat so it doesn't alter the measurement."

Mrs. T.: "O.K., I'll try."

B. You have a patient who cannot tolerate dairy products; they cause diarrhea. What can you teach this patient about planning a diet that contains sufficient calcium?

____

____

____

CHAPTER 4

Care of Preoperative and Intraoperative Surgical Patients

evolve Go to http://evolve.elsevier.com/deWit for additional activities and exercises.

COMPLETION

Preoperative Care

Directions: Fill in the blank with the correct word(s) to complete the sentences.

1. Required tests before surgery include a ________________ and a ____________________________. *(71)*
2. The surgeon should be alerted if a patient's hemoglobin level is below ____________. *(71)*
3. The elderly patient is more prone to fluid and electrolyte imbalances during and after surgery because she is more likely to have ____ ____ ____. *(69)*
4. Before surgery, it is important to know if the patient has any ________________ and if he is taking ______________________________. *(70)*
5. Obese people are at higher risk with surgery because fat contains fewer blood vessels, causing ____________________________ and a greater threat of ____________________. *(73)*
6. The malnourished patient is also at risk because _________________________ is needed to replace blood cells and serum lost during surgery. *(73)*
7. Patients are encouraged to quit smoking before surgery because smoking has a negative effect on _________________________ and ______________________________. *(73)*
8. The diabetic patient is at risk for ________________________________ or ____________________________ during and after surgical procedures. *(73)*
9. Poorly controlled diabetes leads to postoperative complications such as __________________________ and ____________________________. *(73)*
10. Impaired respiration slows down oxygen and carbon dioxide exchange and predisposes the patient to __________________________ and possible ____________________________________. *(73)*

PRIORITY SETTING

Directions: You have finished receiving report and are ready to begin patient care. You are assigned a preoperative surgery patient who is scheduled for surgery at 8:30 AM. How would you prioritize your actions? Number the actions listed below in the order (from 1 to 8) in which you would perform them. ***(79-81)***

______ a. Complete the preoperative checklist.

______ b. Check to see that the patient's signature is on the surgical consent form.

______ c. Check that all diagnostic test results are back and determine if there are any abnormal lab values.

______ d. Have the patient shower, if possible.

______ e. Remind the patient to remain NPO and not to swallow any fluids or food.

______ f. Have the patient remove any metal hairpins and jewelry and all underclothes, leaving on only a clean hospital gown.

______ g. Start the presurgical nurse's notes in the chart which will be finished when the transport person comes for the patient.

______ h. Explain to the family where the surgical waiting room is and how to get there.

MATCHING

Surgical Risk Factors and Their Effects on Recovery

Mr. J. is admitted to the same-day surgery unit for repair of an inguinal hernia. He is 48 years old, has diabetes mellitus for which he takes insulin, is 140 pounds overweight, and smokes one and a half packs of cigarettes a day. He has smoked since age 15 and has chronic bronchitis with a productive cough.

Directions: Match each of Mr. J.'s surgical risk factors with the effect it can have on his recovery from surgery. Note that there may be more than one effect for each risk factor. ***(73)***

1. ______________ Diabetes mellitus
2. ______________ Smoking and chronic bronchitis
3. ______________ Obesity

a. Slower healing and risk of infection because adipose tissue has fewer blood vessels.
b. Decreased lung expansion due to chronic lung disease.
c. Decreased lung expansion due to upward pressure of enlarged abdomen against thorax.
d. Wide variations in blood glucose levels.
e. Potential for wound dehiscence because of added stress on sutures.
f. Accumulations of secretions in air passages.
g. Infection related to less phagocytic action against microorganisms.
h. Reduced level of functional hemoglobin.
i. Abnormal clot formation and obstruction of blood vessels.

COMPLETION

Directions: Fill in the blank with the correct word(s) to complete the statements.

1. The function of the ________________ is important in the surgical patient because this is where anesthetic agents are metabolized. *(71)*

2. The patient's vital signs are taken and recorded prior to surgery to act as a ________________________ for postoperative assessment. *(72)*

3. Surgery is a risk for the malnourished patient because postoperative healing and blood-building requires ____________________. *(71)*

4. In addition to physiologic preparation, most surgical patients have a need for __________________ support. *(70)*

5. As the patient leaves for surgery, family members should be informed about which three things? *(78)*

   a. ____

   b. ____

   c. ____

6. When a patient asks why he can't have anything to eat or drink for 8 hours prior to surgery, how should the nurse respond? *(75)* ____

   ____

APPLICATION OF THE NURSING PROCESS

Scenario: Ms. Thompson, age 48, is to undergo a vaginal hysterectomy for metrorrhagia (excessive bleeding). She will have general anesthesia. She has recently remarried and is concerned about her husband's feelings regarding her surgery.

1. List the nursing diagnoses that would be appropriate for Ms. Thompson in the preoperative period. *(72)*

   ____

   ____

   ____

2. State an outcome objective for each of the above nursing diagnoses. *(72)* ________________________

   ____

   ____

   ____

3. List interventions that you would perform when the transport person comes to take Ms. Thompson to surgery. ***(81)***

____

____

____

4. How would you evaluate the preoperative care given to Ms. Thompson? ***(83)*** ____________________

____

____

____

____

SHORT ANSWER

Intraoperative Care

Directions: Provide a brief answer to each question.

1. Describe autologous blood collection and reinfusion: ***(69)*** ____________________________

____

____

2. What are the advantages of robotic surgery? ***(68)*** ______________________________________

____

3. How is bloodless surgery performed? ***(69)*** ____

____

____

____

4. Can you name three measures that are used to prevent the possibility of surgical infection in the operating suite? ***(84)***

   a. ____

   b. ____

   c. ____

5. Identify the various measures that are used to prevent "wrong patient, wrong site" surgery from occurring. ***(83-84)***

____

____

____

____

6. No matter what type of anesthesia is used, the goals of anesthesia should be kept in mind. They are: ***(84)***

   a. ____

   b. ____

   c. ____

7. Potential complications of anesthesia include the following. Describe an intervention to monitor and/or prevent their occurrence. ***(88-89)***

   a. Infection: ____

   ____

   b. Fluid volume imbalance: ____

   ____

   c. Hypothermia/hyperthermia: ____

   ____

   d. Injury: ____

   ____

NCLEX-PN® EXAM REVIEW

Directions: Choose the best answer(s) for the following questions.

1. The patient who is a heavy smoker is at increased risk of complications after surgery with general anesthesia because: ***(73)***
   1. blood pressure swings may occur when nicotine is withdrawn.
   2. respiratory muscles are weakened, making coughing difficult.
   3. nicotine withdrawal causes considerable nervousness.
   4. irritated lung tissues produce more secretions from inhaled anesthesia.

2. The patient who has liver disease is at increased risk from surgery because: *(Select all that apply.)* ***(71, 72)***
   1. good liver function is needed to metabolize drugs and anesthetics.
   2. the liver helps cleanse the blood of microorganisms.
   3. blood pressure swings are likely when liver function is poor.
   4. clotting times may be affected causing the patient to bleed excessively.
   5. the liver stores extra blood that can be released if the patient becomes hypovolemic.

3. Skin preparation is performed prior to surgery to: *(Select all that apply.)* ***(77)***
   1. provide a better visual field for the surgeon.
   2. sterilize the skin.
   3. help prevent wound contamination.
   4. facilitate postoperative dressing changes.
   5. reduce the number of microorganisms at the surgical site.

4. The patient is scheduled for an exploratory laparotomy for an abdominal mass. The preoperative laboratory results are: ***(71)***
   CBC: Hgb= 14.5 g, RBC 5.1, WBC 8600
   UA: sp. gr. 10.25, glucose negative, ketones negative, WBCs 57 per low power field, casts 10.

   Which test finding would you report to the surgeon? ____________________

5. Which of the following should be covered before a patient signs a surgical consent form? *(Select all that apply.)* ***(74)***
   1. The correct name of the procedure to be performed.
   2. The names and credentials of all surgical assistants.
   3. The potential complications that may occur from the surgery.
   4. The length of time the patient will be in the PACU.
   5. The benefits of the surgery.
   6. Verification that the patient is mentally competent and not coerced into signing the form.

CRITICAL THINKING ACTIVITY

Scenario: Mrs. Holt is scheduled for a colectomy for diverticulosis after many episodes of diverticulitis. She has been feeling much better since she finished the antibiotics for the last episode. You have the preoperative checklist in hand and are preparing her for surgery. She tells you that she has decided she doesn't want the surgery after all, because she is feeling so much better.

1. What do you do? Describe the specific steps you would take in this situation. ***(74)***

2. How would you document this event in her medical record? ***(74)***

STEPS TOWARD BETTER COMMUNICATION

VOCABULARY BUILDING GLOSSARY

Term	Definition
laparoscopic (lap a ro skop' ik)	seen or performed though a laparoscope, an instrument for direct visualization into the peritoneal body cavity
invasive (in va' siv)	involving a puncture or incision of the skin
hemodilution (he' mo di lu' shun)	increase of the fluid content of the blood which decreases its concentration
coercion (co er' shun)	using force or threats to make a person do something

COMPLETION

Fill in the blank in the following sentences with the correct word from the glossary above.

1. Administering too much intravenous fluid may cause ________________________.
2. Telling a patient that she will surely die without the surgery would be ____________________ regarding signing the surgical consent form.
3. Even laparoscopic surgery is ________________________.
4. Gallbladder surgery is often a ______________________________ procedure these days.

GRAMMAR POINTS

Verb Forms—Future Tense

The nurse prepares the patient for surgery by performing preoperative teaching. Instructions to the patient are given using the future tense, such as "You will . . ." or "you should . . .", or "The nurse is going to . . .". For the following set of orders, write out the instruction or explanation you would give to the patient as part of the preoperative teaching.

1. NPO after midnight: ____

   ____

2. Report at 0600 to outpatient surgery unit: ____

   ____

3. Surgical prep: ____

   ____

4. Restoril 30 mg p.o. H.S.: ____

   ____

Directions: Other instructions you would give to the patient might include the following. Fill in the blanks with the proper verb forms.

5. "The nurse ______________________ you to cough and deep breathe every 2 hours."
6. "Turning ______________________ required every 2 hours after surgery."
7. "You will need ________________ for pain medication and should do so before the pain becomes severe."
8. "Your valuable belongings ___________________ locked up in the business office or given to your husband."
9. "You ______________________ your necklace to surgery."
10. "The side rails __________________________ raised after you have been given your preoperative medications."

CULTURAL POINTS

What special items might you need to think about if you are preparing an older patient for surgery?

____

____

____

What information would you give him or her about the items? Write out how you would state that information.

____

____

____

CHAPTER 5

Care of Postoperative Surgical Patients

evolve Go to http://evolve.elsevier.com/deWit for additional activities and exercises.

TABLE ACTIVITY

Anesthesia Implications

Directions: Complete the following table which compares the nursing implications of various types of anesthesia. (86-87)

Type of Anesthesia	Postoperative Nursing Implications
Inhalation (general anesthesia)	
Intravenous drugs (procedural sedation)	
Regional or topical	

SHORT ANSWER

PACU Care

Directions: Provide the answers to the following questions in the blank spaces provided.

1. In the PACU, assessments are performed every ______________________ unless the patient's condition warrants more frequent assessment. ***(93)***

2. If the immediate postoperative patient's breathing seems to be occluded, what would you do? ***(92, 93)***

____

____

3. When discharging a patient from the same-day surgery unit, besides doing postoperative teaching for the patient and family, it is important to: ***(94)***

____

____

Postoperative Care

Directions: Answer the following questions in the spaces provided.

1. What three questions should you ask yourself if you note that a patient returning from surgery has had a tube inserted? ***(92-93)***

   a. ____

   b. ____

   c. ____

2. List five nursing responsibilities regarding the care of active surgical drains. ***(101)***

   a. ____

   b. ____

   c. ____

   d. ____

   e. ____

3. How often should surgical dressings be checked? ***(101)*** ____

____

4. If there is no written order for dressing changes, what should be done? ***(101)*** ____

____

5. What should be recorded on the patient's chart when a dressing is changed and drainage noted? ***(101)***

____

____

6. What signs and symptoms indicate an infected surgical wound? ***(102, 103)*** ____

____

7. What is the correct procedure for the immediate care of a patient who experiences wound dehiscence and evisceration? ***(103, 104)***

____

____

COMPLETION

Directions: Fill in the blanks to complete the statements.

1. Besides checking the rate of respirations, it is important to check both the ____________ and ____________. ***(95)***
2. Besides medicating for pain, measures to promote comfort in the immediate postoperative period include providing ____________ and medicating as needed for ____________. ***(99)***
3. The three initial classic signs of shock resulting from the hypovolemia due to hemorrhage are ____________ ____________. ***(104)***
4. In addition to those above, describe other physical changes that occur with the progression of shock. ***(104)***
   a. Pulse: ____________
   b. Blood pressure: ____________
   c. Respirations: ____________
   d. Skin: ____________
   e. Level of consciousness: ____________
5. Another complication to which the elderly patient is more susceptible is overhydration. Signs that would make the nurse suspect overhydration include: ***(103)***

   ____

   ____
6. A postoperative patient is complaining of shortness of breath and chest pain; he is very anxious and has a rapid pulse and rapid respirations. These could indicate the complication of ____________ ____________. ***(103)***

APPLICATION OF THE NURSING PROCESS

Scenario: Mr. Hope, age 72, has undergone an exploratory laparotomy and appendectomy. He did well through surgery and in the recovery room. He has an IV with D_5NS hanging, an NG tube set to low suction, and a urinary catheter. He has a history of arthritis and hypertension that is well-controlled. He is usually an "active senior," playing tennis and golf a few times each week. He is breathing shallowly when you assess him and is complaining of pain at 7 out of 10 on the pain scale.

1. Choose the top four nursing diagnoses that would appropriate for Mr. Hope during this postoperative period. *(94)*

2. Write at least one expected outcome for each of the above nursing diagnoses.

   a. ______

   b. ______

   c. ______

   d. ______

3. What nursing interventions should be included on the plan of care to monitor for infection? *(102)*

4. What adjunctive measures could you use along with pain medication to treat this patient's pain? *(99)*

5. What measures would you institute to promote good oxygenation and circulation? *(95-96)*

6. What evaluation criteria would tell you that the patient is breathing effectively? *(95)*

7. What evaluation criteria would tell you that the patient's pain is adequately controlled? ***(99)***

____

____

PRIORITY SETTING

You are assigned to care for Mr. H. who is just returning from surgery. He has had an exploratory laparotomy and appendectomy. You receive report from the PACU nurse and settle the patient in the bed. Number the actions listed below in the order (from 1 to 13) in which you would perform them. ***(93-94)***

_______ a. Inspect the surgical dressing

_______ b. Check all tubes and drains for patency

_______ c. Take the vital signs

_______ d. Adjust the IV drip rate to the ordered flow rate

_______ e. Inquire about the patient's pain level

_______ f. Ask the patient to take four deep breaths

_______ g. Hook the NG tube to the suction

_______ h. Document the postoperative assessment

_______ i. Palpate the abdomen gently

_______ j. Verify that the correct IV solution is hanging

_______ k. Provide an additional warmed blanket

_______ l. Allow the family to visit

_______ m. Auscultate the heart and lung

NCLEX-PN® EXAM REVIEW

Directions: Choose the best answer(s) for the following questions.

1. When assessing respiratory function during recovery from anesthesia, the nurse does which of the following? *(Select all that apply.)* ***(93)***
    1. Auscultate the lungs.
    2. Assess the rate of respiration.
    3. Check quality and depth of respiration.
    4. Administer low-flow oxygen.
    5. Place the patient in semi-Fowler's position.
    6. Keep the tongue from occluding the airway.

2. The patient most likely to have pulmonary complications after surgery is the one who has had a(n): ***(95)***
    1. appendectomy.
    2. hysterectomy.
    3. tonsillectomy.
    4. cholecystectomy.

3. Adynamic ileus can occur after anesthesia and abdominal surgery. Signs and symptoms found on assessment include: ***(103)***
   1. high-pitched, frequent bowel sounds in all four quadrants.
   2. diarrhea, cramping, and high-pitched bowel sounds.
   3. absence of bowel sounds in upper quadrants.
   4. abdominal distention, pain, no passage of feces or flatus, and no bowel sounds.

4. Coughing after surgery is evaluated not only by the amount of airflow produced by the cough but also by: ***(95)***
   1. the loudness of the sound made.
   2. the number of coughs produced at one time.
   3. the degree of inspiration prior to the cough.
   4. whether secretions are moved up and out of the bronchial tree.

5. Nursing measures that can be implemented to help a patient void after surgery include: ***(97)***
   1. forcing plenty of fluids.
   2. keeping intravenous fluids running on time.
   3. having a male patient stand to void.
   4. placing pressure over the bladder.

6. When a patient has a nasogastric tube with low suction after abdominal surgery, the tube should be: ***(101)***
   1. irrigated with 100 mL of solution every 2 hours.
   2. looped above the stomach level and not allowed to drop below the level of entry into the drainage container.
   3. looped around the patient's ear and down to the container.
   4. disconnected during meals and then reconnected.

7. The plan of care for the immediate postoperative period should include which one of the following safety measures? ***(95)***
   1. Keeping an emesis basin within the patient's reach.
   2. Positioning the patient on her side until she is alert to prevent aspiration.
   3. Talking to the patient and reorienting her frequently.
   4. Covering the patient with warmed blankets to decrease chilling.

8. Other safety measures for the postoperative patient include which of the following? *(Select all that apply.)* ***(97-100)***
   1. Cautioning the patient not to get out of bed without assistance while receiving narcotic analgesics.
   2. Answering the patient's call light promptly.
   3. Assessing the patient for bladder distention every 8 hours.
   4. Monitoring fluid intake and output closely.
   5. Assessing urine output every 2 hours.
   6. Assessing vital sign trends.

9. The order reads: Infuse D_5W 1000 mL over 6 hours. The IV tubing delivers 15 drops per mL. The drop rate should be _______________ gtts/minute. ***(58)***

10. When assisting the patient to arise from the bed postoperatively, you would have him *first:* ***(99)***
    1. push up from the bed with his elbows.
    2. turn toward the side of the bed from which he is going to exit it.
    3. bend the knees and plant the feet flat on the mattress.
    4. grab the top side rail and push up to a sitting position.

CRITICAL THINKING ACTIVITY

Scenario: Mr. T. has just returned to his room from the PACU. He had a ruptured appendix and an appendectomy was performed. He is receiving IV fluids and antibiotics.

1. On the third postoperative day, he has abdominal distension. He is not passing flatus and no bowel sounds are detected. What complication of surgery might he be experiencing? ***(103)***

 ____

2. An NG tube is inserted and attached to suction. He is placed on NPO status. The last shift assessment found that he is tachycardic, has decreased urine output, poor skin turgor, and his blood pressure has dropped 20 points. What would you suspect is the problem? ***(103)***

 ____

3. Mr. T. improves and is ready for discharge. He will continue oral antibiotics at home. What instructions should he be given? ***(108)***

 ____

 ____

 ____

STEPS TOWARD BETTER COMMUNICATION

VOCABULARY BUILDING GLOSSARY

Term	**Definition**
allay' (ah la')	to calm, to place at rest
induce' (in doos')	to bring on by outside means
grog'gy	unsteady or shaky with an unclear mind
numb (num)	lack of sensation; no feeling
kink'ed	bent sharply so as to block the flow inside
malaise' (mah laz')	general feeling of bodily discomfort

COMPLETION

Directions: Fill in the blank in the following sentences with the correct word from the glossary above.

1. Mrs. P. is awake from anesthesia, but is still very ______________________.
2. The nurse must carefully check each tube and drain after turning a patient to be certain that no tube is ______________.
3. After spinal anesthesia, the patient's legs are ______________ for a few hours.
4. Mr. R.'s wound was healing nicely, but he is suffering from ______________.
5. Certain drugs can sometimes ______________________ anaphylactic shock.

GRAMMAR POINTS

As a nurse, you will be giving postoperative discharge instructions to your patients. Some instructions are about things the patient *should* do; others are about things that she *should not* do. Certain things *must* be done to prevent complications; other things *must not* be done or they may interfere with recovery. Insert the correct instruction before each statement. ***(108)***

You should You should not You must You must not

1. ______________________________ walk for 5–10 minutes three times a day.
2. ______________________________ inspect the incision for signs of redness or drainage every day.
3. ______________________________ scratch the incision if it starts to itch.
4. ______________________________ lift anything heavier than 5 pounds for at least 4 weeks.
5. ______________________________ call the physician if your temperature rises to 100.2° F (38.0° C).

COMMUNICATION EXERCISE

Dialogue Example

Joan, an LVN, is getting Mr. Cox out of bed to sit in the chair for the second time since his surgery yesterday. Note how Joan interacts with Mr. Cox.

Joan: "Mr. Cox, it is time to get you up to sit in the chair for about 20 minutes now. I'll help you sit on the side of the bed and put on your robe."

Mr. Cox: "Do I have to get up now? I just finished breakfast."

Joan: "Yes, your doctor left orders for you to be up in the chair after breakfast."

Mr. Cox: "You won't leave me there too long, will you?"

Joan: "No, I'll be back in about 20 minutes to help you back into bed."

Mr. Cox: "OK."

Joan: "Place your left hand on the side rail and turn toward me." (She raises the head of the bed slightly and helps Mr. Cox to turn on his side and swing his feet over the side of the bed into a sitting position. She helps him put his arms into his robe while he is seated.)

Mr. Cox: "Whee, I feel just a little dizzy."

Joan: "Just sit here for a moment until the dizziness passes."

Mr. Cox: "OK. I feel better now."

Joan: "Let me put your slippers on your feet and then I'll help you to stand up. Place your hands on my shoulders and stand on the count of three." (Joan helps Mr. Cox to stand by supporting him while he rises.)

Mr. Cox: "I made it."

Joan: "That was very good. Now we'll walk over to the chair and turn so that you are ready to sit down."

Mr. Cox: "I don't want to miss the seat when I sit down."

Joan: "Move back so the chair is touching the back of your legs. Place your right hand on the arm of the chair and slowly lower yourself into the chair." (Mr. Cox does this successfully.) "That was great. Would you like a blanket over your legs to keep you warm.?"

Mr. Cox: "No, I'm warm enough. That wasn't as hard as it was yesterday. Thank you."

Joan: "OK. It is 9:10 now, so I'll be back at 9:30."

CHAPTER 6

Infection Prevention and Control

evolve Go to http://evolve.elsevier.com/deWit for additional activities and exercises.

COMPLETION

Directions: Fill in the blanks to complete the statements.

1. All streptococci and staphylococci are gram-____________________ organisms. ***(112)***
2. Chickenpox, influenza, warts, the common cold, and genital herpes infection are all caused by ________________________________. ***(113)***
3. Insufficient hand hygiene by medical staff and other people in contact with patients is a major cause of ________________________________ infections. ***(122)***
4. When inserting a Foley catheter, you should use ____________________________________ technique. ***(125)***
5. Risk of exposure to infection is influenced by ______________, ________________, and ______________________________ status. ***(112, 113)***
6. Pathogens are transmitted by three routes: ______________, ______________, and ______________.
7. Ms. Jones reports giving her child ½ teaspoon of liquid children's fever reducer. How many milliliters (mL) did she give? ________
8. Physician orders 600 mg of acetaminophen. Pharmacy delivers a 3-ounce bottle of acetaminophen 325 mg/10.15 mL. How many mL should be given? _________

SHORT ANSWER

Causes and Symptoms of Infection

Scenario: You are caring for patients on a general medical-surgical unit. Currently, there are several postoperative patients; therefore, you are vigilant for signs and symptoms of infection in these patients. You also have an elderly patient who is fairly immobile, so you are aware of the need to assess her for signs of pneumonia.

Directions: Provide the answers to the following questions.

1. List four specific signs and symptoms that suggest presence of a respiratory infection. *(127)*

   a. ______________________________

   b. ______________________________

   c. ______________________________

   d. ______________________________

2. What are five local signs and symptoms of inflammation? *(118)*

   a. ______________________________

   b. ______________________________

   c. ______________________________

   d. ______________________________

   e. ______________________________

3. Identify seven signs and symptoms of systemic or generalized infection. *(118)*

   a. ______________________________

   b. ______________________________

   c. ______________________________

   d. ______________________________

   e. ______________________________

   f. ______________________________

   g. ______________________________

Nursing Interventions for Patients with Infections

Directions: Provide the answers to the following questions.

1. List three nursing interventions that can be used to reduce high fevers. *(115)*

   a. ______________________________

   b. ______________________________

   c. ______________________________

2. What are three teaching points to help patients avoid spreading respiratory infections to others? *(121)*

   a. ______________________________

   b. ______________________________

   c. ______________________________

3. List five things that you should do to help prevent health care–associated infections. ***(124)***

   a. ______________________________

   b. ______________________________

   c. ______________________________

   d. ______________________________

   e. ______________________________

TABLE ACTIVITY

Changes in Natural Defense Mechanisms that Occur with Age

Directions: Complete the following table by describing the changes that occur with aging in the natural defense mechanisms. ***(117)***

Change	Consequence
Decreased skin turgor and skin fragility	
Decreased elasticity and atherosclerosis of peripheral vessels	
Calcification of heart valves	
Stiffness of thorax, weakened respiratory muscles, decreased ciliary action	
Decreased gastrointestinal tract motility; acid production is decreased	
Prostate changes, bladder prolapse, and urethral strictures	
Immune response decreases, as bone marrow does not produce new blood cells as rapidly	

PRIORITY SETTING

Scenario: You are caring for a patient who was admitted for a leg infection. She needs IV antibiotic medication. She is unsure, but she believes that it will be the first time that she will receive this medication.

*Directions: Prioritize the steps below for safe administration. **(129)***

_______ a. Check the order and know why the patient is to receive an antimicrobial drug.

_______ b. Check that the dosage of the antimicrobial drug is appropriate for the patient.

_______ c. Verify allergies with the patient before administering an antimicrobial drug.

_______ d. Obtain cultures prior to administering the antimicrobial agent.

_______ e. Check to see if serum drug levels or cultures have been ordered.

_______ f. Monitor patient for signs of allergic reaction, such as rash, hives, itching, drug fever, swelling of the mucous membranes, difficulty breathing, or anaphylaxis.

SHORT ANSWER

Sepsis and Septic Shock

Scenario: You are working in an extended care facility. Mr. Amberski is an elderly patient who is generally alert, cheerful, and conversant. Today, you immediately notice a marked change in his behavior and he appears very ill. You are aware that he has been had some urinary symptoms (i.e., frequency and urgency) over the past two days.

Directions: Answer the following questions about sepsis and septic shock.

1. List four signs and symptoms of sepsis. ***(127)***

   a. ______________________________

   b. ______________________________

   c. ______________________________

   d. ______________________________

2. How might these symptoms differ in an elderly person? ***(128)*** ______________________________

   ____

3. List at least six signs and symptoms of septic shock. ***(127)***

   a. ______________________________

   b. ______________________________

   c. ______________________________

   d. ______________________________

   e. ______________________________

   f. ______________________________

4. How is septic shock treated? *(128)* ______________________________

____

____

APPLICATION OF THE NURSING PROCESS

Care of the Patient at Risk for Infection

Directions: Write a short-term and a long-term goal and 4–6 interventions and an example of an evaluation statement for the short-term goal.

Mr. Jones is a 70-year-old gentleman residing in an extended care facility. He has chronic poor circulation to his lower extremities; the skin just above the ankles has a brownish discoloration and is very leathery. He complains of itching and frequently scratches his legs; there are some very faint superficial scratches noted on the right ankle.

Nursing Diagnosis: Risk for infection related to poor circulation and skin ulceration.

Goals/Expected Outcomes	Nursing Interventions	Evaluation

NCLEX-PN® EXAM REVIEW

Directions: Choose the correct answer(s) for the following questions.

1. When a nurse assesses the patient for signs of local infection, which of the following would indicate a local infection? *(Select all that apply.)* ***(118)***
   1. Redness of skin and adjacent tissues
   2. Swelling at the site and surrounding tissues
   3. Pain at the site and surrounding tissues
   4. Limited function of the involved part
   5. Decreased peripheral pulses

2. Inflammation of the tissues is a(n): ***(117)***
   1. response that occurs immediately after an injury.
   2. protective response against injury or damage to cells or tissues.
   3. infection of the cells; no drainage or discharge.
   4. uncommon occurrence in people who do not have a chronic disease.

3. A 10-year-old patient has a staphylococcal infection that developed in an abdominal wound. The dressing must be changed once each shift. The patient is underweight, suffering from malnutrition, and has a fever. Which of the following nursing actions are essential? *(Select all that apply.)* ***(120)***
   1. Assess bowel and urine elimination regularly.
   2. Monitor temperature and promptly report abnormal readings.
   3. Encourage patient to eat well-balanced, nutritious meals.
   4. Strictly adhere to precautions to avoid spreading infection.
   5. Plan active exercise to promote growth and development.

4. A medication likely to be prescribed to combat a staphylococcal infection is: ***(130)***
   1. acetaminophen (Tylenol).
   2. trimethoprim-sulfamethoxasole (Septra).
   3. ketoconazole (Nizoral).
   4. penicillin V (Pen-Vee K).

5. A patient has a hacking cough, a runny nose, and painful swallowing because of a sore throat. He is diagnosed with a streptococcal infection of the throat. The nurse should use gloves for which type of activity? ***(121)***
   1. Taking a radial pulse.
   2. Obtaining a throat swab culture and sensitivity.
   3. Delivering the throat culture tube to the lab.
   4. Reviewing the culture results.

6. To help a patient to avoid spreading his respiratory infection to others, the nurse provides which patient education? *(Select all that apply.)* ***(121)***
   1. Avoid exposing others until after the first dose of medicine.
   2. Use tissues to cover the mouth and blow the nose.
   3. Dispose of contaminated tissues by placing them in a plastic or paper bag.
   4. Avoid going to public places such as crowded stores or theatres.

7. To help a patient recover from a throat infection, he should be advised to do which of the following? ***(118)***
   1. Continue his normal workout routine but to get plenty of rest at night.
   2. Drink 8 ounces of liquid every hour while he is awake.
   3. When the sore throat stops, discontinue prescribed medications.
   4. Take an antipyretic with meals or a snack.

8. The patient comes to the clinic for a chief complaint of burning with urination and urinary urgency. Based on her complaints, what additional assessment data would be most appropriate to obtain *first*? ***(127-128)***
   1. Assess her genitalia for signs of inflammation.
   2. Check her chart for a history of kidney problems.
   3. Check her temperature to assess for a fever.
   4. Ask her about drug and food allergies.

9. While waiting to see the physician for urinary symptoms, the patient tells the nurse that she has to go to the bathroom to urinate. The nurse should: ***(128)***
   1. ask her to delay urination until after the physician has examined her.
   2. instruct her to obtain a clean-catch midstream urine specimen.
   3. get an order for a Foley catheterization to relieve her urinary urgency.
   4. allow her to void freely and wait for the physician's orders.

CRITICAL THINKING ACTIVITIES

Scenario A: You observe that a new nursing assistant has a cough and runny nose. She is assigned to care for a patient with neutropenic precautions. You realize that she maybe be unfamiliar with this type of isolation, or that she may not know how to deal with the situation.

1. What should you do? ______________________________

____

____

Scenario B: You see a laboratory technician drawing blood from a patient. He is not wearing gloves, stating that they are not needed. He appears to be competent and is quickly able to draw the blood without apparent contact with body fluids.

1. Explore how you would handle this situation. ______________________________

____

____

____

____

STEPS TOWARD BETTER COMMUNICATION

VOCABULARY BUILDING GLOSSARY

The following words from Chapter 6 have the long **a** sound, as in *name.* Perhaps you can find others.

Term	**Definition**
survei'lance (ser va'lenz)	continuous watching for something
malaise'(mah laz')	feeling of illness
-phage	eating, swallowing
mac'rophage	large phagocytic cell
phagocyto'sis	surrounding of microorganism by phagocytes
asep'tic	free from bacteria
asep'sis	method to prevent infection, keep bacteria-free

PRONUNCIATION SKILLS

The long "a" sound can be spelled in a number of ways.

Spelling	Examples
a	latent, anal, patient, dangerous, table, dilation, incubation
a–e	invade, isolate, palpate, dilate, lactate, incubate, drape, -phage, make, mistake (silent "e" at end)
ai	brain, pain, malaise, daily, wait, straight
ay	day, say, stay, May
ea	great, break, steak
ei	vein, weigh, nucleic, eight
ey	they, obey

MATCHING

Directions: Match the following terms with their correct definitions.

1. ______	Asepsis	a.	General feeling of illness, not well
2. ______	Malaise	b.	Containing pus
3. ______	Exudate	c.	Watching for
4. ______	Purulent	d.	Keeping free from bacteria
5. ______	Surveillance	e.	Discharge that is composed of tissue, fluid, and dead cells

PRONUNCIATION SKILLS

Directions: In the following sentences, underline the letters in the words that have the long "a" sound.

1. Draping the patient on the table before a procedure protects the patient's privacy and modesty. It helps to maintain aseptic conditions.

2. Ms. Clay has fever and malaise and her wound has green exudate.

3. Mrs. James is not having any pain, but she has gained more than eighteen pounds in weight.

COMMUNICATION EXERCISES

Directions: Write out what you would say for the following situations.

1. Mrs. Compton is admitted for a hysterectomy but has a boil in the axilla. How would you explain the importance of hand hygiene and using clean towels and washcloths to bathe when she goes home?

2. You have a patient with a large infected wound on his shin. How would you explain to him how infection is spread and the precautions that must be taken in caring for him and changing his dressings?

CHAPTER 7

Care of Patients with Pain

evolve Go to http://evolve.elsevier.com/deWit for additional activities and exercises.

TABLE ACTIVITY

Common Terms to Help Patients Describe Their Pain

Directions: Fill in the table with some common terms to help your patient to describe pain. ***(143)***

Degree of pain (from least to most severe)	
Quality of pain	
Frequency of the pain	

COMPLETION

Directions: Fill in the blanks to complete the statements.

1. The body produces ____________________ which can attach to pain receptors and block the pain sensation. ***(137)***

2. Referred pain is defined as pain that is felt in a ____________________ part of body than where it occurs. ***(141)***

3. Rest ________________ pain tolerance and improves response to analgesia. ***(149)***

4. One "rule" to keep in mind is that massage should *not* be used on areas ____________________ ____________________. ***(151)***

5. A dressing change or an uncomfortable procedure can be made less painful if you ask the patient questions and ______________ his attention during the procedure. ***(150)***

6. Repositioning is an important measure in ________________ pain, especially in the elderly. ***(149)***

7. In addition to heat and cold packs, another home remedy useful for relief of certain types of muscle and joint pain is ____________________. ***(152)***

8. Morphine, codeine, and hydromorphone (Dilaudid) are examples of ____________________ analgesics. ***(149)***

9. A measure of the effectiveness of control of chronic pain is how well the patient can accomplish ______________________________. ***(148)***

10. A side effect of long-term narcotic analgesia that you must always keep in mind and treat as it occurs is ______________________________. ***(148)***

11. The complete assessment of a person's pain should include information about: onset and duration, ____________________, ____________________, and quantity. In addition, include data concerning factors that ____________________ the pain, and factors that ____________________ the pain. ***(141)***

SHORT ANSWER

Pain and Pain Management

Directions: Read the scenario and answer the questions that follow.

Scenario: You have been asked to assist the nurse manager to develop an in-service for the nursing staff about pain and pain management. He has asked you to collect some relevant information that can be reviewed with the staff and to make a handout that compares acute and chronic pain.

1. What are five facts that dispel false perceptions about pain? ***(145)***

    a. ______________________________

    b. ______________________________

    c. ______________________________

    d. ______________________________

    e. ______________________________

2. List four nonphysical factors that affect pain tolerance. ***(139)***

    a. ______________________________

    b. ______________________________

    c. ______________________________

    d. ______________________________

3. List at least six nonpharmacologic approaches that can be used as adjuncts to medication. ***(149-151)***

    a. ______________________________

    b. ______________________________

    c. ______________________________

    d. ______________________________

    e. ______________________________

    f. ______________________________

4. Briefly explain how imagery and meditation can assist with pain control. ***(150)***______________________________

    ____

    ____

TABLE ACTIVITY

Acute Versus Chronic Pain

Directions: Fill in the table to compare features of acute and chronic pain. ***(152-153)***

Pain	Acute	Chronic
Duration		
Prognosis for relief		
Cause		
Psychosocial effects		
Effect of therapy		

APPLICATION OF THE NURSING PROCESS

Caring for a Patient with Acute Pain

Directions: Provide the answer to the following questions.

Mr. Poroj was in a motor vehicle accident and was transferred 6 days ago from the ICU to the general medical-surgical unit. He has a broken arm, rib fractures, and soft tissue trauma on both legs. Mr. Poroj has a difficult time verbalizing his pain to the nursing staff and frequently declines medication. He is quiet and withdrawn and often appears very uncomfortable.

1. List at least six physiologic clues that may indicate Mr. Poroj is experiencing pain. ***(140)***

   a. ____________________

   b. ____________________

   c. ____________________

   d. ____________________

   e. ____________________

   f. ____________________

2. List at least five behaviors that may indicate that Mr. Poroj is having pain. ***(139)***

   a. ____________________

   b. ____________________

   c. ____________________

   d. ____________________

   e. ____________________

3. Which of the following diagnoses is a priority for Mr. Poroj? ***(152)***
   a. Knowledge deficit related to pain management
   b. Body image disturbance related to injuries
   c. Pain, acute related to tissue trauma and fractures
   d. Ineffective individual coping related to pain

4. You are reinforcing teaching points to help Mr. Poroj understand pain management. *(Select all that apply.)* ***(148)***
   a. Medication is more effective if taken before pain is too severe.
   b. Taking medication regularly helps control the pain.
   c. Pain actually interferes with wound healing.
   d. Patient addiction to narcotics is usually less than 1%.
   e. Pain tolerance does not vary greatly from one person to the next.

5. List five areas that should be covered in documentation about pain and measures taken for the treatment of pain. ***(145-146)***

   a. ______________________________

   b. ______________________________

   c. ______________________________

   d. ______________________________

   e. ______________________________

PRIORITY SETTING

Directions: Read the scenarios and prioritize tasks and patients' needs appropriately.

Scenario A: You are caring for Mr. Micks. He was admitted for 23-hour observation and cast checks. He sustained a broken ankle with severe soft tissue swelling during a bicycle accident. Initially, he received IV morphine for the procedure. The current order is for 800 mg ibuprofen PO. Prioritize the following nursing responsibilities that are related to giving analgesic medications.

______ Provide analgesic as ordered.

______ Reinforce teaching about medications.

______ Use nonpharmacologic measures such as elevation or ice packs.

______ Report to the physician when measures are not effective.

______ Assess the patient's pain.

______ Check the medication record for last dose.

Scenario B: You are caring for several patients on a busy medical-surgical unit. While you are aware that all patients expect and deserve to receive timely and adequate relief of their pain, you also recognize the need to organize and prioritize your actions. Based on your knowledge of pain and pathophysiology, prioritize the order in which you will attend to the needs of these patients.

______ a. Mr. Jewel is 2 days postoperative for a hernia repair. He complains of pain 8/10 in the lower abdominal area.

______ b. Mrs. Qualle reports pain in the left neck and jaw which radiates down her left arm.

______ c. Mr. Davoudi reports severe pain that started 10 minutes ago, in the area distal to his lower extremity cast.

______ d. Mr. Goldkoen is a diabetic who has continuous neuropathic pain in his lower legs.

NCLEX-PN® EXAM REVIEW

Directions: Choose the best answer(s) for the following questions.

1. The patient is experiencing pain in a limb after amputation. What type of pain is this patient experiencing? ***(138)***
   1. Chronic pain
   2. Phantom pain
   3. Referred pain
   4. Nocieceptive pain.

2. When using a pain scale, it is essential that the patient understands and that the: ***(141)***
   1. nursing staff uses it consistently.
   2. same staff nurse always assesses the patient.
   3. scale is used at the beginning of every shift.
   4. scale is used for patients who can't describe their pain.

3. Which of the following pain scales would be appropriate for a patient who is cognitively impaired? ***(142)***
   1. Visual scale
   2. Color scale
   3. Pieces of pain scale
   4. Behavioral pain scale

4. Gabapentin (Neurontin) is given to relieve which type of pain? ***(147)***
   1. Acute pain
   2. Chronic pain
   3. Neuropathic pain
   4. Nocieceptive pain

5. A patient is undergoing rehabilitative therapy. When would be the best time to give analgesic medication? ***(144)***
   1. Give PRN medications every 4–6 hours.
   2. Give early in the morning before performing ADLs.
   3. Give on a schedule to minimize pain during therapy sessions.
   4. Give whenever the pain is greater than 4/10.

6. The patient is unable to verbalize pain. Of the following patient behaviors, which is the *best* indicator that pain medication is successfully addressing the patient's pain? ***(142)***
   1. Patient sleeps unless aroused by nurse.
   2. Patient watches TV without grimacing.
   3. Patient actively participates in physical therapy.
   4. Patient smiles at friends and family when they visit.

7. The nurse gives the patient a 5mg PO dose of oxycodone HCl (OxyContin) at 8:00 AM. When should the nurse evaluate the effectiveness of the pain control medication? ***(146)***
   1. 8:15 AM
   2. 8:30 AM
   3. 8:45 AM
   4. 9: 00 AM

8. When evaluating the effectiveness of pain medication, in addition to assessing physical body language, the nurse should rely on: ***(146)***
   1. the length of time between requests for pain medication.
   2. how sedated the patient becomes after receiving the medication.
   3. whether the patient experiences nausea from the medication.
   4. what the patient says about his pain relief.

CRITICAL THINKING ACTIVITIES

Scenario: Mrs. Cole, age 54, is admitted to the hospital for a laparoscopic cholecystectomy. She has a history of chronic gallbladder disease with episodes of pain, nausea, and vomiting. During her initial assessment upon admission, you learn that Mrs. Cole has had arthritis of the knees and hips for about 15 years.

1. Which of the following statements most accurately applies to Mrs. Cole's problem of pain?
   a. If she does not mention having pain due to her arthritis, it is because she has gotten used to it over the years and it no longer bothers her much.
   b. Unless some degeneration of the joints is shown by x-rays, there is little reason to believe that a person has pain with arthritis.
   c. You must be careful *not* to administer too many doses of a narcotic analgesic to Mrs. Cole postoperatively because her age and health status make her a good candidate for addiction.
   d. Aspirin, a non-narcotic analgesic, and cold packs applied to her knees help relieve Mrs. Cole's pain at home and could be continued in the hospital.

2. If Mrs. Cole states that she often feels pain under her right shoulder blade when her gallbladder "acts up," you can assume that Mrs. Cole:
   a. probably also has an undiagnosed heart condition.
   b. is feeling referred pain.
   c. is confused about where her pain really is.
   d. is pretending to have pain that does not really exist.

3. The admitting physician has not ordered anything for relief of Mrs. Cole's arthritic pain. In this circumstance, the best nursing action would be to:
   a. explain to Mrs. Cole that whatever she receives for pain after surgery will probably relieve the pain she has in her knees and hips.
   b. ignore the omission of orders because Mrs. Cole's arthritic pain is not as important as her gallbladder disorder.
   c. ask Mrs. Cole what measures she uses at home for relief of her arthritic pain, record the information, institute nursing measures, and ask her physician to order the analgesic she uses.
   d. tell Mrs. Cole nothing can be done about her painful joints because her physician did not write an order for any relief measures.

4. On the evening after her surgery, Mrs. Cole has a long visit with her daughter. During that time, you look in on Mrs. Cole and she seems to be comfortable and happy. After her daughter leaves, Mrs. Cole asks for something for pain. Mrs. Cole's behavior probably indicates that:
   a. she does not have as much real pain as she says she has.
   b. she is afraid to complain in her daughter's presence.
   c. her daughter brought some medication from home to relieve her mother's pain.
   d. her daughter's visit effectively distracted Mrs. Cole and diverted her attention from her pain.

STEPS TOWARD BETTER COMMUNICATION

VOCABULARY BUILDING GLOSSARY

Term	Definition
compounds'	(verb) increases or adds to; makes worse
creep'ing	moving slowly and with difficulty
frail	having delicate health; weak
grim'ace	odd facial expression indicating pain
im'agery	mental pictures
indic'ative	suggesting; pointing out
place'bo	a substance that contains no actual medication
keep a "stiff upper lip"	bear something without an outward show of emotion or body change (slang)
tol'erance	point in drug therapy where the drug no longer works

COMPLETION

Directions: Fill in the blanks with the appropriate words from the Vocabulary Building Glossary above.

1. The use of ____________________ helps patients relax and take a short "mental vacation."
2. The patient was experiencing back pain and was ______________ across the room to the bathroom.
3. When the nurse turned the patient onto his left side, his ______________ indicated that he was experiencing pain.
4. Fatigue ____________________ the problem of pain and makes it more difficult to cope with.
5. The 88-year-old lady had lost 7 pounds and appeared very ____________.
6. Some patients respond well to a ____________ in place of a narcotic analgesic.
7. Mr. Thomas presented a ________________________, not even flinching when the doctor bent his knee after surgery.
8. When a patient frequently complains of pain much sooner than usual after a dose of pain medication, either something is making the pain worse or the patient is developing ______________________ to the pain medication.
9. When a pain medication is no longer effective for the patient, it is ____________________ of the need for a change in the medication order.

MATCHING

Directions: Match the abbreviations with their correct terms.

1. ______	OTC	a.	Transcutaneous electrical nerve stimulation
2. ______	PCA	b.	Over-the-counter
3. ______	TENS	c.	Patient-controlled analgesia

TERMINOLOGY

Evaluating Pain

Directions: Rank (from 1 to 9) the following words for degrees of pain from the least to the worst.

______ moderate

______ minimal

______ extremely severe

______ exquisite

______ mild

______ very severe

______ absent

______ fairly severe

______ severe

MATCHING

Directions: Match the terms indicating the quality of pain on the right with the correct category headings on the left (each category will have more than one term).

1. ______	Heat	a.	Burning
2. ______	Knife	b.	Pulsating
3. ______	Stretching	c.	Dull
4. ______	Vibrating	d.	Twisting
5. ______	Pressure	e.	Tearing
		f.	Throbbing
		g.	Biting
		h.	Searing
		i.	Stabbing
		j.	Crushing
		k.	Tingling
		l.	Pulling
		m.	Sharp

COMMUNICATION EXERCISES

Directions: Read the following scenarios and answer the related questions.

1. Your patient's ordered medication is not controlling the pain for more than 1 hour. You need to call the doctor and ask for the order to be changed. Write out what you would say during the phone call. (Remember you will need to know the current vital signs.) ____________________

____

____

____

____

2. You have given your patient an injection of morphine for pain. An hour later, you notice that the patient's respirations have dropped to 10 per minute. You must notify the charge nurse of the patient's condition. Write out how you would tell the charge nurse this information. ____________________

____

____

____

____

CHAPTER 8

Care of Patients with Cancer

Go to http://evolve.elsevier.com/deWit for additional activities and exercises.

COMPLETION

Directions: Fill in the blanks to complete the statements.

1. Malignant cells often tend to grow much more ________________ than normal cells. ***(158)***

2. A __________________________ is a tumor composed of fibrous tissue. ***(159)***

3. Malignant growths are divided into four main types: ____________________,
____________________, ____________________, and ________________________. ***(159)***

4. TNM staging system identifies cancers by how much the malignancy has spread and includes three basic parts: *T* for ________________________, *N* for ________________, and *M* for ____________________________. ***(160)***

5. ________________, ________________, air and water pollution, and certain ________________________ found in food packaging are all considered to be carcinogens. ***(161)***

6. There are three traditional modes of therapy for malignancies: ______________________,
____________________, and __________________________. ***(169)***

7. Many antineoplastic drugs are ____________________, which can cause tissue damage and severe local injury if they escape from the vein into which they are administered. ***(177)***

8. Suppression of the ________________________________ is the major reason that doses of chemotherapy must be limited. ***(181)***

9. In treating cancer pain, the health care team should continue to seek a combination of interventions or different treatments until the pain ____. ***(183)***

10. Radiation therapy of the abdomen or lower back often produces__________, __________________, and ____________________ starting 7–10 days after the beginning of treatment. ***(180)***

11. The doctor orders hydromorphone (Dilaudid) 4 mg PO liquid for pain. The pharmacy delivers a 90 mL bottle of hydromorphone (Dilaudid) 5 mg/5 mL. How many mL should be given? ______________

MATCHING

Risk Factors for Cancer

Directions: Match each high-risk factor on the left with its associated site of malignancy on the right. ***(165)***

1. ______ Diet heavy in pickled or salted foods	a.	Stomach
2. ______ Frequent sex in early teens	b.	Prostate
3. ______ Early menarche; late menopause	c.	Uterine and endometrial
4. ______ Estrogen therapy	d.	Breast
5. ______ Over age 65; African-American	e.	Uterus and cervix
6. ______ Heavy smoker; asbestos exposure	f.	Lung
7. ______ Use of smokeless tobacco	g.	Mouth

SHORT ANSWER

Interventions for the Side Effects of Chemotherapy

Directions: Read the clinical scenario and answer the questions that follow.

Scenario: You are caring for a patient who is receiving chemotherapy. List at least five nursing activities (assessments or interventions) to include in the care plan of a patient experiencing the common problems related to cancer or the toxic side effects of chemotherapy.

1. Common problem: fatigue ***(182)***

   a. ______________________________

   b. ______________________________

   c. ______________________________

   d. ______________________________

   e. ______________________________

2. Toxic effect: thrombocytopenia ***(181)***

   a. ______________________________

   b. ______________________________

   c. ______________________________

   d. ______________________________

   e. ______________________________

3. Toxic effect: mucositis ***(179)***

    a. ______________________________

    b. ______________________________

    c. ______________________________

    d. ______________________________

    e. ______________________________

4. Toxic effect: immunosuppression ***(181)***

    a. ______________________________

    b. ______________________________

    c. ______________________________

    d. ______________________________

    e. ______________________________

APPLICATION OF THE NURSING PROCESS

Caring for a Patient with Non-Hodgkin's Lymphoma

Directions: Provide the answer to the following questions.

Mrs. Junic is diagnosed with non-Hodgkin's lymphoma. She is receiving combination chemotherapy and radiation. She is trying to be brave and "not bother the nurses or worry her family," but you walk in and find that she is crying. She admits to nausea, vomiting, and diarrhea, "but I know that is just part of the therapy, so I am trying to deal with it."

1. List at least four things to assess for related to Mrs. Junic's vomiting and diarrhea. ***(180)***

    a. ______________________________

    ____

    b. ______________________________

    ____

    c. ______________________________

    ____

    d. ______________________________

    ____

2. Which of the following nursing diagnoses is a priority for Mrs. Junic? ***(180)***
   a. Alteration in nutrition (less than body needs), risk for, related to nausea, vomiting, and diarrhea
   b. Diarrhea related to effects of cancer treatment
   c. Knowledge deficit related to drugs and side effects
   d. Ineffective individual coping related to side effects of treatment

3. List six nonpharmacologic interventions for nausea. ***(180)***

   a. ____________________

   b. ____________________

   c. ____________________

   d. ____________________

   e. ____________________

   f. ____________________

4. List at least five resources that a cancer patient and his or her family might use to help them cope with the problems associated with malignancy. ***(184)***

   a. ____________________

   b. ____________________

   c. ____________________

   d. ____________________

   e. ____________________

5. Which of the following statements by Mrs. Junic indicates that she understands how to deal with the side effects of chemotherapy? ***(178)***
   a. "All drugs, including chemotherapy drugs, have side effects."
   b. "I should report side effects; they could be an adverse response to therapy."
   c. "After I learn to recognize the side effects, I can cope independently."
   d. "A few side effects are okay as long as they don't interfere with activities of daily living."

PRIORITY SETTING

Directions: Read the following scenario and prioritize as appropriate.

Scenario: You are assigned to care for five patients on an oncology unit. You have just received report from the night shift nurse. *Prioritize the order in which you will attend to the needs of these patients.*

_______ a. Ms. Altnu needs her AM dose of Megace.

_______ b. Mrs. Jwa needs assistance with eating breakfast.

_______ c. Mr. Lain's laboratory report shows a platelet count of 20,000/mm^3.

_______ d. Mr. Nezzer is asking for a PRN pain medication.

_______ e. Ms. Decoux wants information about cancer support groups.

NCLEX-PN® EXAM REVIEW

Directions: Choose the best answer(s) for the following questions.

1. When assessing the effect of anorexia on maintaining ideal body weight, a significant loss of weight would be: ***(179)***
    1. 1 pound per month.
    2. 0.5 pound per week.
    3. 2 pounds per month.
    4. 2 pounds or more per week.

2. The nurse directs the nursing assistant in safety measures to be used while caring for a patient undergoing radiation therapy with a sealed implant. Which of the following is appropriate to include? ***(175)***
    1. Use ordinary standard precautions, but nothing else is required.
    2. Limit total time in patient's room to 60 minutes/8-hour shift.
    3. Wear a radiation detection badge to detect the amount of radiation exposure.
    4. Wear a lead apron to decrease exposure to radiation.

3. The principles of radiation protection when working with patients undergoing internal radiation are to coordinate: ***(174)***
    1. needs, care, and priorities.
    2. time, distance, and shielding.
    3. supplies, food, and procedures.
    4. treatments, meals, and medications.

4. When evaluating the patient's response to chemotherapy, which assessment finding is the greatest immediate concern? ***(181-182)***
    1. Constipation and straining
    2. Bleeding after brushing teeth
    3. Alopecia or change in hair color
    4. Fatigue and irritability

5. The patient is newly diagnosed with cancer and faces enormous stress. Which response by the nurse would be the most useful in helping the patient cope? ***(185)***
    1. "The doctor will give you all the information you need to know."
    2. "Tell me what the doctor told you and maybe I can help to clarify things."
    3. "Try to read or watch television. Just keep your mind busy."
    4. "Don't worry about chemotherapy, my aunt had it and she did just fine."

6. Tamoxifen is currently used to treat: ***(178)***
    1. prostate cancer.
    2. leukemia.
    3. breast cancer.
    4. lung cancer.

7. Alopecia resulting from chemotherapy is: ***(182)***
    1. temporary.
    2. irreversible.
    3. treatable.
    4. preventable.

8. The nurse gives the patient an oral dose of morphine 30 mg. The response to the mediation should be assessed in: ***(183)***
   1. 15 minutes.
   2. 20 minutes.
   3. 30 minutes.
   4. 60 minutes.

9. Which of the following statements by the family indicates an understanding of palliative care? ***(185)***
   1. "We want him to be comfortable, so oral medications are preferred."
   2. "We should encourage water and other nourishment as much as possible."
   3. "He'll feel short of breath and we'll hear the "death rattle."
   4. "He'll continue with his cancer treatments if they don't cause side effects."

10. The patient is having diarrhea secondary to radiation therapy of the pelvic area. Which of the following statements by the patient indicates a need for additional teaching about the diarrhea? ***(180)***
    1. "I will cleanse the rectal area and apply petroleum jelly."
    2. "I will report an increase in the number and frequency of bowel movements."
    3. "I will avoid eating foods such as bananas and cheese."
    4. "I may need to have my electrolytes checked if the diarrhea is severe."

CRITICAL THINKING ACTIVITIES

Scenario: Mr. Long is scheduled to begin receiving external radiation therapy to his chin and neck for cancer of the mandible.

1. Select all of the correct teaching points to share with Mr. Long about his therapy. ***(172-173)***
   a. Local skin irritation may not appear immediately, but may appear later.
   b. The treatment will be delivered in divided doses over many days.
   c. He must avoid contact with others to avoid exposing them to radiation.
   d. Written instructions are provided to help manage the expected side effects.
   e. Skin damage will be permanent, but the area will be very small.

2. Which of these side effects is most likely to occur as a result of radiation to the neck? ***(173)***
   a. Thrombocytopenia
   b. Loss of taste
   c. Alopecia
   d. Leukopenia

3. Choose measures that would be included in the care plan for Mr. Long. *(Select all that apply.)* ***(172-173)***
   a. Increased fluid intake
   b. Artificial saliva to be used as needed
   c. Minimal brushing of teeth to reduce irritation
   d. Avoid spicy food and alcohol
   e. Limited protein intake

4. To minimize damage to the skin exposed to radiation, Mr. Long should be instructed to do which of the following? ***(173)***
   a. Wear a tight-fitting scarf around his neck to protect it from sunlight.
   b. Wash the skin gently with mild soap, tepid water, and a soft washcloth.
   c. Avoid applying any lotions or powders unless prescribed by physician.
   d. Examine the condition of his skin weekly and report any blistering.

5. Mr. Long becomes unusually angry and demanding after his third treatment. You recognize that: ***(185)***
   a. he had a bad experience with the radiation therapy team.
   b. anger is one of the normal stages in the grieving process.
   c. the physician should be notified to prescribe an anxiolytic drug.
   d. confusion and personality changes are side effects of therapy.

6. In helping Mr. Long to deal with his anger, choose the most therapeutic response. ***(185)***
   a. "Everything will be okay, Mr. Long. Let me sit with you for awhile."
   b. "You don't seem like your usual self. Tell me what happened."
   c. "Those treatments are really tiring. Just rest for awhile."
   d. "I can see that you are upset. Why are you acting this way?"

STEPS TOWARD BETTER COMMUNICATION

VOCABULAR BUILDING GLOSSARY

Term	Definition
ad'juvant	serving to help or assist; used in addition to (another treatment)
be'nign	not malignant; gentle or kind
carcin'ogen	substance that tends to produce a cancer
depletes'	uses up; seriously decreases the supply
immunocom'petent	able to develop immunity
in si'tu	contained within the original site
intrin'sic	naturally belonging to or within something
malig'nant	uncontrolled growth that is harmful and may cause death
metas'tasis	spread of cancer cells to other parts of the body
oc'cult	hidden; not readily detectable
transforma'tion	change in nature, character, or appearance
ves'icant	agent that causes severe irritation and can cause blisters

WORD ATTACK SKILLS

Combining Forms: Prefixes

adeno-	gland
carcino-	cancer
melano-	black
fibro-	fiber; refers to connective tissue
leio-	smooth muscle
leuko-	white blood cell; white
lipo-	fat; lipid
lympho-	lymphocyte (clear tissue fluid)
osteo-	bone
radio-	radiant energy waves such as in radiation therapy

Combining Forms: Suffix

-oma	tumor

Word Families

metas'tasis:	(noun) invasive spread of tumor cells
metas'tasize:	(verb) to spread throughout the body
metasta'tic:	(adjective) capable of spreading throughout the body
carcino'ma:	(noun) malignant tumor of epithelial tissue
carcin'ogen:	(noun) agent that may cause cancer
carcinogen'ic:	(adjective) capable of causing cancer

PRONUNCIATION SKILLS

Directions: Look at the accent mark on each of the following words and practice their pronunciations.

mes en chy' mal (*ch* sounds like "k")

ma lig' nant

per i to ne' al

car cin o gen' ic

mi cro scop' ic ally (*ically* sounds like "ikly")

prog no' sis

car cin no' ma

car cin' o gens

de oxy ribo nu cle' ic

COMPLETION

Directions: Fill in the blanks with the appropriate words from the Vocabulary Building Glossary to complete the statements.

1. Chemotherapy drugs that are highly irritating are administered into a vein that has a high blood flow; such drugs may cause blisters and are termed ____________________.
2. A tumor whose cells reproduce in an uncontrolled, nonstructured pattern is called a ____________________ tumor.
3. If a malignant tumor occurs in the gastrointestinal tract, the only early symptom may be ____________________ bleeding.
4. When certain body cells are exposed to a ____________________ repeatedly over time, the cells may undergo malignant changes.
5. When chemotherapy or radiation is effective on a solid tumor, the cells in the tumor undergo a ____________________ and the tumor shrinks or stops growing.
6. A brain tumor may be ____________________ and still be life-threatening.

7. The excessive malignant growth of a tumor places a strain on the body and ______________________ nutritional stores.

8. The use of tamoxifen is a(n) ______________________ therapy added to surgery, radiation, and/or chemotherapy for breast cancer.

9. A normal, healthy body has the ______________________ ability to fight and kill beginning cancer cells.

10. Poor nutrition, exposure to toxic substances, chronic illness, and long periods of excessive stress make the body less ______________________ and may contribute to the growth of cancer.

11. When found ______________________, cervical cancer has a very good cure rate.

12. Breast cancer, as well as many other types of cancer, tends to ______________________ to other parts of the body if not caught and treated early.

Types of Tissues

Directions: From what type of tissue does each of the following tumors arise? ***(159)***

1. Adenocarcinoma: ______________________
2. Leiomyoma: ______________________
3. Lymphoma: ______________________
4. Melanoma: ______________________
5. Osteosarcoma: ______________________
6. Fibroma: ______________________

COMMUNICATION EXERCISE

Mr. Tomm, age 72, has metastatic prostate cancer. He is to undergo radiation therapy. Practice what you would say in the remainder of the dialogue.

Nurse: "Good morning, Mr. Tomm. How do you feel this morning?"

Mr. Tomm: "Pretty good, I guess. I woke up a lot last night."

Nurse: "Were you worrying about this morning's radiation treatment?"

Mr. Tomm: "I am a bit anxious, yes."

Nurse: *(Continue with statements by both the nurse and Mr. Tomm.)*

CHAPTER 9

Chronic Illness and Rehabilitation

evolve Go to http://evolve.elsevier.com/deWit for additional activities and exercises.

SHORT ANSWER

Chronic Illness and Immobility

1. The knowledge base and skills of the nurse who works with a patient who has a chronic illness must include: ***(190)***

   a. ______________________________

   b. ______________________________

   c. ______________________________

   d. ______________________________

2. One of the biggest problems for a person with a chronic illness who has lost functions and is no longer able to do everyday activities as easily is ______________________________ ______________________________. ***(191)***

3. The patient with a chronic illness often feels ______________________________. ***(191)***

4. The patient must develop new ____________ mechanisms in order to effectively deal with the changes the illness or situation has brought. ***(191)***

5. Five disorders that may cause immobility are: ***(191)***

   a. ______________________________

   b. ______________________________

   c. ______________________________

   d. ______________________________

   e. ______________________________

6. Patients who are on bedrest for just a few days are still at risk for the ____________ of immobility. ***(191)***

7. Early effects of immobility are: ***(191)*** ____________________

____

____

____

8. The elderly are more susceptible to the complications o immobility. It is especially important to monitor an elderly immobile patient for signs of: ***(191)***

   a. ____________________
   b. ____________________
   c. ____________________
   d. ____________________
   e. ____________________

TABLE ACTIVITY

Directions: Complete the following table with the measures used to prevent complications within the particular body system. ***(205)***

Body System	Measures to Prevent Complications
Musculoskeletal	
Gastrointestinal	
Cardiovascular	
Neurologic	
Renal/urinary	
Respiratory	
Integumentary	

COMPLETION

Directions: Fill in the blanks to complete the statements.

1. When working with a rehabilitation patient, the nurse must recognize that the patient is the ________________________ team. ***(203)***

2. The rehabilitation team often consists of the physician, nurse, vocational counselor, and the ________________________, ________________________, ________________________, and ________________________ therapists. ***(203)***

3. The basis of the philosophy of rehabilitation nursing is recognition of ________________________ ________________________. ***(200)***

4. The three components of a respiratory rehabilitation program are: ***(203)***

   a. ________________________

   b. ________________________

   c. ________________________

5. The first step in the prevention of falls is recognition of which ________________________ ________________________. ***(196)***

6. The second step in the prevention of falls is recognition of ________________________ ________________________ that could precipitate a fall. ***(196)***

7. Encouraging elderly residents of long-term care facilities to ________________________ to pick up something and ________________________ to dry the feet helps prevent dizziness or loss of balance and a fall. ***(197)***

8. When a resident is placed in a restraint, the nurse must visually check him every 30 minutes to ensure that ________________________ and that there are no problems. ***(198)***

9. When dealing with a confused patient, it is best to limit the ________________________ that the patient must make during an activity. ***(198)***

10. Sensory deficits such as impaired ________________________ or ________________________ may add to a patient's confusion and anxiety at night. ***(198)***

11. Residents who are taking diuretics must be constantly monitored for ________________________ ________________________ which might cause confusion. ***(196)***

12. A major part of promoting independence in patients is for the staff to ______________________________

____

____________________. ***(199)***

13. The goal of home care is to keep the patient ______________________________ and enable her to ____. ***(208)***

14. A difference between hospital and home care that must influence the philosophy of the home care nurse is that the ______________________________________. ***(208)***

NCLEX-PN® EXAM REVIEW

Directions: Choose the best answer(s) for the following questions.

1. It is important for the LPN/LVN to have knowledge about chronic illness as there are about ____________________ people in the United States with chronic illnesses or disabilities that interfere with normal function. ***(190)***

2. Within the long-term care environment, the LPN/LVN usually functions in the capacity of: ***(195)***
   1. supervisor of the facility.
   2. admission nurse with Medicare paperwork duties.
   3. basic caregiver.
   4. charge nurse guiding the care team.

3. The goals of care for the long-term or extended care facility are to: *(Select all that apply.)* ***(195)***
   1. provide a safe environment.
   2. promote individual independence.
   3. instruct in new hobbies.
   4. provide sufficient fluids for hydration.
   5. allow maintenance of autonomy.
   6. assist to maintain or attain as much function as possible.

4. Restorative care programs are beneficial in preventing falls. A restorative program focuses on: *(Select all that apply.)* ***(196)***
   1. restoring skin integrity.
   2. muscle strengthening.
   3. maintaining functionality.
   4. balance.
   5. ambulation.

5. When working with a rehabilitation patient, the nurse's function is to assist her to achieve an optimal state of health as: ***(200)***
   1 agreed upon by the health care team.
   2. defined by the physician.
   3. defined by the patient.
   4. defined by the nurse and physical therapist.

6. An appropriate expected outcome for the nursing diagnosis of impaired physical mobility for the resident who is right-handed and who has right-sided hemiparesis from a stroke is: ***(204)***
   1. bedrest will be maintained at all times.
   2. resident will begin crutch walking within 4 weeks.
   3. resident will comb hair and brush teeth by the end of 4 weeks.
   4. resident will show no signs of infection at time of discharge.

7. When assigning a task to an unlicensed assistive person, as the charge nurse, you must: ***(195)***
   1. be sure it is acceptable to the resident for the person to perform the task.
   2. ask the unlicensed person if he or she knows how to perform the task.
   3. be certain that competence in performing the task has been documented for the unlicensed person.
   4. test the unlicensed person for competence.

8. A nursing intervention that can help prevent ambulatory residents from falling at night on the way to the bathroom is to: ***(197)***
   1. leave a small light on in the room at night.
   2. instruct the patient not to get up without assistance.
   3. place the patient's slippers within reach at the bedside.
   4. place the call bell within reach.

9. A nursing measure to decrease wakeful behavior for a resident during the night is to: ***(198)***
   1. leave bright lights on in the room.
   2. listen to the patient and try to determine possible causes of unrest or fear.
   3. remind the patient of the day and date frequently.
   4. prevent napping during daylight hours.

10. When working with a confused resident on dressing, it is best to gain cooperation by: ***(198)***
    1. providing a variety of choices of what to do when.
    2. limiting choices and the need to make decisions.
    3. decreasing as much sensory input as possible.
    4. keeping the resident engaged in activities during the day.

CRITICAL THINKING ACTIVITIES

Scenario A

J.T., age 22, was in a motorcycle accident. He fractured his left leg, cervical spine (nondisplaced), and sustained a head injury. He is in the rehabilitation institute for rehabilitative care. He is in halo traction, has a leg brace, and is alert, but has some cognitive problems such as aphasia and memory loss.

1. What services would you expect to be included in J.T.'s care? ***(200)***

2. What specific interventions should be on his interdisciplinary care plan related to his skin? ***(206)***

3. What measures would be on the plan to preserve and promote mobility? ***(195)***

Scenario B

Ms. O.P., age 78, suffered a cerebrovascular accident (CVA, stroke). She has left-sided hemiparesis and is undergoing rehabilitation in the long-term care facility. She had been living at home alone. She is beginning to show improvement in use of her extremities.

1. What do you think would be the overall goals for this resident? ***(198-200)***

2. What therapies would have the highest priority? ***(196)***

3. What physical concerns should be addressed within her care plan? ***(194)***

STEPS TOWARD BETTER COMMUNICATION

VOCABULARY BUILDING GLOSSARY

Term	**Definition**
ascertain' (as er tan')	(verb) make certain or sure
co'ping (ko'ping)	(verb) dealing with difficulties and problems and attempt to overcome them
op'ti'mal	the best, as in *the best treatment*
peo'ple skills	social abilities that help a person get along well with other people
sub'op'ti'mal	less than ideal
sundowning	(noun) when a person becomes confused as the sun goes down

COMPLETION

Directions: Fill in the blanks with the appropriate words from the Vocabulary Building Glossary.

1. The nurse and social worker work with the patient to improve his ____________________ skills.

2. Mr. Jones exhibited ________________________ by becoming very agitated on the evening shift.

3. Sometimes the nurse must ______________________ what is preventing the patient from making progress toward his goals.
4. Mr. Otong achieved an ______________________ recovery from his stroke as he can walk quite well.
5. To work well on a rehabilitation team, the nurse must develop very good ______________________.
6. Mrs. Krause has not regained use of her arm after her stroke and her recovery is considered ______________________.

PRONUNCIATION SKILLS

The consonant blend **th** in English is difficult for many people, especially since it has two different sounds. To make the **th** sound, such as in "**th**ank you" and "**th**ree," put your tongue between your front teeth and blow out air between your tongue and top teeth. Practice the following words:

ar**th**ritis	**th**anks
ba**th**	**th**igh
bir**th**day	**th**in
brea**th**	**th**irst
mon**th**	**th**ree
mou**th**	**th**umb
tee**th**	**Th**ursday

To make the voiced **th** sound, such as in "**th**ere" and "**th**ey," make the **th** sound but use your voice. Compare the following:

Noun	**Verb**
ba**th**	ba**th**e
tee**th**	tee**th**e
brea**th**	brea**th**e

Notice that the silent **e** makes the preceding vowel sounds long. Practice the following words having voiced **th** sounds:

ba**th**e	**th**ere
brea**th**e	**th**ese
o**th**er	**th**ey
than	**th**is
that	**th**ose
the	toge**th**er

COMMUNICATION EXERCISES

1. Read the following communication. Circle every **th** sound, and put a line under every voiced **th** sound.

   The therapist will come to see you on Thursday. We will come together. I hope your arthritis is better by then. Take your bath and brush your teeth before we come. These are the breathing exercises that you need to practice. They will help you feel better. Thanks for being such a good sport.

2. You are working in a long-term care facility. Write out what you would say when you ask another nurse to cover your assigned patients while you are at lunch.

CHAPTER 10

The Immune and Lymphatic Systems

evolve Go to http://evolve.elsevier.com/deWit for additional activities and exercises.

COMPLETION

Review of Anatomy and Physiology

Directions: Fill in the blanks to complete the statements.

1. The ______________, ____________________, and ____________________ all provide external barriers to foreign substances and organisms. ***(213)***
2. The _________________________ process is the first step in the body's defense mechanisms. ***(213)***
3. Both ___________ cells and ___________ cells are necessary for a normal immune response to occur. ***(214)***
4. ______________ and _____________ are lymph tissue that guard the airway from inhaled microbes. ***(214)***
5. The neutrophils and macrophages of the hematologic system assist the immune system by ____________________ when an antigen is encountered. ***(215)***
6. Protective proteins that are activated in the inflammatory response include the ________________________________ of proteins. ***(215)***
7. When the body produces an immune response to a "self" cell or tissue this causes an ___________________ disorder. ***(216)***
8. Antibodies are specifically designed to do battle with ________________. ***(217-218)***
9. ______________________ are antibodies that are a kind of protein synthesized by plasma cells. ***(218)***
10. An antibody can either destroy or inactivate its particular antigen by _______________ it, activating a complement system, or causing the release of chemicals that affect the environment of the antigen. ***(218)***
11. An antitoxin is a specific type of antibody that acts through the process of _________________. ***(218)***
12. The major function of the humoral (antigen-antibody) response is to provide protection against ____ diseases. ***(218)***

SHORT ANSWER

Directions: Write brief answers for the following questions.

1. List at least five circumstances that indicate a need to postpone routine immunizations. ***(222)***

   a. ______________________________

   b. ______________________________

   c. ______________________________

   d. ______________________________

   e. ______________________________

2. List four nonpharmacologic measures to reduce hyperpyrexia. ***(231)***

   a. ______________________________

   b. ______________________________

   c. ______________________________

   d. ______________________________

Caring for a Patient with an Immune Disorder

Directions: Read the clinical scenario and answer the questions that follow.

Scenario: You are caring for Mr. Watson. He has an immune disorder and the doctor orders protective isolation. Mr. Watson appears very apprehensive when you first meet him and he tells you that he is not sure why he is isolated, or what to expect, or what he should be doing to help himself.

1. Explain the purpose of protective isolation to Mr. Watson: ***(258)*** ______________________________

   ______________________________.

2. Share three goals of nursing care with Mr. Watson to help him understand the plan of care. ***(253)***

   a. ______________________________

   b. ______________________________

   c. ______________________________

3. What are two psychosocial concerns for a patient who has an immune disorder? ***(249)***

   a. ______________________________

   b. ______________________________

4. Name three important teaching points for Mr. Watson to help him understand things he can do to help himself after he is discharged from the hospital. ***(253-254)***

   a. ______________________________

   b. ______________________________

   c. ______________________________

PRIORITY SETTING

Directions: Read the scenario and prioritize as appropriate.

Scenario: You are preparing to do a physical assessment on Mr. Stevens. He reports having some generalized fatigue and intermittent tenderness in "my neck, just underneath my ears." He was referred to the clinic for a immunologic workup. *Prioritize the order of the elements below that are part of the physical assessment.* ***(249)***

_______ a. Inspect the skin for color, turgor, texture, and presence of lesions.
_______ b. Palpate lymph nodes in the neck to identify enlargement or tenderness.
_______ c. Take vital signs, noting if there is an increase in temperature or pulse rate.
_______ d. Auscultate lung fields and assess work of breathing.
_______ e. Inspect extremities for edema.
_______ f. Analyze lab results such as CBC, C-reactive protein, and antibody screening tests.

APPLICATION OF THE NURSING PROCESS

Caring for a Patient with an Allergic Reaction

Directions: Provide the answer to the following questions.

Ms. Roman comes to the clinic for a rash after eating peanuts several days ago. She also reports, "This has never happened to me before and this really itches! Is this going to happen to me again?"

1. While you are examining Ms. Roman's skin, what assessments and observations are you making? ***(262)***

____

____

____

2. Write a patient-centered goal for the following diagnosis: Risk for impaired skin integrity secondary to irritation and scratching. ***(263)***

____

3. List five interventions to use for Ms. Roman's risk for impaired skin integrity. ***(251)***

a. ____
b. ____
c. ____
d. ____
e. ____

4. Which of the following evaluation statements indicates that Ms. Roman has understood the patient education regarding allergy testing? *(Select all that apply.)* ***(259-260)***
   a. A scratch test may be done by dropping extracts of allergens into scratches made on the skin.
   b. Intradermal injection of allergens is used to detect peanut allergies.
   c. Patches containing allergens can reduce peanut allergies.
   d. Inflammation and itching identify those allergens that provoke the immune system.
   e. Allergy testing is not necessary, because her immune reaction was typical for peanut allergies.

NCLEX-PN® EXAM REVIEW

Directions: Choose the best answer(s) for the following questions.

1. Which of the following are necessary for the immune system to function properly? ***(216)***
   1. Detect the absence of a foreign agent when it leaves body cells.
   2. Overcome the process of inflammation.
   3. Inhibit phagocytosis and the membrane-attack complex.
   4. Remember a particular foreign agent if it appears in the body a second time.

2. Having a case of chickenpox provides a person with which type of immunity? ***(220)***
   1. Passive artificial immunity
   2. Active naturally acquired immunity
   3. Active artificially acquired immunity
   4. Natural (innate) immunity

3. Why are immunizations given in divided doses to children? ***(221)***
   1. The immunizing agent is too potent to be given in a single dose.
   2. There is no production of antibody until three contacts with its antigen.
   3. Exposure to the diseases for which the vaccines are given is not likely to occur before the child is 1 year old.
   4. First exposure initiates antibody production and subsequent exposures cause production of more potent antibodies.

4. What is the purpose of giving "booster doses" of an immunizing agent, such as tetanus toxoid? ***(221)***
   1. Provides an immediate supply of antibody when a person is in danger of contracting the disease.
   2. Provides active immunity for a short period until any danger of the person developing the disease is past.
   3. Stimulates the memory of plasma cells and thereby stimulates synthesis of greater quantities of antibody.
   4. Boosts the synthesis of antibodies by sensitizing the immune cells for the first time.

5. Which group is at high risk for infection due to an immature immune system? ***(222)***
   1. Elderly
   2. Neonates
   3. Transplant recipients
   4. AIDS patients

6. The patient has a fever. Which of the following tasks would be appropriate to assign to the nursing assistant? *(Select all that apply.)* ***(4)***
   1. Help the patient remove excess clothing.
   2. Ask the patient about fever and chills.
   3. Obtain an antipyretic from the medication room.
   4. Take the temperature with an oral thermometer.
   5. Talk to the patient about over-the-counter fever reducers.
   6. Get the patient a popsicle.

CRITICAL THINKING ACTIVITIES

Scenario A: Mrs. Sanderson brings her newborn in for a well-baby check. She is a new mother and is very conscientious and interested in learning about childcare and doing the best for her baby. She tells you that she is reluctant to have her child receive any routine immunizations.

1. What types of questions would you ask her? ______________________________

____

____

2. What information would be appropriate to give this mother? ______________________________

____

____

3. If she continues to refuse, despite your best efforts, what will you do next? ______________________________

____

____

____

____

Scenario B: You are working with a new nursing assistant and you have asked her to carefully monitor vital signs for a patient with a fever. She appears eager and willing to help you.

1. What specific directions should you give to the nursing assistant about this task? ______________________________

____

____

____

____

____

STEPS TOWARD BETTER COMMUNICATON

VOCABULARY BUILDING GLOSSARY

Term	Definition
bad'ger	harass, annoy, or pester
con sti tu' tion	health or disposition (also structure or organization)
im mu no glob' ulin	protein that functions as an antibody
jog	nudge as a reminder (also run at a slower pace)
mi' grate	move around
neu' tral ize	make safe or to reduce the effect
pre dis pose'	to be inclined toward
sur veil'lance (ser va'lenz)	watch or monitor

COMPLETION

Directions: Fill in the blanks with the appropriate words from the Vocabulary Building Glossary to complete the statements.

1. There are five classes of ____________________ (Ig): IgA, IgD, IgE, IgG, and IgM.
2. Antivenins that contain antibodies may ____________________ snake venom.
3. Living in close proximity to others (i.e., homeless shelters, long-term care facilities) may ____________________ an individual to infectious disease.
4. Advise your patient, that although he may have a naturally strong ____________________, adequate nutrition, immunizations, and healthy lifestyle habits will help to prevent immune disorders.
5. The Centers for Disease Control performs ____________________ for infectious disease, such as West Nile virus.
6. When supervising nursing assistants, give instructions and feedback about performance, but do not ____________________ them about minor mistakes.
7. Cancer cells can ____________________ to different locations in the body.
8. Taking a review course will help to ____________________ your memory before you take the test for licensure.

WORD ATTACK SKILLS

Prefixes and Suffixes

A *prefix* is attached to the beginning of a word or root to change the meaning. A vowel is used when needed to connect the prefix to the word.

a-, an-	no, not, without, absence of
anti-	against
auto-	self
hyper-	excessive, more than normal; high
hypo-	decreased, less than normal; low
immun/o-	provide immunity
in-	not, or into
lymph/o-	lymph, lymphatic
lys/o-	destruction

A *suffix* is attached to the end of a word or root to change the meaning.

-cyte	cell
-penia	deficiency of
-genic	produced by

COMPLETION

Directions: Complete the sentences with the correct prefix or suffix.

1. If sterile technique is not used for Foley catheter insertion, the patient may develop an **iatro-** ________________________________ infection.
2. Lupus erythematosus is an example of an ________________ **-immune** disorder.
3. In a person with a normally functioning immune system, the presence of an antigen in the body will cause formation of an ________________ **-body.**
4. Patients with **neutro-**________________ need reverse or protective isolation.

WORD ATTACK SKILLS

Word Families

Actor	Verb	Process	Result
pro tec' tor	pro tect'	pro tec ' tion	
med' ia tor	me d' iate	me dia' tion	
re ac' tor	re act'	re ac' tion	
al' ler gen			al'ler gy

Singular and Plural Forms

Singular	**Plural**
serum	sera
diagnosis	diagnoses

PRONUNCIATION SKILLS

The following words have the long **e** sound, as in the word "he." Notice the sound can be written with e, ee, ea, ei, i, or y.

me 'diate
diagno'ses
proc e 'dure
re' nal
secr e' tions
tech ni que'
fe'ver
deep bre ath'ing
decr e ase'/incr e ase'

Directions: Underline the letters in the words that make the long "e" sound.

1. Please use standard precautions for handling body secretions.
2. Her fever has increased, but she is breathing deeply.
3. Does he know the procedure for keeping the needles clean?

GRAMMAR POINTS

Active Versus Passive

Immunizations can be active or passive, and the English language can be active or passive, too. In acquired immunity, a person can either actively produce his own antibody or passively receive antibodies that have been produced by another person or animal. In English, when the subject of a sentence or clause does the action, the sentence or clause is called *active.*

Examples: *The housekeeper cleans the room.*
A nurse takes vital signs several times a day.
People produce their own antibodies.

The housekeeper, the nurse, and people do the action, so these are active sentences.

Passive sentences or clauses are used when it is not known or it is less important who or what does the action.

Examples: *The bed is made.*
Vital signs are taken in the morning and evening.

The bed and vital signs do no action (some other agent does it), so these are passive sentences.

Scientific writing often uses the passive form because there may not be an actor, or there may be no action, only a state of being. However, it is preferable to use active voice whenever possible.

Examples: *Allergies are divided into three major groups.*
Antibodies are found in the serum of blood.

Who or what divides or finds is not important.

If the agent of the action must be included, a "by" or "through" phrase is usually used to tell who or what does the acting.

Examples: *Temperatures and blood pressures are taken by a nurse.*
The bed is made by the housekeeping staff.
Antibodies are produced by the plasma cells.
Trends can been seen by taking vital signs on a regular schedule.
Vaccination became accepted though the efforts of Edward Jenner.
AIDS is caused by transmission of the HIV.
Edema is characterized by tight, shiny skin.

The action is not done by the subjects of these passive sentences, but rather by the nouns in the underlined phrases.

A *passive verb* is formed by using the verb "to be" in any form (am/is/are, was/were, have/has been, will/would be, and so on) followed by a past participle. The *past participle* of a regular verb is its *-ed* form, such as *divided, prepared,* and *used.* Other past participles are irregular, such as *found, taken, seen, made,* and *known.*

CHAPTER 11

Care of Patients with Immune and Lymphatic Disorders

evolve Go to http://evolve.elsevier.com/deWit for additional activities and exercises.

SHORT ANSWERS

Immune Deficiency

Scenario A: You are working in a HIV/AIDS clinic that provides testing, information, referrals, and outpatient care. The clinic also takes an active role in the community to provide health information seminars and to be a resource for families.

Directions: Write brief answers for the following questions.

1. List at least five of the initial symptoms of AIDS *(237)*

   a. ____________________

   b. ____________________

   c. ____________________

   d. ____________________

   e. ____________________

2. Identify four modes of transmission for HIV. *(235)*

   a. ____________________

   b. ____________________

   c. ____________________

   d. ____________________

3. When collecting data and taking a history for patients who may have an immune deficiency, identify at least six factors that should be assessed. *(235-236)*

   a. ____________________

   b. ____________________

   c. ____________________

   d. ____________________

   e. ____________________

   f. ____________________

4. Describe in your own words the diagnostic testing for HIV. ***(237)***

5. Identify at least four teaching points for persons who are HIV positive that should be included according to *Healthy People 2010* Goal 13 HIV. ***(236)***

   a.

   b.

   c.

   d.

6. List four important things to assess for a patient with AIDS-related dementia. ***(249)***

   a.

   b.

   c.

   d.

APPLICATION OF THE NURSING PROCESS

Disorders of Inappropriate Immune Response

Directions: Read the scenario and write brief answers for the following questions.

Scenario: Janice Euway suspects that she may have allergies to environmental allergens. She reports runny nose, sneezing, and watery eyes that seems to be unassociated with a fever or cold.

1. Which of the following nursing diagnoses is the priority for Ms. Euway today?
   a. Knowledge deficit related to self-care
   b. Risk for ineffective breathing related to systemic reaction to allergens
   c. Anxiety related to new health condition
   d. Altered nutrition related to food restrictions

2. List four drug classifications that are used to alleviate systemic reactions to allergens. ***(260)***

   a. ______________________________

   b. ______________________________

   c. ______________________________

   d. ______________________________

3. The doctor suggests that she initially try an over-the-counter medication. List five common side effects of medication such as diphenhydramine (Benadryl). ***(260)***

   a. ______________________________

   b. ______________________________

   c. ______________________________

   d. ______________________________

4. List six suggestions that will help Ms. Euway control environmental allergens. ***(262)***

   a. ______________________________

   b. ______________________________

   c. ______________________________

   d. ______________________________

   e. ______________________________

   f. ______________________________

PRIORITY SETTING

Directions: Read the scenario and prioritize nursing actions as appropriate.

You are working in a smaller clinic and you hear one of the x-ray technicians calling for help. The patient is having an anaphylactic reaction to IV contrast dye and the radiologist asks you to help. The patient has a patent IV line and the emergency equipment is in the room. *Prioritize these five measures used to treat anaphylaxis.*

_______ a. Provide psychological support

_______ b. Administer oxygen

_______ c. Establish a patent airway

_______ d. Administer antihistamine (diphenhydramine hydrochloride, Benadryl)

_______ e. Administer aqueous epinephrine

NCLEX-PN® EXAM REVIEW

Directions: Choose the best answer(s) for the following questions.

1. Opportunistic infections occur when: ***(240)***
   1. the body is weakened or the immune system is suppressed.
   2. heavy exposure to tuberculosis occurs.
   3. another infection is already present in the body.
   4. antiviral therapy has affected the immune system.

2. Which of the following is a common sign of Kaposi's sarcoma? ***(248)***
   1. A lung infection
   2. A central nervous system infection
   3. Blisters on the skin
   4. A "bruise" or large area of plaque on the skin

3. Which of the following statements by an elderly patient indicates a need for additional patient teaching about risk for HIV? ***(236)***
   1. "Condoms are not needed because pregnancy is not an issue."
   2. "There is a decline in functioning of the immune system for elderly people."
   3. "I may have to remind my health care provider to ask about sexual health."
   4. "Skin and mucous membranes are more fragile in the elderly person."

4. A patient is diagnosed with herpes zoster. Which is the drug of choice for herpes? ***(245)***
   1. Acyclovir (Zovirax)
   2. Foscavir (Foscarnet)
   3. Valganciclovir (Valcyte)
   4. Cidofovir (Vistide)

5. Why is additional intravenous normal saline administered when giving cidofovir (Vistide) and foscarnet (Foscavir)? ***(245)***
   1. To counteract the nephrotoxic effects.
   2. To prevent hepatotoxic effects
   3. To decrease irritation to the veins
   4. To flush the medication from the IV line

6. The patient comes to the clinic for a physical examination and HIV testing. He tells the nurse that he thinks he may have been recently exposed to HIV. Which of the following assessment items should be included at this point? *(Select all that apply.)* ***(235-236)***
   1. Sexual history
   2. IV drug use
   3. Current medications
   4. Vital signs
   5. Presence of anasarca
   6. Change of mental status

7. The doctor orders several diagnostic tests including an HIV test for a patient. Appropriate patient information includes which of the following? ***(237)***
   1. Use of an FDA-approved home test for HIV is adequate and confidential.
   2. He will first have an enzyme-linked immunospecific assay (ELISA).
   3. He will have the Western Blot test as the first initial screening for HIV.
   4. He must fast after midnight and return in the early AM for specimen collection.

8. The patient should be advised that if the first test is negative, a second test must be conducted. When should the second test be conducted? ***(237)***
   1. 1–3 months later
   2. 4–6 months later
   3. 6–12 months later
   4. 3–6 weeks later

9. The patient becomes very angry when he is told that there is a waiting period between the first and second tests. "I can't believe that you won't give me a simple straight answer!" Best response is: ***(8-11)***
   1. "Try to calm down and I'll have the doctor give you more information."
   2. "I can see you are angry, but there is nothing I can do about it."
   3. "This is really frustrating. Let's talk about what you should do in the interim."
   4. "Just wait for the test results. I'm sure that everything will be okay."

10. Allergy symptoms are caused by the release of: ***(258)***
    1. histamine.
    2. antibodies.
    3. immune globulins.
    4. atopy.

11. Which group of drugs commonly tends to cause allergies in many people? ***(259)***
    1. Antihypertensives, diuretics, and antiarrhythmics
    2. Aspirin, barbiturates, anticonvulsants, and antibiotics
    3. Vitamin and mineral supplements and electrolyte replacements
    4. Antibiotics, antianginals, sedatives, and antipychotics
    6. Urinary frequency

12. Which test used to identify allergens involves putting a small amount of the allergen on the surface of the skin and covering with an airtight dressing? ***(260)***
    1. Scratch test
    2. Intradermal test
    3. Patch test
    4. Wheal test

13. The use of antihistamines in aging males sometimes causes problems with which of the following? ***(260)***
    1. Hesitancy and urinary retention
    2. Orthostatic hypotension and dizziness
    3. Angina and cardiac arrhythmias
    4. Depression and general malaise

14. A patient was recently diagnosed with systemic lupus erythematosus. Which of the following signs and symptoms would the nurse expect to find documented in this patient's medical record? *(Select all that apply.)* ***(267)***
    1. Painful or swollen joints
    2. Red rash usually on the face
    3. Fatigue and weakness
    4. Nausea, vomiting, and diarrhea
    5. Unexplained fever
    6. Sensitivity to the sun

15. Which medications are likely to be prescribed for a patient with systemic lupus erythematosus? ***(267)***
    1. NSAIDs and prednisone
    2. Doxorubicin (Adriamycin) and vincristine (Oncovin)
    3. Isoniazid (INH) and rifampin (Rifadin)
    4. Lamivudine (Combivir) and ethambutol (Myambutol)

16. The nurse is giving skin care instructions to a patient with systemic lupus erythematosus. Which of the following instructions is appropriate? ***(268)***
    1. Use alcohol-based skin care products for the antibacterial action.
    2. Avoid use of cosmetics, moisturizers, and soaps.
    3. Wear long pants, a long-sleeved shirt, and a hat when in the sun.
    4. Apply over-the-counter hydrocortisone cream as needed.

17. During the routine physical, the nurse notices that a patient has some swollen lymph glands. On further questioning, the patient admits to pain in the lymph nodes after bouts of excessive drinking. This is significant to report because this type of pain is diagnostic for: ***(268)***
    1. Hodgkin's.
    2. non-Hodgkin's.
    3. lymphedema.
    4. AIDS.

18. The physician recommends that a patient be scheduled for a diagnostic test to detect presence of Reed Sternberg cells in the tissues to rule out lymphatic cancer. Which of the following diagnostic tests will detect these cells? ***(268)***
    1. Computed tomography
    2. Biopsy of the lymph nodes
    3. Biopsy of the bone marrow
    4. Positron emission tomography

19. The patient begins to cry. "I am really scared. Am I going to die of cancer? Why is this happening to me?" Which of the following is the best response? ***(8-11)***
    1. "Let me get your wife and the two of you can have some privacy."
    2. "You should not be using your energy to be worried right now. You should wait until the doctor verifies the diagnosis."
    3. "I'd be scared too. My aunt had cancer and I know just how you feel."
    4. "I can tell you're scared and I don't know why this is happening, but we are here to give you support and information."

20. The patient asks the nurse to explain some of the differences between Hodgkin's and Non-Hodgkin's. Which of the following is correct? *(268)*
    1. Hodgkin's is more widespread through the lymphatic tissues.
    2. Hodgkin's is less widespread through the lymphatic tissues.
    3. Hodgkin's identified as B cell and T cell lymphoma.
    4. Hodgkin's has a lower survival rate and a worse prognosis.

CRITICAL THINKING ACTIVITIES

Scenario A

1. You are working in walk-in clinic. The physician orders an antibiotic injection for a patient. You give the medication as ordered. Almost immediately after receiving the medication, the patient tells you, "I feel kind of funny. Maybe a little short of breath. Is that normal?" What should you do? *(264-265)*

____

____

____

____

____

____

2. List four signs and symptoms that may indicate an anaphylactic reaction. *(263)*

    a. ____

    b. ____

    c. ____

    d. ____

Scenario B

The physician orders postmedication IV hydration for a patient. The current maintenance IV is infusing at 125 mL/hour per pump. The order is to increase the IV fluid to 200 mL/hour X 3 hours then resume previously ordered rate. It is now 8:00 AM. *(58)*

a. What volume should the patient have received at the end of 3 hours? ____________________.

b. At 8:00 AM, you should set the pump to deliver how many mL/hour? ____________________.

c. At 11:00 AM, you should reset the pump to deliver how many mL/hour? ____________________.

STEPS TOWARD BETTER COMMUNICATION

VOCABULARY BUILDING GLOSSARY

Term	Definition
CDC	Centers for Disease Control
gay	homosexual
myth (mith)	traditional belief or ancient story
opportunis'tic	to use an opportunity; (medical field) a microorganism that normally does not cause disease but may do so when the immune response is impaired
pro'drome	symptom indicating the onset of a disease

PRONUNCIATION AND MEANING

When you encounter long medical words, try breaking them down into smaller parts. This will help you with their meanings.

Example: antiretroviral = anti (against) + retro (backward) + viral (relating to a virus)

It will also help you to pronounce the words correctly.

Examples:

cryptococcosis	krip' to kok o' sis
disseminate	di sim' in at
immunosuppression	im' u no sa pre' shun
cytomegalovirus	si' to meg' ah lo vi' rus

COMPLETION

Directions: Fill in the blanks in the sentences with the correct terms from the Vocabulary Building Glossary.

1. In someone with a suppressed immune system, an infection caused by an organism that normally would not cause infection is called an ____________________ infection.

2. There have been many cases of AIDS transmitted from partner to partner among the ______________________________ population in this country.

3. Guidelines for infection control are compiled and published by the ______________________________ ____________________.

4. Difficulty breathing in the AIDS patient may be the ____________________ of an opportunistic infection affecting the lungs.

5. The belief that elderly adults are unlikely to contract AIDS is a ___________.

TERMINOLOGY

Directions: Name the organ or structure to which each condition below is related. (Hint: each word contains a part that means a specific organ or structure.)

1. Retinitis: ______________________________
2. Meningitis: ______________________________
3. Encephalopathy: ______________________________
4. Nephrotoxicity: ______________________________
5. Mucocutaneous: ______________________________
6. Neuralgia: ______________________________
7. Lymphoma: ______________________________
8. Neutropenia: ______________________________

MATCHING

Directions: Match the acronym (abbreviated term) on the left with what it stands for (meaning) on the right.

1. ______	HIV ***(235)***	a.	Personal protective equipment
2. ______	KS ***(248)***	b.	Cytomegalovirus
3. ______	CDC ***(235)***	c.	Acquired immune deficiency syndrome
4. ______	HSV ***(244)***	d.	Centers for Disease Control
5. ______	PCP ***(247)***	e.	*Mycobacterium avium* complex
6. ______	AIDS ***(235)***	f.	*Herpes simplex* virus
7. ______	CMV ***(245)***	g.	Opportunistic infection
8. ______	MAC ***(246)***	h.	*Pneumocystis carinii* pneumonia
9. ______	PPE	i.	*Herpes zoster* virus
10. ______	HZV ***(244)***	j.	Kaposi's sarcoma
11. ______	OI ***(240)***	k.	Human immunodeficiency virus

CHAPTER 12

The Respiratory System

evolve Go to http://evolve.elsevier.com/deWit for additional activities and exercises.

REVIEW OF ANATOMY AND PHYSIOLOGY

Terminology

Directions: Match the term on the left with the correct statement, function, or definition on the right.

1. ______ Bronchioles *(278)*
2. ______ Pleural cavity *(278)*
3. ______ Cilia *(278)*
4. ______ Macrophages *(279)*
5. ______ Cough reflex *(292)*
6. ______ Central nervous system *(278)*
7. ______ Receptors in brain stem *(279)*
8. ______ Receptors in arteries *(279)*
9. ______ Inspiration and expiration *(279)*

a. Controls involuntary and voluntary respiration
b. Carry air to alveoli
c. Hairlike projections that trap and help expel inhaled foreign particles
d. Reside in alveoli to dispose of inhaled bacteria and other foreign particles
e. Respond to high CO_2 and hydrogen ion levels in cerebrospinal fluid, signaling nerves to increase respiratory rate
f. When depressed, secretions are retained and pneumonia may occur
g. Pressure within is less than that of outside atmosphere
h. Respond to low levels of arterial oxygen, signaling nerves to cause lungs to inflate more fully
i. Controlled by movement of diaphragm and muscles in chest wall

Completion

Directions: Fill in the blank(s) to complete the following sentences.

1. ____________________ decreases surface tension on the alveolar wall, allowing it to ____________ more easily with _________________ and preventing alveolar collapse upon ________________. *(279)*
2. Two conditions that can interfere with oxygen and carbon dioxide exchange are ____________ surfactant and interstitial __________________. *(279)*
3. Respiratory gases are carried mostly in the bloodstream by the __________________________. *(280)*
4. Oxygen attaches to the _____________ portion of the ___________________ carried by the ___________________, forming _________________________. *(280)*

5. Carbon dioxide combines with ____________ within the red blood cell, forming
__________________________. *(280)*

6. A large percentage of carbon dioxide is transported in the blood plasma in the form of
______________________ ions. *(280)*

7. In the lung, bicarbonate ions disassociate into ________________ and ______________________
______________ and the ____________________________ diffuses across the alveolar membrane. *(280)*

SHORT ANSWER

Age-related Changes Affecting the Respiratory System

Directions: Provide a short answer to the following questions. ***(280)***

1. Why are the elderly more susceptible to respiratory infections?______________________________

____

2. Why is the potential for aspiration greater in the elderly person? ____________________________

____

____

3. What is the effect of lessened ciliary action in the airways? ________________________________

____

____

4. What alveolar changes affect respiration in the elderly person? ______________________________

____

____

5. The sum of the above changes that occur with aging mean that elderly people, particularly those over 70, may have:

____

____

TERMINOLOGY

Assessment

Directions: Match the terms on the left with the statements on the right that best describe them. (There may be more than one answer for each.)

1. ______ Assessment of mouth and pharynx *(287)*
2. ______ Indirect laryngoscopy *(285)*
3. ______ Direct laryngoscopy *(285)*
4. ______ Laryngography *(285)*
5. ______ Throat culture *(287)*

a. Simple removal of polyps can be done during this procedure.
b. Endoscope is passed to visualize interior of larynx.
c. Patient is NPO until gag reflex returns.
d. Patient is instructed to cough after procedure to remove oil from air passages.
e. Usually performed to confirm infection with streptococcus.
f. Tracheostomy set and resuscitative equipment must be at hand during recovery from procedure.
g. Examiner uses warm laryngeal mirror, head mirror, and light source.
h. Examiner uses tongue blade and light source.
i. Biopsy can be taken during examination.
j. Food and liquids withheld 6–8 hours before procedure.

SHORT ANSWER

Directions: Provide a short answer to the following questions.

1. What would be two particular findings indicative of pharyngitis? *(282)*

   a. ______________________________

   b. ______________________________

2. Why is obtaining a history of smoking and alcohol intake pertinent to a respiratory assessment? *(282)*

   ____

   ____

3. What can skin color tell you that is pertinent to a respiratory assessment? *(283)* ______________

   ____

   ____

4. What might frothy, pinkish, or blood-tinged sputum indicate? *(283)* ______________________________

____

5. What is the best position in which to place the patient for lung auscultation? *(283)* ______________________________

____

PRIORITY SETTING

Directions: Indicate the order of priority in which you would begin actions for the following scenario. ***(286)***

Your patient is to undergo a bronchoscopy. You will provide pre- and post-test care.

_____ a. Check the gag reflex before allowing fluids by mouth.
_____ b. Administer pretest sedation if ordered.
_____ c. Verify that the patient understands the procedure.
_____ d. Monitor for bleeding and dyspnea.
_____ e. Check to see that the consent form is signed.
_____ f. Auscultate the lungs for a baseline assessment.
_____ g. Raise the head of the bed to 30 degrees.
_____ h. Take the vital signs for a baseline assessment.
_____ i. Position the patient with the head turned to the side until alert.
_____ j. Auscultate the lungs.
_____ k. Monitor oxygen saturation by pulse oximetry.
_____ l. Keep patient NPO for 6 hours.

NCLEX-PN® EXAM REVIEW

Directions: Choose the best answer(s) for the following questions.

1. Evaluation of the effectiveness of deep breathing and coughing is best done by: *(282)*
   1. auscultating the lungs bilaterally both before and after.
   2. assessing the color and amount of secretions produced.
   3. observing the respiratory rate and quality afterward.
   4. asking the patient whether he is breathing more easily.

2. When performing a respiratory assessment, which of the following should be performed? *(Select all that apply.) (282)*
   1. Inquire about exposure to respiratory inhalants.
   2. Check the heart rate and rhythm.
   3. Auscultate the lungs bilaterally.
   4. Assess the temperature of the skin.
   5. Assess color of mucous membranes.
   6. Assess the rate and quality of respirations.
   7. Check for use of accessory muscles.
   8. Look for signs of anxiety or restlessness.

3. Increasing fluid intake when the patient has chest congestion is helpful because: *(Select all that apply.)* ***(282)***
   1. fluid helps decrease the cough reflex.
   2. coughing may cause dehydration.
   3. it helps thin secretions.
   4. it decreases the chance of infection.
   5. it may make secretions easier to cough up.
   6. it increases comfort of breathing.

4. When a patient is short of breath when lying down and breathes better sitting up, the condition is called: ***(293)***
   1. paroxysmal nocturnal dyspnea.
   2. bradypnea.
   3. orthopnea.
   4. tachypnea.

5. Which of the following is an objective sign of long-term decreased oxygenation? ***(283)***
   1. Chest pain with deep inspiration
   2. Paroxysmal nocturnal dyspnea
   3. Rapid respiratory rate
   4. Clubbed fingers

6. Which of the following positions is best for the patient undergoing a thoracentesis? ***(288)***
   1. Sitting up, leaning forward on an overbed table
   2. Side-lying, affected side up, head slightly raised
   3. Side-lying, affected side down, head flat
   4. High Fowler's position

7. An elderly patient with a severe respiratory infection is seen in the emergency department. The physician orders an IV of D_5½NS 1000 mL over 12 hours. The IV tubing delivers 10 drops per mL. At what drip rate should this IV be administered? ________________

8. Indicate on the diagram where you would place the stethoscope to begin the respiratory assessment. ***(284)***

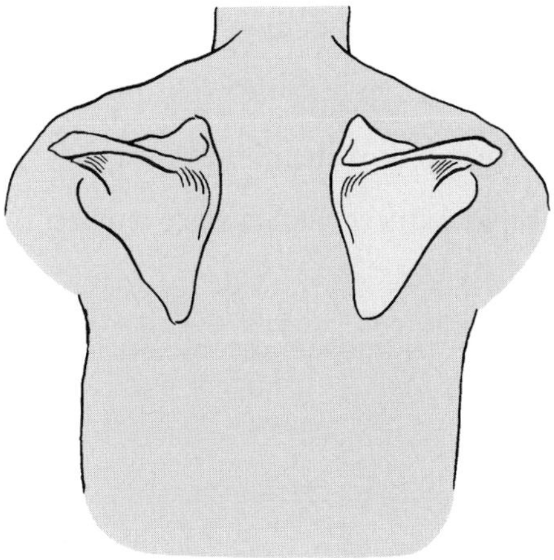

9. When a patient is scheduled for a lung ventilation and perfusion scan, which of the following nursing actions is pertinent? *(286)*
   1. Keep the patient NPO for 6 hours before the test.
   2. Assess for allergy to iodine or shellfish.
   3. Be certain the patient is well hydrated pretest.
   4. Inform the patient that he will be isolated until the radioactive substance is completely excreted.

CRITICAL THINKING ACTIVITIES

1. Describe particular ways you would adjust your teaching for an elderly patient who needs to be taught to use an incentive spirometer and cough effectively.

2. Within your extended family, determine the risk factors for respiratory disorders.

STEPS TOWARD BETTER COMMUNICATION

VOCABULARY BUILDING GLOSSARY

Term	**Definition**
malaise'	(noun) general feeling of bodily discomfort
refrain'	(verb) to avoid doing something
dysphag'ia (dis fa' jee ah)	(noun) difficulty swallowing
hypocapnea	deficiency of carbon dioxide in the blood
hypercapnea	excess of carbon dioxide in the blood
surfactant	an agent that reduces fluid surface tension
naris, *plural* nares	nostril
adventitious	accidental, occasional; abnormal, outside of the usual place

COMPLETION

Directions: Complete the following sentences using the glossary words above.

1. You may hear ______________________________ sounds that are abnormal.

2. The elderly patient seemed to have a general feeling of ______________________________.

3. A ______________________________ is used to make soaps more effective, as well as being found naturally in the body.

4. Please ______________________________ from smoking near the entryway.

MATCHING

Directions: Match the combining form or abbreviation on the left with its meaning on the right.

1. ______	-itis	a.	magnetic resonance imaging
2. ______	-oscopy	b.	computed tomography
3. ______	MRI	c.	inflammation
4. ______	CT	d.	process of visually examining

TERMINOLOGY

Directions: Identify the correct term for each definition.

1. Examination of the larynx: ______________________________
2. Sinuses next to the nose: ______________________________
3. Abnormal lung sounds: ______________________________
4. Oxygen-deficient: ______________________________
5. Difficulty breathing: ______________________________

PRONUNCIATION

Directions: Practice saying these words with a partner.

1. "l" as the initial sound: (Curl the tip of your tongue and place it against the back of your front teeth. Air will flow around the sides of your tongue.)

laryngi'tis	le'sions	lung
larynx	lined	

2. "l" as the final sound

cell	na'sal	tonsil
fron'tal	or'al	vo'cal
muco'sal	skull	

COMMUNICATION EXERCISE

A. With a partner, practice an explanation to an elderly person of the steps she should take to avoid contracting a URI (immunization, staying out of crowds, prompt treatment of any symptoms, avoid youngsters with coughs and colds, maintain adequate rest and nutrition, good handwashing).

B. Switch roles and explain to a youngster how to avoid catching and spreading respiratory diseases (covering coughs—cough into elbow, disposing of tissues, handwashing—sing the ABC song 2–3 times to expand alveoli, don't go to school or parties when you are sick or contagious, stay away from crowded places).

CHAPTER 13

Care of Patients with Disorders of the Upper Respiratory System

evolve Go to http://evolve.elsevier.com/deWit for additional activities and exercises.

SHORT ANSWER

Directions: Provide a short answer for the following questions.

1. List three common symptoms of sinusitis. ***(300)***

   a. ______________________________

   b. ______________________________

   c. ______________________________

2. List three common symptoms of pharyngitis. ***(301)***

   a. ______________________________

   b. ______________________________

   c. ______________________________

APPLICATION OF THE NURSING PROCESS

Upper Respiratory Disorders

Directions: Provide a short answer for the following questions.

1. Write one expected outcome for each of the following nursing diagnoses.

   a. Impaired verbal communication related to inability to speak due to tracheostomy

   ____

   b. Risk for aspiration related to impaired swallowing

   ____

   c. Ineffective airway clearance related to physical alteration in airway (tracheostomy)

   ____

2. List two nursing interventions for each of the following nursing diagnoses for a patient who has undergone a laryngectomy. ***(308-309)***

   a. Ineffective airway clearance related to throat surgery: ____________________

   ____

   b. Impaired verbal communication related to loss of voice: ____________________

   ____

   c. Risk for injury related to aspiration: ____________________

   ____

COMPLETION

Directions: Fill in the blanks to complete the statements.

1. A nursing intervention to help promote drainage in the patient with acute sinusitis is ____________________. ***(300)***

2. Warning signs of cancer of the larynx include ____________________. ***(304)***

3. Tonsillectomy is usually considered if the patient has more than ______ episodes of tonsillitis in 1 year. ***(302)***

4. The nurse's chief concern for the postoperative tonsillectomy patient is ____________________. ***(302)***

5. One way to detect postoperative bleeding in the tonsillectomy patient is to observe for frequent ____________________. ***(302)***

6. A newer surgical option for cancer of the larynx is ____________________. ***(305)***

7. A total laryngectomy is required when the tumor has reached the point of ____________________. ***(305)***

8. If a radical neck dissection must be performed, a ____________________ is performed at the same time. ***(305)***

9. When suctioning a tracheostomy, the nurse must use totally ____________________ technique. ***(309)***

10. When cleaning the tracheostomy site and tube, the nurse must be careful not to allow ____________________. ***(311)***

PRIORITY SETTING

1. You are assigned the following patients:
   - M.S., a preoperative patient scheduled for for surgery at 10:00 AM.
   - O.T., an early tonsillectomy (adult) who was admitted due to excessive bleeding.
   - M.R., a postlaryngectomy patient with a tracheostomy who is first day postoperative.

Directions: Indicate the order of priority in which you would do the following: (Use 1, 2, 3.)

_______ Assess O.T.'s status.

_______ Assess M.R.'s status.

_______ Provide preoperative care for M.S. including the preoperative checklist.

2. Which patient should be your first priority? ____________
   a. The patient with the tracheostomy who is having considerable difficulty breathing.
   b. The postoperative patient just arriving on the unit from surgery.
   c. The radical neck dissection patient who is complaining of considerable pain.

NCLEX-PN® EXAM REVIEW

Directions: Select the best answer(s) or fill in the blank with the correct word(s) for the following questions.

1. The priority assessment for any patient with any problems of the upper airway is: ***(307)***
   1. anxiety and pain.
   2. adequacy of oxygenation.
   3. presence and thickness of nasal and oral secretions.
   4. signs of dyspnea.

2. A patient comes to the emergency department with a nosebleed. Which is the appropriate action? ***(301)***
   1. Applying ice to the back of the neck.
   2. Having the patient tip the head way back, hyperextending the neck.
   3. Packing the nose with gauze.
   4. Applying pressure to the nose with the thumb and forefinger.

3. When drugs are prescribed for treatment of rhinitis and sinusitis, which of the following classes of drugs would be included? *(Select all that apply.)* ***(300)***
   1. Decongestants
   2. Bronchodilators
   3. Antihistamines
   4. Antitussives
   5. Antipyretics
   6. Mucolytics

4. Which of the following is a true statement regarding rhinitis and the elderly patient? ***(299)***
   1. Complementary and alternative therapies are ineffective in the older adult.
   2. Antihistamines and decongestants should be used with caution.
   3. Antipyretics and antibiotics are not used because of risk of allergic reactions.
   4. Viral rhinitis is self-limiting and comfort measures are sufficient.

5. An appropriately chosen nursing diagnosis for the patient with acute pharyngitis is "Risk for: ***(302)***
   1. fluid volume deficit related to reluctance to drink."
   2. impaired tissue perfusion related to infection."
   3. pain related to inflammation."
   4. alteration in cardiac output."

6. Symptoms of chronic sinusitis include: *(Select all that apply.)* ***(300)***
   1. headache.
   2. chronic productive cough.
   3. hoarseness.
   4. malaise.
   5. high fever.
   6. purulent nasal drainage.

7. The patient with sinusitis should increase fluid intake to at least ____________ per day to help thin secretions and assist the sinuses to drain. ***(300)***

8. In the immediate postoperative period after a tonsillectomy, which one of the following is of highest priority? ***(302)***
   1. Pain control
   2. Adequate hydration
   3. Prevention of aspiration
   4. Treatment of nausea

9. A patient undergoing sinus surgery (Caldwell-Luc procedure) has a preoperative piggyback of cefazolin (Ancef) ordered. 500 mg of the drug is dissolved in 50 mL of IV solution. The powdered drug was mixed with 10 mL of sterile water before it was added to the IV solution. The drug is ordered to be administered over 20 minutes. The IV tubing delivers 10 drops per mL. The IV should run at ______________ per minute. ***(58)***

10. When suctioning a tracheostomy, infection control guidelines indicate that you should use: *(Select all that apply.)* ***(310)***
    1. sterile glove(s).
    2. sterile drape.
    3. mask.
    4. face shield.
    5. sterile water.
    6. sterile suction catheter.

CRITICAL THINKING ACTIVITIES

A 76-year-old male patient possibly has laryngeal cancer. He is to undergo diagnostic testing and then, if cancer is diagnosed, he will have a laryngectomy.

1. What diagnostic tests would most likely be done for this patient? ***(305)***

2. If the patient has a laryngectomy and a tracheostomy, how would you provide a means of communication? *(314)*

3. What criteria would you use to determine when the patient's tracheostomy needs suctioning? *(311)*

4. What are the two most important principles to be observed when suctioning? *(314)*

STEPS TOWARD BETTER COMMUNICATION

VOCABULARY BUILDING GLOSSARY

Term	Pronunciation	Definition
diligent	dil' ah jent	(adj.) hardworking, dedicated at all times
vigilant	vij' ah lent	(adj.) watchful, alert to danger
prevalent	prev'a lent	(adj.) commonly occurring, widespread
susceptible	sus cep'ti ble	(adj.) easily affected by something—physical or emotional
prone	prohn	(adj.) 1. lying face down 2. likely to do or feel something

COMPLETION

Directions: Fill in each blank with the appropriate word from the Vocabulary Building Glossary to complete the statement.

1. Mr. Soares was especially ____________ to upper respiratory infections due to his uncontrolled pollen allergies.

2. To prevent a respiratory infection in a tracheostomy patient, the nurse must be ____________________ with hand hygiene before suctioning .

3. The elderly are very __________________________ to upper respiratory infections.

4. When a patient suffers from dysphagia, the nurse must be ____________________ for signs of aspiration when the patient is eating or drinking.

5. The idea of the value of immunization is very ____________________ in Western culture.

SHORT ANSWER

Directions: Write the word to match the definition.

1. nosebleed: ***(301)*** ______________________________
2. removal of the adenoids: ***(302)*** ______________________________
3. inflammation of the sinuses: ***(300)*** ______________________________

IDIOMATIC USAGES

"Catching" a cold means getting a viral infection.

"Stuffier" means becoming more congested.

"Dull" can mean mentally slow, as well as referring to sound or sight. The opposite would be "sharp, clear" for all of these meanings.

A "magic slate" is a board covered with wax and a plastic sheet on top that can be written on with a stylus. The words show, but are erased when the sheet is lifted so that it can be reused indefinitely.

PRONUNCIATION

In English, the consonant sound **"l"** is found at the beginning, middle, or end of words. It is made by putting the tip of the tongue against the back of the top front teeth with the lips open a little. The tongue lies in the bottom of the mouth and the air comes out on both sides. The voice is used.

Directions: Practice saying these words with a partner.

1. **"l"** as the middle sound:

air-filled	irregular'ity	physiol'ogy
al'lergy	malig'nant	plaque
car'tilage	max'illary	pol'yps
cil'ia	mobil'ity	re'flex
cold	mus'cle	swal'lowed
eld'erly	olfact'ory	swell'ing
epiglot'tis	pa'late	til'ted
flu	pal'lor	ulcera'tion
glot'tis	pal'pate	
inflamma'tion	par'ticles	

2. **"l"** is silent:

calm	half	talk
could	should	would

SPELLING AND PRONUNCIATION SKILLS

ph = f

When the letters **"ph"** occur in the same syllable in English, they are pronounced like **"f."** They may occur at the beginning, middle, or end of words. The sound is made by touching the top teeth with the bottom lip. Air is blown out between the lip and the teeth.

Directions: Practice saying the following words.

dysphagia	esophageal	facial	
esophagus	larynx	lymph	frontal

Directions: Take the words in the pronunciation exercises above and place them in the column for the category to which each belongs. (Some words do not fit in these categories.)

Parts of the Body	Symptoms or Diseases	Descriptions or Locations	Verbs
larynx	*laryngitis*	*oral*	*lined*

CHAPTER 14

Care of Patients with Disorders of the Lower Respiratory System

evolve Go to http://evolve.elsevier.com/deWit for additional activities and exercises.

REVIEW OF ANATOMY AND PHYSIOLOGY

Terminology

Directions: Match the term on the left with its best description on the right. ***(282)***

1. ______	Diffusion	a.	Deficient oxygenation of blood
2. ______	Elastance	b.	Ability of lung to distend in response to inhaled air
3. ______	Lung compliance	c.	Amount of gas either inhaled or exhaled with each breath
4. ______	Hypoxia	d.	Extent to which lungs can return to their original position after being barely stretched
5. ______	Hypoxemia	e.	Prevents collapse of lung by stabilizing alveoli and decreasing capillary pressure
6. ______	Resistance	f.	Oxygen deficit
7. ______	Perfusion	g.	Takes place between gas in alveolar space and blood in capillaries of lung
8. ______	Surfactant	h.	Amount of gas in air one can exhale after maximal inhalation
9. ______	Ventilation	i.	Amount of air or gas lung can hold at end of maximal inspiration
10. ______	Total lung capacity	j.	Passage of fluid through vessels of an organ
11. ______	Vital capacity	k.	Movement of air from outside body to alveoli
12. ______	Tidal volume	l.	Chiefly determined by radius or caliber of airway

APPLICATION OF THE NURSING PROCESS

Directions: List specific nursing actions that could be planned for a patient according to the following data obtained during history-taking.

1. Describe each of the following abnormal breath sounds. ***(284)***

   a. Wheezes: ____

   b. Stridor: ____

   c. Rhonchi: ____

   d. Crackles: ____

2. Give a possible cause for each of the following characteristics of sputum. ***(283)***

    a. Sticky, rust-colored: ____________________

    b. Frothy, pinkish, or blood-tinged: ____________________

    c. Yellow-green, foul-smelling: ____________________

    d. Very thick, viscous: ____________________

3. List four points to include in the assessment of a patient with a cough. ***(292)***

    a. ____________________

    b. ____________________

    c. ____________________

    d. ____________________

Directions: Provide a nursing action to alleviate the problem.

4. Data: "My husband coughs as hard as he can, but he just can't get the phlegm up from his lungs." ***(292)***

    Nursing action: ____________________

5. Data: "It seems that I have to come to the hospital at least twice a year for an infection in my lungs. I suppose there is nothing I can do about it now that I have chronic bronchitis and emphysema." ***(330)***

    Nursing action: ____________________

6. Data: "I get short of breath just trying to take a bath and put on my clothes. Here at the hospital, there is someone wanting to do something to me every time I turn around. I wish I could get some rest." ***(295)***

    Nursing action: ____________________

SHORT ANSWER

Directions: Describe the nursing action to be implemented for each of the following.

1. Anxiety about a scheduled bronchoscopy. ***(286)***

    Nursing action: ____________________

2. A patient tells you his sputum is streaked with blood following his bronchoscopy. ***(286)***

    Nursing action: ____________________

SHORT ANSWER

Directions: Answer the following questions in the spaces provided.

1. You are asked to assist with a thoracentesis and pleural biopsy and to watch the patient after the procedure. *(288)*

   a. How would you prepare the patient? ______________________________

   ____

   b. How would you monitor the patient after the procedure? ______________________________

   ____

2. List four signs or symptoms that are helpful to data collection when caring for a patient with a lower respiratory disorder. *Example: Sits leaning forward with shoulders elevated.* ***(283)***

   a. ______________________________

   b. ______________________________

   c. ______________________________

   d. ______________________________

COMPLETION

Directions: Fill in the blanks to complete the statements.

1. Expectorant cough medicines help ____________________ mucus from the bronchial tree. ***(332)***
2. Many respiratory infections are spread by ______________________________. ***(319)***
3. Name three reasons why problems of nutrition and hydration are common in patients with respiratory disease. ***(295)***

   a. ______________________________

   b. ______________________________

   c. ______________________________

4. The fatigue that is often present in patients with respiratory disease is usually caused by a deficit in the ____________________ supply to the tissues. ***(296)***
5. Excessively high concentrations of inhaled oxygen can bring about collapse of the alveoli because of an interruption in production of ____________________, which stabilizes the alveoli. ***(279)***
6. List five signs of respiratory alkalosis. ***(52)***

   a. ______________________________

   b. ______________________________

   c. ______________________________

   d. ______________________________

   e. ______________________________

7. Name four interventions that can help prevent pneumonia. *(322)*

a. ______________________________

b. ______________________________

c. ______________________________

d. ______________________________

PRIORITY SETTING

Directions: It is 7:15 AM. Your patients have the following needs. In what order would you try to meet them? Number in order of priority.

______ a. A patient post-thoracotomy is complaining of pain in spite of using his PCA pump.

______ b. A patient needs clean gown and towels to shower. She is scheduled for surgery at 8:00 am

______ c. A patient with pneumonia did not get his breakfast tray and is asking for it.

______ d. A nursing assistant has just told you that a patient is suddenly febrile.

______ e. A patient with a tracheostomy needs suctioning.

NCLEX-PN® EXAM REVIEW

Directions: Select the best answer(s) or fill in the blank with the answer for the following questions.

1. Safety factors for administering oxygen to the patient with chronic obstructive pulmonary disease (COPD) include: *(331)*
   1. auscultating the lungs once during each shift.
   2. keeping oxygen flow below 2 L per minute.
   3. placing the patient in a high Fowler's position.
   4. filling the humidifier with warm tap water.

2. A nursing intervention that can *best* help prevent respiratory failure in the patient with compromised lung function is to: ***(338-339)***
   1. encourage at least 3000 mL of fluid intake per day.
   2. assist with all activities of daily living (ADLs) to prevent excess fatigue.
   3. have the patient turn, cough, and deep breathe at least every 2 hours.
   4. administer an expectorant to help clear airways.

3. Evaluation of the effectiveness of deep breathing and coughing is done by: *(Select all that apply.)* ***(292)***
   1. auscultating the lungs bilaterally both before and after.
   2. assessing the color and amount of secretions produced.
   3. observing the respiratory rate and quality afterward.
   4. asking the patient whether he is breathing more easily.
   5. assessing the pulse oximetry reading.
   6. listening to the character of the patient's voice.

4. When assessing the patient for early stage emphysema, the nurse would particularly look for: *(Select all that apply.)* ***(330)***
   1. clubbed fingers.
   2. pale skin color.
   3. yellow, tenacious sputum.
   4. rapid, pounding pulse.
   5. barrel-shaped chest.
   6. pursing of lips upon expiration.

5. When evaluating the effective functioning of a chest tube after a thoracotomy, the nurse assesses the: *(Select all that apply.)* ***(347)***
   1. amount of drainage in the collection chamber.
   2. ease of the patient's breathing.
   3. color of the drainage in the collection device.
   4. increase in breath sounds as the lung re-expands.
   5. decreasing complaints of pain.
   6. fluctuation of fluid within the tube in the water seal chamber.

6. Symptoms of tuberculosis may include: *(Select all that apply.)* ***(325)***
   1. cough.
   2. afternoon low-grade fever.
   3. copious, thin, clear sputum.
   4. anorexia and weight loss.
   5. barrel-shaped chest.
   6. pink tinge to skin.
   7. night sweats.
   8. hemoptysis.

7. Your pneumonia patient is encouraged to increase his fluid intake. He had 340 mL at breakfast, 60 mL with pills, 280 mL midmorning, 410 mL with lunch, and 240 mL midafternoon. How much more fluid does he need to reach the goal of 3000 mL for the day? ________________ ***(323)***

8. When administering respiratory medications to your patient, which one of the following would you administer *last*? ***(320)***
   1. Albuterol (Proventyl)
   2. Montelukast (Singulair)
   3. Robitussin cough syrup
   4. Advair discus

9. One of the main problems with lung cancer is that it: ***(338)***
   1. rarely responds to chemotherapy.
   2. has metastasized from cancer elsewhere in the body.
   3. is resistant to radiation therapy.
   4. has often metastasized by the time it is discovered.

10. A major intervention to prevent further lung damage in the patient with chronic airflow limitation (CAL) is: ***(337)***
    1. institute a plan to balance rest and activity.
    2. convince the patient to quit smoking.
    3. teach proper breathing techniques.
    4. teach ways to maintain optimal health.

CRITICAL THINKING ACTIVITIES

A patient who had been living in Southeast Asia for the past 2 years has just been diagnosed with tuberculosis. He is complaining of night sweats, fatigue, and weight loss. He has a cough. ***(324-325)***

1. Therapy for tuberculosis consists of several medications. What medications would you expect to be prescribed? What teaching points are especially important for this patient?

2. At what point will this patient no longer be considered contagious?

3. What are the reasons that tuberculosis is increasing in the United States?

STEPS TOWARD BETTER COMMUNICATION

VOCABULARY BUILDING GLOSSARY

Term	Definition
re'coil	to move back quickly; to return with force to an original position
flar'ing	getting wider
pursed (purst)	rounded, gathered together (as when lips are ready to blow out a candle or to whistle)
adventi'tious (ad ven ti' shus)	abnormal
foul	very bad, as a bad odor
tet'any (tet' ah nee)	muscle spasm or cramp
due to	caused by
suscep'tible (su sep' ti bel)	likely or probably will be affected
aggres'sive care	vigorous, strong; frequent care that follows all guidelines
cor'relate	link together two or more things; fit together into a pattern (e.g., *correlate* the symptoms with the disease)
ag'gravate	to cause to increase
paradox'ical (par ah dok' si kel)	something that looks contradictory but is true; two things that are working opposite of usual
hall'mark	sign, criteria
prone	leaning toward, susceptible to something, such as an idea or disease
predispos'ed	ready for, susceptible to
"gold standard"	(slang) the best
fluc'tuate	to change, vary up and down
cal'ibrate	to measure exactly, usually with markings
occlud'ed	blocked

PRONUNCIATION OF DIFFICULT TERMS

Directions: Practice pronouncing the following words:

Term	Pronunciation	Definition
kyphosis	ki fo' sis	abnormal outward curvature of the spine; hunchback
Kussmaul's	koos mowlz'	pattern of respiration
scoliosis	sko lee o'sis	S-type curvature of the spine
rales	rahlz	fine crackles in the lungs
rhonchi	rong' ki	loud rattling sounds in the lungs
apneusis	ap nu' sis	long inspiration unrelieved by expiration
empyema	em pie ee' ma	accumulation of pus in a body cavity
hemoptysis	he mop'ti sis	coughing and spitting of red, frothy blood
hematemesis	hem ah tem'e sis	vomiting of blood

COMPLETION

Directions: Fill in the blanks with the appropriate words from the Vocabulary Building Glossary to complete the statements.

1. Learning to breathe with _______________ lips helps decrease dyspnea for the patient with emphysema.
2. People with CAL are more _______________ to respiratory infections than the general public.
3. When a chest tube is functioning properly, the fluid in the water seal chamber will _______________ with each breath.
4. Bronchitis is usually evident upon auscultation of the lungs because _______________ sounds are present.
5. When several ribs are fractured, _______________ chest motion will be observed.
6. When respiratory distress is occurring, the nurse may observe _______________ of the patient's nostrils.
7. A _______________ of acute respiratory distress syndrome (ARDS) is respiratory failure.
8. Mechanical ventilation is the _______________ of care for respiratory failure.
9. When turning a patient who is attached to a ventilator, the nurse must be careful to check to see that the ventilator tubing is not _______________.
10. Patients with severe _______________ or _______________ of the spine often have restrictive lung disease.

WORD ATTACK SKILLS

Directions: Look at the word elements defined below and then break the listed words into their word parts using vertical lines. Write the meaning of each word.

-oid:	resembling
-megal/o:	enlargement
-osis:	condition
anti-	against

1. Cytomegalovirus: ______________________________
2. Immunocompromised: ______________________________
3. Immunosuppressive: ______________________________
4. Antiinfective: ______________________________
5. Coccidioidomycosis: ______________________________

COMMUNICATION EXERCISE

Directions: Here is an example of what you would say to teach a patient ways to prevent the spread of a respiratory infection.

"You can help prevent the spread of your respiratory infection by washing your hands frequently with soap and warm water. Cover your mouth when you cough or sneeze. Throw away used tissues immediately and wash your hands again. Be careful not to touch objects after coughing or sneezing before you wash your hands. Try to sit and stand several feet away from other people while your nose is running and you are coughing and sneezing. Stay out of crowded places."

Directions: With a peer, practice performing a respiratory assessment.

Take and record the respiratory history. Document your physical assessment findings. Ask your instructor to review your documentation of the assessment.

____
____
____
____
____
____
____
____
____
____

CHAPTER 15

The Hematologic System

evolve Go to http://evolve.elsevier.com/deWit for additional activities and exercises.

REVIEW OF ANATOMY AND PHYSIOLOGY

Completion

Directions: Fill in the blanks to complete the statements.

1. The type of blood cell responsible for the transport of oxygen is the ______________________________ ______________________________. *(362)*

2. Erythropoiesis must continue throughout life because the average life span of a red blood cell is ______________________________. *(362)*

3. Excessive production of erythrocytes results in a condition called ______________________________. *(362)*

4. The major functions of leukocytes take place in the ______________________. *(362)*

5. The formed elements most important in preventing hemorrhage are the ______________________________ ______________________________. *(363)*

6. The three major plasma proteins are __________________, ______________________, and ______________________. *(361)*

7. The storage and release of blood and the removal of old blood cells are major functions of the ______________________________. *(362)*

COMPLETION

Age-related Changes Affecting the Hematologic System

Directions: Complete each of the following statements.

1. A problem that might be encountered by the decrease in plasma volume after age 60 is ***(363)***

____

____.

2. The elderly are at greater risk for infection because ______________________________ ______________________________. *(363)*

3. Anemia, when it occurs, takes longer to resolve in the elderly because ______________________________ ______________________________. ***(363)***

4. Changes in blood coagulation make the elderly person more at risk for ______________________________ ______________________________. ***(363)***

SHORT ANSWER

Causes and Prevention of Hematologic Disorders

Directions: Provide a short answer for each of the following questions.

1. Inherited disorders that interfere with normal blood function are: ***(360)***

   a. ______________________________

   b. ______________________________

   c. ______________________________

2. Four iatrogenic causes of blood dyscrasias or loss are: ***(364)***

   a. ______________________________
   ____

   b. ______________________________
   ____

   c. ______________________________
   ____

   d. ______________________________
   ____

3. Some drugs within which drug classifications may cause blood dyscrasias? ***(364)***

   a. ______________________________

   b. ______________________________

   c. ______________________________

   d. ______________________________

4. Nutritional deficiencies that may interfere with erythropoiesis are: ***(364)*** ______________________________
____

5. Lifestyle factors that can help prevent anemia are: ***(366)*** ______________________________
____
____

6. You can help prevent excessive blood loss by: ***(365)*** ____________________

____

7. Two ways you can help prevent blood dyscrasias are: ***(366)***

   a. ____________________

   ____

   b. ____________________

   ____

SHORT ANSWER

Assessment and Diagnostics

Directions: Briefly answer the following.

1. List the five kinds of data that should be obtained during history-taking for assessment of a patient with a blood disorder. ***(369)***

   a. ____________________

   b. ____________________

   c. ____________________

   d. ____________________

   e. ____________________

2. State the possible cause or condition usually associated with each of the following. *(Example: tarry stools—intestinal bleeding)*

   a. Jaundice: ***(368)*** ____________________

   b. Bruises and petechiae: ***(368)*** ____________________

   c. Plethora: ***(370)*** ____________________

   d. Sore and bleeding gums: ***(369)*** ____________________

   e. Smoky, brownish urine: ***(370)*** ____________________

   f. Swollen and painful joints: ***(370)*** ____________________

   g. Weakness and intolerance to physical activity: ***(370)*** ____________________

   h. Irritability, dizziness, and difficulty concentrating: ***(370)*** ____________________

3. Inquiring about occupation and hobbies is important to a hematologic history because: ***(369)***

____

____

4. If during assessment, a patient states that he or she bruises easily, it could indicate: ***(369)***

____

5. List two nursing responsibilities in the care of a patient following bone marrow aspiration. ***(368)***

   a. ____

   b. ____

6. When blood collection is performed, nursing responsibilities are to: ***(366)***

   a. ____

   b. ____

   c. ____

7. On the blood count differential, allergy may be indicated by the presence of ____________________ ____________________. ***(363)***

8. A normal platelet count is ____________________. ***(363)***

PRIORITY SETTING

Directions: You have been asked to obtain a blood sample for a CBC from a patient in the ambulatory clinic. Number the following tasks in the order in which you would perform them. Consider that a task may be performed more than once. ***(366)***

______ a. Obtain the needed supplies.
______ b. Place the label the specimen tube.
______ c. Don latex gloves.
______ d. Write the information on the specimen label.
______ e. Send the specimen to the laboratory.
______ f. Perform the venipuncture.
______ g. Cover the wound.
______ h. Identify the patient using two identifiers.
______ i. Remove the gloves.
______ j. Fill out the laboratory requisition slip.
______ k. Stop bleeding at the site.
______ l. Perform hand hygiene.
______ m. Explain what you are going to do to the patient.

NCLEX-PN® EXAM REVIEW

Directions: Choose the best answer(s) for the following questions.

1. Plasma proteins are important to maintain osmotic pressure. A laboratory test that indicates whether proteins in the blood are sufficient is: ***(361)***
   1. serum albumin.
   2. serum bilirubin.
   3. hemoglobin.
   4. platelets.

2. Erythropoiesis cannot occur normally if: *(Select all that apply.)* ***(362)***
   1. bone marrow activity is suppressed.
   2. there is a lack of vitamin K.
   3. there are insufficient amino acids available.
   4. the diet does not include sufficient green and yellow vegetables.
   5. vitamin E is insufficient.
   6. linoleic acid is not present.

3. The normal range for hemoglobin in adults is ____________________ g/dL. ***(362)***

4. The elderly who live alone are at high risk of poor nutrition due to problems with: *(Select all that apply.)* ***(365)***
   1. cooking ability.
   2. vision or arthritis.
   3. financial means.
   4. mobility.
   5. chronic diseases that cause fatigue.
   6. cooking equipment.

5. When gathering assessment data you would: (*Place the choices in proper sequence.*) ______________ ***(369)***
   1. Inspect the skin for abnormal color.
   2. Inquire about family hereditary diseases.
   3. Check scleral and conjunctival color.
   4. Inquire about headaches or palpitations.
   5. Inquire about ease of bleeding.
   6. Measure vital signs.
   7. Check for swollen or painful joints.
   8. Check condition of fingernails and hair.

6. Yellowed skin or sclera and conjunctiva may occur from: *(Select all that apply.)* ***(368)***
   1. anemic state.
   2. excess bilirubin in the blood.
   3. inadequate platelet function.
   4. hemolysis.
   5. excess consumption of carrots.

7. Lymph node enlargement can be found during a bath if one palpates: ***(363)***
   1. behind the knees.
   2. under the arms.
   3. below the clavicles.
   4. around the ankles.

8. When a patient is anorexic, things that may interfere with eating are: *(373)*
   1. providing socialization during meals.
   2. odors in the room.
   3. serving small frequent meals and snacks.
   4. providing mouth care before each meal.

9. People who have a blood abnormality may be prone to bleeding problems and ______________. *(373)*

10. When a patient has a prolonged clotting time, after drawing blood, you should: *(372-373)*
    1. apply pressure for 2 full minutes.
    2. have the patient apply pressure to the site until the bleeding stops.
    3. apply pressure for 5–10 minutes.
    4. use a styptic pencil to stop the bleeding.

CRITICAL THINKING ACTIVITIES

1. If you came upon an auto accident, stopped to help, and found someone on the ground spurting blood from the upper thigh, what would you do first? After that, what would you do? *(373)*

2. You have been assigned to a recent postoperative patient who has just had a thoracotomy. You know that postoperative hemorrhage is always a potential complication. What would you specifically assess to assure yourself as best you can that a postoperative hemorrhage is not occurring? *(372)*

STEPS TOWARD BETTER COMMUNICATION

VOCABULARY BUILDING GLOSSARY

Term	Definition
ag'gregate	(verb) bring separate parts together in a group, clump together
brought on	caused to occur, induced
clot	a thickened mass of liquid, especially of blood
perni'cious (per nish' us)	having a very harmful effect
pleth'ora	red complexion caused by excessive blood

COMPLETION

Directions: Fill in the blanks with the appropriate words from the Vocabulary Building Glossary above to complete the statements.

1. When a cut occurs and a blood vessel is damaged, platelets ______________ as part of the clotting process.

2. ______________________ anemia is caused by an inability of the body to absorb vitamin B_{12} from the intestinal tract.

3 Fibrinogen is another factor in addition to platelets that works to form a blood _________________.

4. Patients suffering from polycythemia vera often display _______________________.

5. Lymphedema may be__________________________ by the lymph node extraction that accompanies a radical or modified mastectomy.

PRONUNCIATION

Directions: With a peer, practice pronouncing the following words. Use each word in an appropriate sentence.

Term	Pronunciation	Definition
dyscra'sia	dis kray' zee ah	imbalance in the elements of something
erythropoi'etin	a rith' ro poi' e tin	hormone that stimulates red blood cell production
erythropoie'sis	a rith' ro poi ee' sis	red blood cell production
fatigue'ed	fa teeg' d	very tired, exhausted
parenterally	pah ren' ter a lee	by a route other than the digestive tract
pete'chia	pa tee' ki a	round red spot
splenomeg'aly	splen' o meg' a lee	enlargement of the spleen
throm'bocytope'nia	throm' bo si to pee' ne ah	decrease in the number of platelets

MATCHING

Directions: Match the prefix or suffix on the left with its correct meaning on the right.

1. ______	-cyte	a.	have affinity for
2. ______	-chrom	b.	normal, usual
3. ______	-phils	c.	negative prefix (not)
4. ______	a-	d.	white
5. ______	normo-	e.	cell
6. ______	gran-	f.	large, long
7. ______	neo-	g.	color
8. ______	mono-	h.	sole, one
9. ______	macro-	i.	grain, particle
10. ______	leuko-	j.	new, young
11. ______	erythro-	k.	red

SHORT ANSWER

Directions: Write the meaning of each word, referring to the word elements in the exercise above. Use your dictionary as needed.

1. Macrophage: ______________________________
2. Monochrome: ______________________________
3. Leukocytosis: ______________________________
4. Erythropoietin: ______________________________
5. Granulocyte: ______________________________
6. Neutrophil: ______________________________
7. Agranulocyte: ______________________________
8. Normochromic: ______________________________

CHAPTER 16

Care of Patients with Hematologic Disorders

evolve Go to http://evolve.elsevier.com/deWit for additional activities and exercises.

COMPLETION

Hematologic Disorders

Directions: Fill in the blanks to complete the statements.

1. An individual with pernicious anemia does not produce ________________________, which is essential to the production of erythrocytes. ***(377)***
2. Treatment of pernicious anemia consists of ______________________________. ***(377)***
3. The primary difficulty caused by anemia is failure to meet the ________________________________ ___________________________. ***(376)***
4. Sickle cell trait occurs when the individual has ____________________________. ***(384)***
5. When both parents have sickle cell trait, the chances of their children having sickle cell disease rise to ______%. ***(384)***
6. The symptoms suffered during a sickling crisis are the result of ________________________________ ________________________________. ***(384)***
7. Leukemias are characterized by ____ ______________________. ***(386)***
8. The most common cause of death in leukemia patients is ______________________. ***(388)***
9. There is a hereditary link for __________________________________ leukemia. ***(388)***
10. Patients who have undergone splenectomy are at risk for ______________________. ***(398-399)***
11. Management of classic hemophilia is by transfusion of ______________________. ***(392)***
12. When a patient has an iron-deficiency anemia, treatment consists of ____________________________ ____ ____. ***(378)***
13. Oxygen therapy is indicated when a patient has an arterial oxygen level below ______________________ ____________________. ***(398)***
14. Side effects of oral iron therapy include ____ ____. ***(380)***

15. Aplastic anemia is a disorder in which ______________________________ ______________________________. *(382)*

16. A blood loss of as little as ________ mL can cause hypovolemic shock. *(376)*

17. The classic signs and symptoms of hypovolemic shock are ______________________________ ______________________________ ______________________________. *(377)*

18. The patient experiencing hypovolemic shock is positioned ______________________________ ______________________________.

19. Nutritional anemia is caused by inadequate ________________, ________________, or ______________________________. *(377)*

APPLICATION OF THE NURSING PROCESS

Directions: Write an expected outcome and list three nursing measures for each of the following nursing diagnoses commonly found in patients with blood disorders.

1. Altered tissue perfusion related to decreased red blood cells and hemoglobin

   Expected outcome: ______________________________ ______________________________

   a. ______________________________

   b. ______________________________

   c. ______________________________

2. Risk for infection related to decreased or abnormal white blood cells

   Expected outcome: ______________________________ ______________________________

   a. ______________________________

   b. ______________________________

   c. ______________________________

3. Activity intolerance related to fatigue and weakness

   Expected outcome: ______________________________ ______________________________

   a. ______________________________

   b. ______________________________

   c. ______________________________

4. Risk for injury related to possible hemorrhage

   Expected outcome: ______________________________

   ____

   a. ______________________________

   b. ______________________________

   c. ______________________________

5. List interventions you would place on the teaching plan for the 35-year-old female patient who has iron deficiency anemia. *(379)*

   ____

   ____

   ____

   ____

   ____

   ____

PRIORITY SETTING

Your patient is to receive a transfusion of packed red cells. Place the following actions in the order in which you would do them. (See both the text chapter and the procedure for administration of blood products on the CD-ROM with the text.) ***(393-394)***

______ a. Prime the filter and IV tubing with normal saline.

______ b. Hook up the unit of packed cells to the IV tubing.

______ c. Check the orders.

______ d. Stay with the patient.

______ e. Obtain the blood bag from the blood bank.

______ f. Check the size of the IV cannula that is in place already.

______ g. Check the patient's identification with the blood bag and the relevant papers.

______ h. Establish that the IV site is patent.

______ i. Verify the blood unit numbers and the patient's blood bracelet with another nurse.

______ j. Set the correct drop rate for the blood to flow for the first 15 minutes.

______ k. Take the baseline vital signs.

______ l. Inquire if the patient has ever had a transfusion reaction.

______ m. Perform hand hygiene.

______ n. Don impermeable gloves.

______ o. Attach the blood IV tubing to the IV cannula.

______ p. Take the vital signs again.

______ q. Reset the drop rate to the calculated flow rate.

NCLEX-PN® EXAM REVIEW

Directions: Choose the best answer(s) for the following questions.

1. An important part of assessment of the patient with an iron deficiency anemia is: (*Select all that apply.*) ***(382)***
   1. determining if there is a family history of this type of problem.
   2. determining if there is abnormally high blood loss with menstruation.
   3. asking if the patient takes any vitamins.
   4. determining if the patient is a strict vegetarian.
   5. checking to see if any drugs that cause hemolysis are being taken.
   6. obtaining a thorough dietary history of what the patient normally eats.

2. Independent care for the patient admitted with severe anemia should include: ***(379)***
   1. interventions to conserve the patient's energy.
   2. obtaining blood specimens for diagnostic testing.
   3. administering ordered blood products.
   4. assessing the patient for signs of depression.

3. When the nurse administers a form of iron to the anemic patient, she keeps in mind that iron: ***(380)***
   1. comes in many different forms and strengths.
   2. should be given through a straw if in liquid oral form.
   3. usually leaves a bad aftertaste in the mouth.
   4. is more quickly effective in the intravenous form.

4. When assessing the elderly patient who is anemic, the nurse remembers that in this age group: ***(381)***
   1. anemia is a normal result of the aging process.
   2. anemia is most often a result of occult bleeding.
   3. the problem is most often due to poor nutrition.
   4. malignancy is the most likely cause of the anemia.

5. The patient who has polycythemia vera must be observed for the complication of ______________. ***(386)***

6. A treatment often used for polycythemia vera is: ***(386)***
   1. iron therapy.
   2. vitamin C.
   3. phlebotomy.
   4. aspirin.

7. Nursing interventions for the patient with idiopathic thrombocytopenia purpura must include measures to: ***(390)***
   1. prevent spontaneous bleeding.
   2. increase the number of red blood cells.
   3. prevent health care–associated infection.
   4. encourage better nutrition.

8. Nurses can help prevent aplastic anemia by: (*Select all that apply.*) ***(382)***
   1. monitoring the blood counts of all patients.
   2. teaching patients proper nutrition to build blood cells.
   3. explaining why a room should be well-ventilated when using household chemical cleaners for tile.
   4. carefully monitoring patients who are receiving drugs that can potentially cause this disorder.
   5. teaching people to avoid skin exposure to garden chemicals and weed killers.
   6. explaining how to avoid exposure to toxic substances that cause the disorder.

9. A high-priority goal for the planning of care for the patient with aplastic anemia is: *(382)*
   1. prevention of fatigue.
   2. assistance with activities of daily living (ADLs).
   3. prevention of infection.
   4. alleviation of pain.

10. When assessing the patient with possible leukemia, the nurse knows that the most common symptoms are: *(387)*
    1. excessive bleeding, headaches, and chills.
    2. exposure to known toxic agents that cause the disorder.
    3. fatigue, malaise, and frequent infections.
    4. viral infection, nausea, and decreased hemoglobin.

11. One of the first signs of disseminated intravascular coagulation is: *(393)*
    1. blood clotting that interferes with circulation in the extremities.
    2. chest pain from tiny blood clots throughout the lungs.
    3. continued bleeding from an injection site, ecchymoses, and petechiae.
    4. bleeding from the mouth, nose, and other body orifices.

12. When administering more than one unit of blood by transfusion, the nurse must: *(395)*
    1. change the filter for each new unit to be transfused.
    2. wait at least 1 hour between administration of units.
    3. allow the second unit to warm to room temperature before hanging it.
    4. administer at least 250 mL of normal saline between units given.

13. Subtle signs of a transfusion reaction may be: *(395)*
    1. somnolence and confusion.
    2. bradycardia and increased blood pressure.
    3. backache and a feeling of anxiety.
    4. irritability and headache.

14. Leukapheresis is performed to: *(396)*
    1. wash antigens from the bloodstream.
    2. separate neutrophils from the blood.
    3. treat all types of leukemia.
    4. treat certain types of immune disorders.

15. Which one of the following statements is true about bone marrow transplant? *(397-398)*
    1. There is a 50% chance of HLA match between siblings.
    2. 200 mL of bone marrow is needed for the transplant.
    3. A potential complication for the donor is excessive blood clotting.
    4. Engraftment of the transplanted bone marrow takes 2–5 weeks.

16. A common blood disorder among the elderly is ________________. *(377)*

17. The basis for having elderly adults take a low-dose aspirin daily is: *(388)*
    1. the blood of the elderly tends to coagulate more easily.
    2. aspirin stimulates the bone marrow to produce new cells.
    3. aspirin assists the uptake of iron from the intestinal tract.
    4. aspirin helps prevent the ecchymoses common in the elderly.

18. The order is to infuse 2 units of packed red cells over 2 hours. One unit contains 210 mL and the other contains 200 mL. The blood is to infuse over 2 hours. The blood IV tubing setup delivers 10 gtts/mL. At what rate should the infusion run? ________________

CRITICAL THINKING ACTIVITIES

Scenario A

S.T. is a 37-year-old black man who has sickle cell disease. He has frequent episodes of pain. His anemia has been managed with transfusions on several occasions. He has signs of chronic renal failure. He has been prescribed pentoxifylline (Trental), oxycodone/acetaminophen (Roxicet), and folic acid (Folvite). At the hematology clinic this morning, his Hgb was 6.9 g/dL. He was transfused with 2 units of packed red cells over 3 hours and then sent home. About an hour and a half later, he developed dyspnea. His wife called 911 and he arrived at the emergency department with oxygen by mask.

1. How would you describe sickle cell disease? How is it related to race? ***(384)***

2. What is the mechanism by which patients with sickle cell disease develop anemia? ***(384)***

3. Why should the admitting nurse inquire about his pain and the need for medication? ***(385)***

Scenario B

P.W., age 12, has hemophilia B (Christmas disease). His mother brought him to the emergency department because of considerable pain and swelling in his left knee. He states that he bumped the knee on a desk at school. A CBC shows Hgb of 10.4 g/dL and a deficiency of clotting factor IX.

1. Describe how this X-linked recessive trait for hemophilia is transmitted. ***(392)***

2. Explain why this patient has a bleeding problem when injured. ***(392)***

3. What is the expected treatment for P.W.? ***(392)***

STEPS TOWARD BETTER COMMUNICATION

VOCABULARY BUILDING GLOSSARY

Term	Definition
clump	(noun) a cluster, group of pieces
	(verb) pieces gather or stick together in a group
dire (dīr)	very serious
enhance'	increase, improve
har'vest	to collect something for use
meti'culous	extremely careful
mit'igate	(verb) reduce, lessen, alleviate
modal'ity, -ies	a particular system or arrangement, a method
sic'kle	a crescent shape, like a new moon; a farm tool with a curved blade

COMPLETION

Directions: Fill in the blanks with the appropriate words from the Vocabulary Building Glossary above to complete the statements.

1. When extensive bleeding occurs during surgery, extra fluids are given to ________________ the effect of the blood loss.
2. When a patient develops leukopenia, the nurse must use ________________________ aseptic technique to prevent infection.
3. When an injury occurs to tissue, platelets ________________ to help stop bleeding.
4. An oxygen deficit will cause red blood cells to ________________ in patients with sickle cell disease.
5. When leukemia is diagnosed, the patient and physician must choose an appropriate ____________________ of treatment.
6. When a leukemia patient suffers an episode of bleeding, the consequences may be ________________.
7. Using strict asepsis when caring for a patient with a blood dyscrasia will ______________________ the chances of preventing infection.
8. Before a bone marrow transplant, the physician must ____________________ marrow from a matching donor.

GRAMMAR POINTS

The word **"by"** + the **-ing** form of a verb is often used when talking about how something happens, or the method of doing something. An object or phrase is usually required to complete the sentence.

Example: Nurses help patients by teaching about drug side effects.

Directions: Complete each sentence using "by" plus the -ing forms of the following verbs:

cautioning	undergoing
reporting	following
asking	suppressing
using	destroying
wearing	administering

1. After giving a narcotic, nurses help prevent patient falls ________________ patients not to get up without assistance.
2. Patient information is relayed to the oncoming shift ________________ on the condition, treatments, and complaints of patients by the nurses leaving.
3. A thorough history is obtained ________________ the patient several specific questions.
4. A nurse complies with Standard Precautions ________________ gloves whenever contact with body fluids is likely.
5. The nurse is protected from contamination ________________ a waterproof gown, gloves, and goggles when irrigating a wound.
6. A patient fights leukemia ________________ chemotherapy treatment.
7. The immunosuppressed patient prevents infection ________________ strict guidelines to avoid contact with pathogens.
8. Many types of chemotherapy work ________________ replication of the malignant cells.
9. Radiation therapy works ________________ malignant cells.
10. Hypovolemic shock is treated ________________ fluids and blood.

COMMUNICATION EXERCISE

Directions: With a partner, make a list of the most important points to use in teaching the patient and the family about 1) prevention of infection, 2) prevention and treatment of bleeding episodes, and 3) appropriate nutrition. Then orally "teach" your partner about these issues.

____

____

____

____

CULTURAL POINT

Be aware that some religions prohibit blood transfusions, and other people are very suspicious of the procedure. Approach a patient carefully to determine his or her feelings about transfusions.

CHAPTER 17

The Cardiovascular System

evolve Go to http://evolve.elsevier.com/deWit for additional activities and exercises.

REVIEW OF ANATOMY AND PHYSIOLOGY

Labeling

Structures of the Circulatory System

Directions: On the figure below, label the structures of the circulatory system. Then, using arrows, indicate the pathway that blood follows through the system. Explain the diagram and pathway to a partner. ***(404)***

superior vena cava	inferior vena cava	pulmonary artery
pulmonary vein	mitral valve	tricuspid valve
pulmonic valve	aortic valve	right atrium
right ventricle	left atrium	left ventricle
aorta		

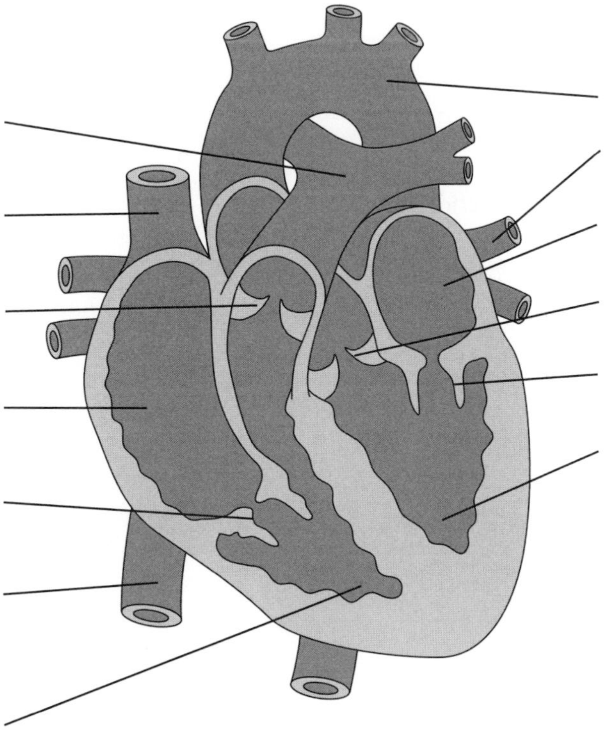

COMPLETION

Directions: Fill in the blanks to complete the statements.

1. Cardiac output depends on the heart ________________, the amount of blood returning to the ____________________, the strength of ________________, and the ______________________ to the ejection of the blood. ***(404)***
2. The left atrium receives ___________________ blood from the pulmonary veins. ***(403)***
3. ________________________ equals the amount of blood pumped out of the heart each minute. ***(405)***
4. _______________________ is the condition where fibrous plaque with fatty deposits form in the interior layers of the arteries, causing narrowing. ***(406)***
5. A _________________________ is the difference between the apical and radial pulse rates when they are counted at the same time. ***(420)***
6. A weight gain of 3 lbs. or more in a _______________________ period indicates fluid retention. ***(428)***
7. The doctor orders furosemide (Lasix) oral liquid 20 mg PO every morning. The pharmacy delivers a 100 mL bottle of furosemide with a concentration of 40 mg/5 mL. How many mL should you give the patient? _____________ mL ***(58)***

SHORT ANSWER

Risk Factors and Assessment for Cardiac Disorders

Directions: Read the clinical scenario and answer the questions that follow.

Scenario: Mr. Blue is a 55-year-old construction worker. He reports that he was having difficulty performing his job because of fatigue and shortness of breath. He tells you, "At first, I thought it was just stress and being sort of overweight and just smoking, drinking, and eating too much. I decided to make an appointment because my wife reminded me that we have heart disease and diabetes in the family."

1. You are collecting information about cardiac risk factors from Mr. Blue. What are four unmodifiable risk factors related to the development of heart disease? ***(419)***

   a. ____

   b. ____

   c. ____

   d. ____

2. List five modifiable risk factors that Mr. Blue has just reported in the scenario. What information can you give him about modifying the factors that he has just mentioned? ***(409-410)***

   a. ____

   b. ____

   c. ____

   d. ____

   e. ____

3. Write at least five questions that you could ask Mr. Blue to get additional information about his shortness of breath. ***(419)***

   a. ____

   b. ____

   c. ____

   d. ____

   e. ____

4. List at least six things that should be included in the physical assessment of a patient like Mr. Blue, who may have a cardiac disorder. ***(419)***

   a. ____

   b. ____

   c. ____

   d. ____

   e. ____

   f. ____

COMPLETION

Diagnostic Testing for Cardiac Disorders

Directions: Fill in the blanks to complete the statements.

1. Ultrasound Doppler flow studies are conducted to detect a ________________ in the vessel or to determine the ______________________________ of the vessel. ***(414)***

2. Coronary angiography requires injection of a __________________________. ***(414)***

3. The purpose of a venogram is to detect ______________________________ ______________________________. ***(414)***

4. Explain to the patient that during impedance plethysmography, he may feel some discomfort related to ______________________________. ***(414)***

5. Myoglobin level is performed to detect damage to the ____________________ from a ____________________ infarction. ***(416)***

APPLICATION OF THE NURSING PROCESS

Changes with Aging

Directions: Read the scenario and provide the answers to the following questions.

Scenario: You are working in an extended care facility and Mrs. Wiabo is one of your elderly patients. Mrs. Wiabo is in stable condition, but she has several chronic health problems, including hypertension and occasional problems with fluid retention.

1. List at least six changes in the cardiovascular system associated with aging. ***(407-408)***

   a. ______________________________

   b. ______________________________

   c. ______________________________

   d. ______________________________

   e. ______________________________

   f. ______________________________

2. List at least five interventions (including assessments) to use with patients like Mrs. Wiabo who have fluid retention. ***(427-428)***

   a. ______________________________

   b. ______________________________

   c. ______________________________

   d. ______________________________

   e. ______________________________

   f. ______________________________

3. Which of the following nursing diagnoses is top priority for Mrs. Wiabo? ***(428)***
   a. Chronic low self-esteem related to activity intolerance
   b. Knowledge deficit related to disease process, medications, and self-care
   c. Imbalanced fluid volume, risk for, related to heart failure
   d. Impaired social interaction related to being away from family

4. Which of following is the best indicator that Mrs. Wiabo is not having any problems with fluid retention? *(428)*
   a. Urinates freely without pain or discomfort.
   b. No signs of pitting edema in the sacral area.
   c. Breath sounds are clear on auscultation.
   d. Shows no change in daily weight.

PRIORITY SETTING

Directions: Read the scenario and prioritize the steps to perform the procedure. ***(421)***

Scenario: You are preparing to take a routine blood pressure on an ambulatory patient at a clinic. You have never taken a blood pressure on this patient before and the patient does not remember his last blood pressure reading. You must use an ordinary manual blood pressure cuff (i.e., not a blood pressure machine). Put the following steps in the correct order to perform the procedure.

_______ a. Palpate the brachial artery.

_______ b. Select the correct cuff size.

_______ c. Center the bladder cuff over the brachial artery.

_______ d. Listen until the sounds stop.

_______ e. Report abnormal findings to the RN or MD.

_______ f. Release cuff and wait 30–60 seconds.

_______ g. Deflate cuff slowly and smoothly to obtain a correct diastolic reading.

_______ h. Record your findings as soon as you obtain the reading.

_______ i. Support the patient's arm, on which the cuff is placed, at heart level.

_______ j. Ensure the patient has not smoked or had caffeine for the past 30 minutes.

_______ k. Place the bell of your stethoscope over the brachial artery.

_______ l. Tighten the screw clamp; inflate cuff 30 mm above the palpated pressure.

_______ m. Obtain a palpated systolic blood pressure.

NCLEX-PN® EXAM REVIEW

Directions: Choose the best answer(s) for the following questions.

1. The patient has diabetes. In order to lessen the risk of atherosclerosis, she should be advised to keep the blood sugar consistently below: ***(411)***
   1. 80 mg/dL.
   2. 110 mg/dL.
   3. 120 mg/dL.
   4. 200 mg/dL.

2. The nurse knows that in order to correctly perform the procedure for taking an apical pulse, the pulse must be counted for: ***(420)***
   1. 15 seconds.
   2. 30 seconds.
   3. 1 minute.
   4. 2 minutes.

3. The nurse has observed that the patient's jugular veins are prominent when the patient is in an upright position. This finding is associated with which of following cardiovascular disorders? ***(409)***
   1. Congestive heart failure
   2. Cardiac dysrhythmia
   3. Angina pectoris
   4. Aortic aneurysm

4. When obtaining a patient's blood pressure, the nurse knows that if the blood pressure cuff is too narrow, the blood pressure will be: ***(421)***
   1. unaffected by the equipment.
   2. falsely elevated.
   3. lower than expected.
   4. the same in both arms.

5. The nurse should report a positive Homans' sign because this may indicate: ***(422)***
   1. intermittent claudication.
   2. arterial occlusion.
   3. edema and fluid retention.
   4. deep vein thrombosis.

6. The nurse is evaluating the patient's peripheral pulses. Which of following should be included in a routine assessment? ***(420)***
   1. Note rate and rhythm and mark the location.
   2. Take radial pulse on the patient's dominant side.
   3. Compare pulses bilaterally; note volume and strength.
   4. Elevate the extremity and check the pulse.

7. Which of the following is considered the best indicator of fluid buildup? ***(428)***
   1. Pitting edema
   2. Decreased urinary output
   3. 3 lbs. weight gain in 24 hours
   4. Low serum sodium

8. The patient is experiencing acute anginal pain. Which group of drugs is the physician most likely to prescribe to treat this condition? ***(474)***
   1. Cardiotonic and antilipemic
   2. Nitroglycerin and morphine sulfate
   3. Diuretic and ACE inhibitor
   4. Anxiolytic and antihypertensive

9. When planning nursing care, the nurse knows that many heart medications need to be given as close to the prescribed time as possible. The best rationale for this practice is to: ***(474)***
   1. complete shift duties in a timely fashion.
   2. prevent adverse response to medications.
   3. avoid confusing your elderly patients.
   4. maintain a steady blood level of the drug.

10. Which statement by the patient's wife indicates a need for further discussion about modifiable risk factors for cardiac disorders? ***(410)***
    1. "He can't lose weight because his parents were obese."
    2. "He could have up to two alcoholic drinks per day."
    3. "He could take a relaxation or meditation class for stress."
    4. "His blood pressure should be lower than 120/80."

11. The nurse is caring for a patient with Activity intolerance related to chronic heart failure. Which of the following activities would be best to assign to the nursing assistant? *(425)*
    1. Observe the patient for fatigue and shortness of breath when ambulating.
    2. Assist the patient with limited morning hygiene such as washing face and brushing teeth.
    3. Explain to the family why taking long walks on the hospital grounds is not feasible at this time.
    4. Obtaining assistive devices that would help the patient to conserve energy and strength.

CRITICAL THINKING ACTIVITIES

Scenario: Mrs. Reno is an elderly female who comes to the clinic after experiencing some mild chest pain. She is accompanied by her husband. You are attempting to perform the PQRST for pain assessment. Mr. Reno keeps answering for his wife, even though she is alert and oriented and seems capable of answering for herself. She sits quietly and smiles at you, but allows her husband to do the talking despite your best efforts.

1. What is the PQRST pain assessment? *(420)* ____________________

   ____

   ____

   ____

2. Could Mr. Reno provide correct answers to any of the PQRST pain assessment questions? If so, which questions might he be able to accurately answer? *(420)*

   ____

   ____

   ____

3. What are your personal feelings about this type of situation? ____________________

   ____

   ____

4. What factors (i.e., cultural, social, age, psychological) might help to explain Mr. and Mrs. Reno's behavior?

   ____

   ____

   ____

   ____

   ____

   ____

STEPS TOWARD BETTER COMMUNICATION

VOCABULARY BUILDING GLOSSARY

Term/Phrase	Pronunciation	Meaning
a whooshing or purring sound	whoosh' ing	a sound like quickly moving air
equipment used should be calibrated	cal' i brated	marked with correct units of measure
appear pale and mottled	mot' tled	marked with irregular patches of color
condition indicative of gangrene	in dic' a tive	showing signs of, suggesting
excoriations	ex co ri a' tions	scratches or abrasions on skin
it is a good gross assessment	gross as sess' ment	general and broad, not specific
circulation is occluded by constriction	oc clud' ed	blocked
assessment and staging of edema	stag' ing	determining the extent or phase of a disease or condition
dependent edema	de pen' dent	hanging down, which can cause swelling
impede, impedence	im pede'	to block, to get in the way of
precipitate; precipitating event	pre cip' i tate	to cause to start
assess mentation	men ta' tion	mental activity
collaborate with patients/colleagues	col lab' o rate	to work together with in both planning and action

COMPLETION

Directions: Using the vocabulary above, prepare five sentences. Leave the vocabulary word space blank, and ask a classmate to complete the sentence with the correct word.

1. ______________________________

2. ______________________________

3. ______________________________

4. ______________________________

5. ______________________________

VOCABULARY EXERCISE

Descriptors, Descriptive Terms, Special Uses

Directions: The words listed below are used to describe the quality and character of a patient's pulse. If you are not sure of the meaning of some of the words, ask your instructor to explain, or to let you hear an example.

Descriptors of pulse qualities: full, strong, weak, thready, bounding, rapid, slow, fast, irregular, regular, erratic, diminished, distant, barely palpable, absent, hammer-like, normal, fleeting, moderate, 1+, 2+, 3+, 4+ (designates strength)

Directions: Evaluate the expected pulse of the following three people and write out your assessment findings using the descriptive terms.

Person 1: Radial pulse of someone who has just run a race: ______________________________

____

Person 2: Pedal pulse of someone with arterial vascular disease: ______________________________

____

Person 3: Apical pulse of a patient with heart disease who has a dysrhythmia: ______________________

____

COMMUNICATION EXERCISE

History-Taking and Documenting Assessment

1. What are the things you would need to ask about in history-taking that would provide information about a cardiovascular patient? What objective observations could you make that would also provide information?

   ____

   ____

   ____

2. With a peer, practice cardiac assessment using the questions in Table 17-1 of the textbook. Write out the questions you will use. Take turns asking and then answering the questions. Take notes and document your assessment findings. Ask your partner or the instructor to critique your documentation.

   ____

   ____

   ____

   ____

   ____

   ____

COMMUNICATION EXERCISE

Directions: With a partner, discuss some things you would say to a patient in each of these cases.

1. The patient is in pain and you want to interact therapeutically with active listening.

____

____

____

____

____

____

2. Mr. Johnson wants a hot water bottle on his feet because they are cold.

____

____

____

3. Miss Bennett does not want anything to eat or drink, but her medications are to be taken with food.

____

____

____

4. Explain to a family which risks to cardiac health cannot be controlled or modified and which can be.

____

____

____

CULTURAL POINT

Black people and women have different experiences with heart conditions and symptoms than those usually described for white males. Be sure that you learn what these differences are and pay attention to the symptoms of these people.

CHAPTER 18

Care of Patients with Hypertension and Peripheral Vascular Disease

evolve Go to http://evolve.elsevier.com/deWit for additional activities and exercises.

COMPLETION

Hypertension

Directions: Fill in the blanks to complete the statements.

1. Hypertension can indirectly affect the heart by causing ________________________ changes in the blood vessels. ***(434)***

2. The three organs most likely to be damaged by a consistently high blood pressure are the ________________, ______________________, and ______________________. ***(435)***

3. Hypertension can be secondary to and symptomatic of other diseases, such as those affecting the blood supply to the__________________ and _________________. ***(434)***

4. Nicotine has a major impact on blood vessels and blood pressure by producing ____________________________. ***(434)***

5. Hypertension is diagnosed when an elevated blood pressure is taken at least _______________ and averaged on two different occasions, ___________ weeks apart. ***(433)***

6. The physician examines blood vessels in the ______________________ to detect signs of persistent hypertension. ***(435)***

SHORT ANSWER

Hypertension

Directions: Read the following scenario and answer the questions that follow.

Scenario: You are participating in a health fair that includes blood pressure screening for hypertension and dispensing information about healthy lifestyle habits. In addition, interested people are inquiring about how to recognize potential symptoms and various types of treatment, including medication for hypertension.

1. List four specific ways in which a person with mild hypertension might help reduce his blood pressure without taking any antihypertensive drugs. ***(438)***

   a. ______________________________

   b. ______________________________

   c. ______________________________

   d. ______________________________

2. List subjective symptoms and objective data that would be significant in the assessment of a patient with hypertension. ***(434-435)***

   a. Subjective symptoms: ______________________________

   ____

   b. Objective data: ______________________________

3. The target is to maintain a blood pressure at or below ____________________. ***(436)***

4. List specific patient information in each of the following areas: self-care and keeping blood pressure under control.

   a. Limiting sodium intake: ***(440)*** ______________________________

   ____

   ____

   ____

   ____

   ____

   ____

   ____

   b. Limiting caffeine and nicotine intake: ***(440)*** ______________________________

   ____

   ____

5. List three drug classifications that may be used in the treatment of hypertension and give an example of each classification. ***(437)***

   ____

   ____

   ____

APPLICATION OF THE NURSING PROCESS

Caring for a Patient with Arterial Insufficiency

Directions: Read the scenario and provide the answers to the following questions.

Scenario: Mrs. Rodriguez reports that she recently joined a fitness center. She noticed leg cramps when she started jogging on the treadmill, but states that the cramps resolved within several minutes after she stopped jogging. She denies pain or discomfort if walking at a regular pace. The physician tells her that she may have a mild arterial insufficiency that can be treated with exercise and possible medication if her symptoms worsen.

1. List three contributing factors in the development of arterial insufficiency. ***(442)***

   a. ______________________________

   b. ______________________________

   c. ______________________________

2. List five signs and symptoms that would indicate diminished *arterial* blood flow in the peripheral vessels. ***(442)***

   a. ______________________________

   b. ______________________________

   c. ______________________________

   d. ______________________________

   e. ______________________________

3. You are assessing Mrs. Rodriguez and checking the "5 Ps." What are the "5 Ps"? ***(442)***

   a. ______________________________

   b. ______________________________

   c. ______________________________

   d. ______________________________

   e. ______________________________

4. The doctor tells Mrs. Rodriguez that she has intermittent claudication. You explain to her that intermittent claudication is characterized by: ***(442)***
   a. edema of the lower legs.
   b. cramping pain that eases with rest.
   c. warm, reddened areas on the lower legs.
   d. pale, cold feet.

5. What are three major nursing goals for patients like Mrs. Rodriguez? ***(444-445)***

 a. ______________________________

 b. ______________________________

 c. ______________________________

6. List five self-care measures that could be taught to Mrs. Rodriguez to help her cope with impaired peripheral circulation and to avoid stasis ulcers and possibly gangrene. ***(445)***

 a. ______________________________

 b. ______________________________

 c. ______________________________

 d. ______________________________

 e. ______________________________

7. Write evaluation criteria that would indicate that the interventions are successful and the expected outcome is being met for Mrs. Rodriguez for the following patient goal: ***(446)***

 Patient will verbalize at least three self-care measures to protect tissues from injury due to decreased arterial flow, after patient teaching session.

 a. ______________________________

 b. ______________________________

 c. ______________________________

PRIORITY SETTING

Directions: Read the scenario and prioritize as appropriate.

Scenario: You are caring for Mr. Ebuto, who has been admitted for a diagnosis of deep vein thrombosis, and he is currently on bedrest and receiving IV heparin. He has anti-embolism (TED) hose in place, with sequential compression devices (SCDs).

1. In the morning, you enter Mr. Ebuto's room and you find that the IV heparin has been turned off. Mr. Ebuto tells you that "somebody came in during the evening and took the IV pump away." What is your priority action? ***(445-446)***
 a. Quickly obtain a new pump and restart the heparin.
 b. Report the incident to the charge nurse.
 c. Obtain a physician's order for partial thromboplastin time (PTT) and activated partial thromboplastin time (aPTT).
 d. Check the physician's orders to see if heparin was discontinued.

2. Mr. Ebuto is lying in bed. His TED hose are in place, but the SCDs are at the bottom of the bed. He tells you that the new nursing assistant removed them during morning hygiene. What is your priority action? ***(445-446)***
   a. Replace the SCDs; talk to the nursing assistant about the purpose of SCDs.
   b. Instruct the nursing assistant on how to replace the SCDs.
   c. Teach the patient how to replace them and to call for assistance as needed.
   d. Report the incident to the nursing educator and the charge nurse.

3. While you are assessing Mr. Ebuto after lunch, you note several abnormal findings. Which assessment finding is the priority? ***(445-446)***
   a. Bleeding of the gums and petechiae
   b. Dyspnea and tachypnea
   c. Increasing pain in the calf
   d. Pitting edema of the affected limb

4. Based on your determination of the priority assessment finding (#3 above), which action will you take first? ***(445-446)***
   a. Check the PTT and aPTT results.
   b. Obtain equipment to give oxygen.
   c. Assess the quality/onset of calf pain.
   d. Measure the circumference of the limb.

NCLEX-PN® EXAM REVIEW

Directions: Choose the best answer(s) for the following questions.

1. When assessing a patient for possible peripheral vascular disease (PVD), which one of the following is a prime contributing factor? ***(441)***
   1. History of structural defects in the arteries
   2. History of excessive alcohol intake
   3. History of inflammation of the veins
   4. History of cigarette smoking

2. A nursing intervention that is important in the care of a patient with a deep vein thrombosis is to assess for complications of: ***(445)***
   1. infection.
   2. gangrene.
   3. embolus.
   4. severe pain.

3. The most common cause of peripheral arterial disorders is: ***(441)***
   1. arteriosclerosis.
   2. a sedentary lifestyle.
   3. rheumatic fever.
   4. hypertension.

4. The nurse should teach patients with chronic venous stasis to sit with their legs: ***(446)***
   1. crossed.
   2. straight.
   3. elevated.
   4. dependent.

5. The nurse is teaching the patient about dietary sources of potassium. Which of following food groups is the best dietary source for potassium? ***(438)***
   1. Milk, cheese, and eggs
   2. Beef, turkey, and tomatoes
   3. Whole grain bread and cereals
   4. Lettuce, cabbage, and onions

6. An acute sign of inadequate blood supply to the feet is: ***(442)***
   1. excessive hair growth.
   2. reddened, warm skin.
   3. brittle, thick toenails.
   4. pale, cool, mottled skin.

7. The patient is taking digoxin and a thiazide diuretic. This combination of medications increases the risk for cardiac dysrthymias related to: ***(438-439)***
   1. hypokalemia.
   2. hypotension.
   3. hyperkalemia.
   4. hypertension.

8. When evaluating continuous intravenous heparin therapy for a patient with a deep vein thrombosis, the nurse assesses for: ***(457)***
   1. the degree of discomfort the patient is experiencing.
   2. the results of the prothrombin time laboratory test.
   3. signs of internal and external bleeding.
   4. nausea and anorexia due to the medication.

9. An important safety factor in planning the care for a patient with a deep vein thrombosis is to: ***(457)***
   1. apply heat packs to the affected leg.
   2. handle the leg gently to prevent dislodgment of the clot.
   3. keep the leg straight and at hip level to prevent edema.
   4. maintain the heparin drip so that the clotting time is three times that of the control.

10. Upon assessment, signs of abdominal aortic aneurysm include: ***(448)***
    1. higher blood pressure in the legs than in the arms.
    2. bounding popliteal pulses and warm, pink skin.
    3. an enlarged abdomen with decreased bowel sounds.
    4. back pain and possibly a visible pulsation of the abdomen.

11. Which of following assessment findings would be most likely to be found in the documentation of a patient admitted for a cerebral aneurysm? ***(448)***
    1. Pressure sensation in the back
    2. Difficulty breathing
    3. Visible pulsation of the abdomen
    4. Impaired speech and confusion

12. When providing postoperative care for a patient following a carotid endarterectomy, which of following assessment findings is the priority concern? ***(444)***
    1. Increasing hoarseness
    2. Loss of appetite
    3. Presence of a bruit
    4. Nausea

13. When a patient is receiving intravenous heparin, the diagnostic test performed to monitor its effectiveness is: *(457)*
    1. serum heparin level.
    2. activated partial thromboplastin time or partial thromboplastin time.
    3. platelet aggregation test.
    4. prothrombin time and International Normalized Ratio value.

CRITICAL THINKING ACTIVITIES

Scenario: You are working with several patients who are to receive heparin. Perform the following math calculations to determine the correct dose or to verify the setting of the IV infusion. *(58)*

1. The patient is on an IV heparin drip for treatment of a deep vein thrombosis. The IV heparin bag (25,000 units/250 mL) is in place with a pump. It is set to infuse at 8 mL/hour. The physician has ordered 800 units/hour. Is the pump setting correct or incorrect? ________________________

2. The doctor orders 5000 units SQ heparin for postoperative prophylaxis. The pharmacy delivers a 10 mL vial of heparin sodium (5000 units/mL). How many mL should you give? ________________________

3. The pharmacy delivers a premixed bag of heparin 25,000 units/500 mL. How many units are in 1 mL? ________________________

4. The patient is on an IV heparin drip. The IV heparin bag (10,000 units/100 mL) is in place with a pump. It is set to infuse at 10 mL/hour. The physician has ordered 1000 units/hour. Is the pump setting correct or incorrect? ________________________

STEPS TOWARD BETTER COMMUNICATION

VOCABULARY BUILDING GLOSSARY

Term	Pronunciation	Definition
bar'orecep'tor	bar o re cep' tor	sensory receptor stimulated by changes in pressure
claudica'tion	klaw di kay' shun	pain in leg muscles, limping or lameness
depen'dent	de pen'dent	hanging down
incom'petent	in com'pe tent	not able to perform the function or job
ischemia	is kee' me a	insufficient blood in a part
periph'eral	pa rif' ah ral	on the outer edges
poten'tiated	po ten' shee a ted	made more powerful (two drugs may react together to be more powerful)
synco'pe	sing ko' pee	temporary loss of consciousness, fainting
tor'tuous	tor' tu ous	twisted, winding
viscos'ity	vis cos' i ty	thickness of a liquid
noncompli'ant	non com pli'ant	does not follow instructions
"silent" symptoms		symptoms that the patient is unable to observe or feel
side effect		result of a treatment or medication in addition to the intended effect

COMPLETION

Directions: Fill in the blanks with the appropriate words from the Vocabulary Building Glossary to complete the statements.

1. When taking a blood pressure, the arm should be at the level of the heart rather than ________________ ______________________________.
2. When the nurse assessed the patient's arm before trying to start an intravenous infusion, the veins were found to be __________________________________.
3. The patient who is polycythemic has increased blood ____________________.
4. The patient with swollen, dusky feet probably has _____________________ vascular disease.
5. Many hypertensive patients are ___________________________ with therapy because they do not notice any symptoms of high blood pressure.
6. The patient who has peripheral arterial vascular disease often experiences _________________________ ____________________ when walking.
7. A ______________________ signals the brain about changes in blood pressure.
8. When a vein develops varicosities, it becomes _________________________.
9. The effect on blood pressure is _______________________________ when an antihypertensive is combined with a diuretic medication.
10. Hypertension often causes only ___________________________________.
11. When a thrombosis occurs in a vessel, ________________________ develops distal to it.
12. Carotid occlusion may cause __________________________ in the patient.
13. Hypokalemia is a _________________________________ of many diuretics.

WORD ATTACK SKILLS

Combining Forms

These combining forms are used in words found in Chapter 18 of the textbook:

angi/o	vessel, channel
vaso	vessel, duct
sclero	hard, hardening
ven/o	vein
thromb/o	blood clot
sta/	make stand, stop
sten/	narrow, compressed

Directions: Write the meanings of the following words constructed from the combining forms above. Use your dictionary as necessary.

1. Vasospasm: ______________________________
2. Vasodilator: ______________________________
3. Vasoconstriction: ______________________________
4. Vasopressor: ______________________________
5. Vasomotor: ______________________________
6. Sclerosis: ______________________________
7. Venogram: ______________________________
8. Venous: ______________________________
9. Thrombectomy: ______________________________
10. Thrombosis: ______________________________
11. Thrombus: ______________________________
12. Stasis: ______________________________
13. Stent: ______________________________

CHAPTER 19

Care of Patients with Cardiac Disorders

evolve Go to http://evolve.elsevier.com/deWit for additional activities and exercises.

COMPLETION

Cardiac Disorders

Directions: Fill in the blanks to complete the statements.

1. A(n) ______________________ is used for patients who have repeated episodes of life-threatening ventricular fibrillation or cardiac asystole (arrest). ***(479)***

2. The signs and symptoms of mitral valve disorders are ______________, ______________, ______________, and ______________. ***(483)***

3. ______________________ is the most common cause of cardiac inflammation in children who do not have congenital cardiac abnormalities. ***(479)***

4. For women, the main symptom of a heart attack may be diffuse chest pain, which may be mistaken for ______________________. ***(463)***

5. Valve surgery is performed on the dysfunctional valve when the person's ______________________. ***(482)***

6. A sign of pericarditis that can be heard during auscultation of the heart is ______________________. ***(481)***

7. ______________ imbalances may cause serious cardiac dysrhythmias. ***(470)***

APPLICATION OF THE NURSING PROCESS

Care of the Patient with Congestive Heart Failure

Directions: Read the scenario and provide the answers to the following questions. ***(467-468)***

Scenario: Mrs. Santo, age 63, has moderate congestive heart failure. She has been admitted to the hospital for complaints of severe dyspnea, generalized edema, weakness, and fatigue. Her physician has ordered bedrest, up to bathroom PRN, in chair for 30 minutes three times a day, and oxygen PRN for dyspnea. Mrs. Santo is also receiving digoxin (Lanoxin) 0.250 mg daily, hydrochlorothiazide (a diuretic), and Isordil (a venous dilator). Her daily sodium intake is limited to 1000 mg.

1. List objective and subjective data that would help assess Mrs. Santo's status with regard to dyspnea, edema, and peripheral circulation.

   a. Dyspnea: Subjective data: ______________________________

   ____

   Objective data: ______________________________

   ____

   b. Edema: Subjective data: ______________________________

   ____

   Objective data: ______________________________

   ____

   c. Peripheral circulation: Subjective data: ______________________________

   ____

   Objective data: ______________________________

   ____

2. Upon admission, which of the following nursing diagnoses is a priority for Mrs. Santos? ***(467)***
   a. Activity intolerance related to decreased perfusion
   b. Risk for injury related to complications of CHF
   c. Decreased cardiac output related to ineffective cardiac muscle
   d. Dyspnea, gas exchange, impaired related to fluid in lung tissue

3. List three nursing actions you would expect to find on Mrs. Santo's nursing care plan during her hospitalization. ***(468-469)***

   a. ______________________________

   b. ______________________________

   c. ______________________________

4. An appropriate task to assign to the nursing assistant would be to:
   a. ask the patient if she needs extra pillows to prevent orthopnea.
   b. assist the patient to turn every 1–2 hours.
   c. determine if Mrs. Santo needs partial or full assistance with ADLs.
   d. check the sacral area for edema and skin breakdown.

5. Mrs. Santo lives with her husband, daughter, and four grandchildren. Before she is discharged, she will need instruction in self-care and her family will need instruction so they can give her support and encouragement. She has been told by her physician to walk at least 1 mile per day, to continue taking her digoxin and diuretic, to stay on her sodium-limited diet, and to lose 25 pounds. Identify at least five points that should be included in the teaching plan for Mrs. Santo and her family so that she can remain relatively symptom-free once she returns home. ***(467)***

a. ______________________

b. ______________________

c. ______________________

d. ______________________

e. ______________________

6. Which of the following statements by Mrs. Santos indicates that she understands the implications of digoxin toxicity? *(474)*
   a. "I will report nausea, vomiting, and anorexia."
   b. "I can eat bananas and citrus to counteract side effects."
   c. "I can skip a dose if I experience side effects."
   d. "I should carry digoxin immune (Digifab) as an antidote."

7. Mrs. Santo is prescribed digoxin 0.250 mg daily. The pharmacy delivers a bottle with 50 Lanoxin tablets; 125 mcg/tablet. Has the pharmacy delivered the correct medication? ______________ If so, how many tablets should Mrs. Santo take? ______________

PRIORITY SETTING

Directions: Read the scenario and prioritize as appropriate.

Scenario: You are caring for Mr. Ducas, an elderly gentleman who was admitted for congestive heart failure. During the morning assessment you find that his condition seems to have deteriorated compared to yesterday. You find several abnormalities. *(467-468)*

1. Which of the following assessment findings is the priority?
   a. Absent peripheral pulses
   b. Frothy sputum and orthopnea
   c. Confusion and irritability
   d. Fever and tachycardia

2. Based on your assessment findings, Mr. Ducas appears to be having complications due to congestive heart failure and he is exhibiting the signs and symptoms of acute pulmonary edema. Which of following is the priority action? *(470)*
   a. Immediately report your findings to the RN/physician.
   b. Check for standing orders for oxygen and morphine.
   c. Place the patient in a high Fowler's position.
   d. Stay with the patient until the code team arrives.

NCLEX-PN® EXAM REVIEW

Directions: Choose the best answer(s) for the following questions.

1. Which of the following should the nurse expect to note with a diagnosis of atrial fibrillation? *(472)*
   1. Low blood pressure
   2. Headaches and fatigue
   3. Feelings of palpitations
   4. An irregular pulse rate

2. Medications that the nurse might administer to patient with atrial fibrillation include: ***(475)***
   1. digoxin and Coumadin.
   2. potassium and Tenormin.
   3. lidocaine and calcium.
   4. aspirin and Isordil.

3. A patient is receiving digoxin. To evaluate the effectiveness of the medication, the nurse would check: ***(474)***
   1. pulse rate and breath sounds.
   2. digoxin and potassium laboratory values.
   3. blood pressure and respirations.
   4. weight loss and appetite.

4. Early signs of congestive heart failure include: ***(467)***
   1. weight gain and dyspnea on exertion.
   2. a wet cough and severely swollen ankles.
   3. cyanosis, fatigue, and dyspnea.
   4. an irregular pulse rate and elevated blood pressure.

5. When the nurse is administering digoxin, she should always first: ***(474)***
   1. assess the amount of weight gain or loss.
   2. question the patient about fatigue and dizziness.
   3. check for signs of hypokalemia.
   4. be certain that the patient has a full stomach.

6. A patient with atrial fibrillation is taking an oral anticoagulant. The patient should be taught to have a follow-up appointment for: ***(477)***
   1. prothrombin time (PT) and international normalized ratio (INR).
   2. partial thromboplastin time (PTT) and activated partial thromboplastin time (aPTT).
   3. complete blood count (CBC) and hematocrit (Hct).
   4. cardiac enzymes.

7. A patient who has modifiable risk factors must be taught to: ***(466)***
   1. eat regular meals, drink sufficient amounts of water, and avoid caffeine.
   2. exercise 20 minutes per day at least twice a week.
   3. limit alcohol consumption to two drinks per week.
   4. keep blood pressure < 120/80 mm Hg.

8. The postoperative care of a patient who has received a permanent pacemaker includes which of the following? *(Select all that apply.)* ***(482)***
   1. Monitor heart rate and rhythm and check vital signs.
   2. Perform dressing changes and care for the insertion site.
   3. Check peripheral pulses proximal to the insertion sites.
   4. Check level of consciousness frequently in the immediate postoperative period.
   5. Teach the patient to count his pulse for a full minute.
   6. Teach patient that full recovery takes about 12 weeks.

9. When planning care for a patient who needs dietary modifications to improve heart health, the nurse would include teaching to: ***(484)***
   1. include 12 grams of fiber in diet each day.
   2. include foods that contain trans-fats.
   3. avoid drinking any coffee or iced beverages.
   4. eat six or more servings of whole grain products each day.

CRITICAL THINKING ACTIVITIES

Scenario

You are assigned to work on a telemetry unit. There is a telemetry technician who is monitoring the patients from a remote location; however, there is a monitor at the nurse's station that is displaying the EKG rhythm for each patient. Although the technician will call if he notes a problem, the nurses are responsible to also be able to recognize arrhythmias and respond accordingly.

Directions: Identify the EKG rhythms and answer the related questions. ***(471-473)***

1. Rhythm strip #1

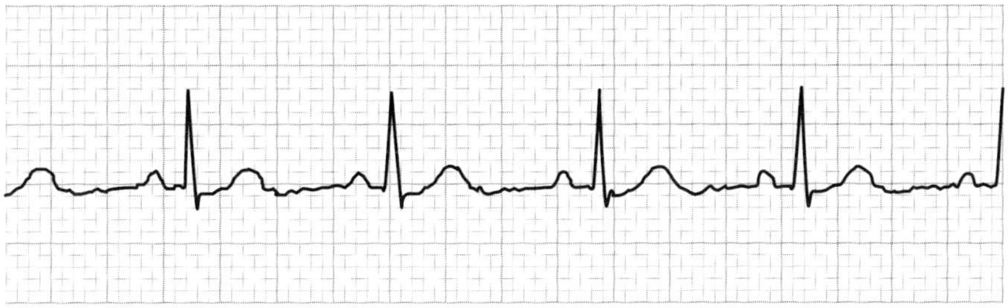

   a. Identify this rhythm. ____________________

   b. What is the appropriate action to take? ____________________

   ____

2. Rhythm strip # 2

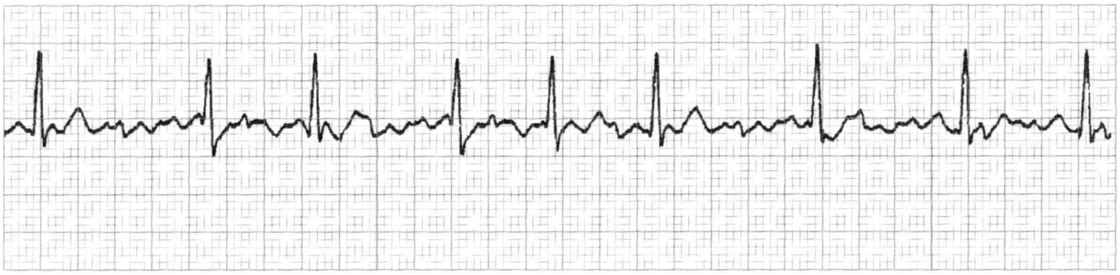

   a. Identify this rhythm. ____________________

   b. Explain why patients who have this arrhythmia may be on Coumadin.

   ____

   ____

3. Rhythm strip # 3

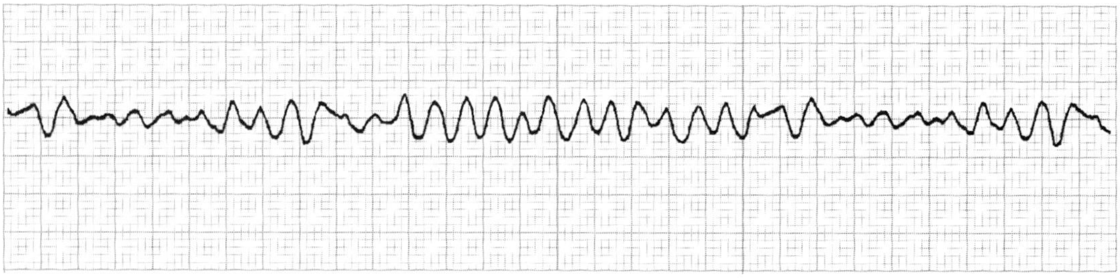

a. Identify this rhythm. ____________________

b. What is the appropriate action to take? ____________________

____

4. Rhythm strip # 4

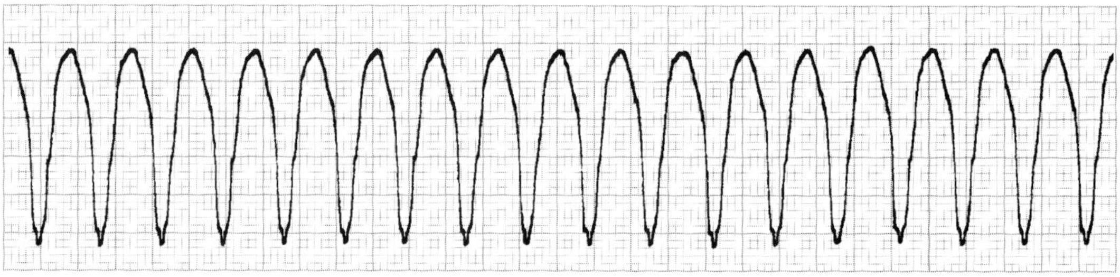

a. Identify this rhythm. ____________________

b. What are two medical treatments that could be ordered to treat this arrhythmia?

____

____

5. Rhythm strip # 5

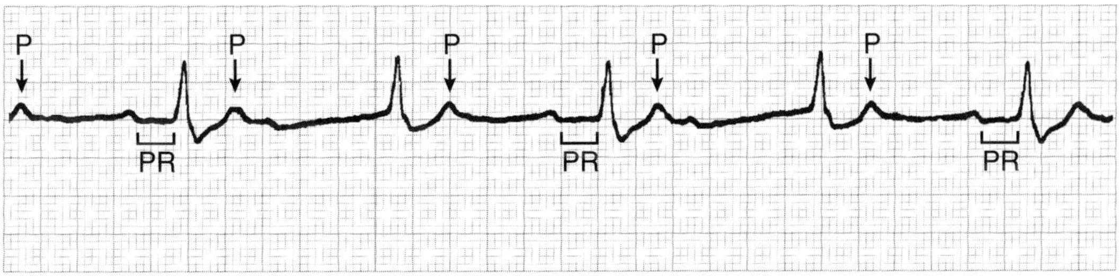

a. Identify this rhythm. ______________________________

b. Explain in your own words why this rhythm may cause your patient to have a change in mental status.

____

____

STEPS TOWARD BETTER COMMUNICATION

VOCABULARY BUILDING GLOSSARY

Term	Pronunciation	Definition
inva'sive	in va'sive	involving the puncture or cutting of the skin, or putting an instrument into the body
telem'etry	te lem' e try	measuring data with radio waves and electronic equipment
engorg'ed	en gorj' d	filled to the limit; swollen
bloated	blo' tid	to be swollen, larger than normal
quiver	kwiv' er	to vibrate with a small, rapid motion
hyper'trophy	hi per' tro fee	extra growth, thickened
cardiomyop'athy	kar dee o mi op' ah thee	disorder of heart muscle that prevents it from pumping effectively
a'trioventric'ular	a' tree o ven trik' u lar	relating to an atrium and ventricle of the heart
fib'rilla'tion	fib' ri la' shun	small, rapid, irregular muscle contractions; quivering
intersti'tial	in ter stish' al	spaces in the tissue between the cells

COMPLETION

Directions: Fill in the blanks with the appropriate words from the Vocabulary Building Glossary to complete the statements.

1. During ventricular fibrillation, the heart ________________________.
2. The patient whose heart rate is being monitored is hooked up to a ____________________________ unit that transmits the EKG pattern to the monitor in the nurse's station.
3. ______________________ or increased growth of left ventricle muscle may be hereditary.
4. When congestive heart failure occurs, the lung vessels become ______________ with blood and fluid leaks into the interstitial spaces.
5. A cardiac catheterization is a(n) ____________________________ type of test.
6. The major problems exhibited by patients with __________________ are heart failure and dysrhythmias.
7. If the SA node fails to pace the heart, the ________________________ node may take over.
8. Patients can be treated for chronic atrial ___________________________, but ventricular ___________________________ is life-threatening.
9. The patient who experiences right-sided congestive heart failure develops a swollen liver and may feel ___________________________.
10. Edema results if body fluids in the intravascular fluid compartment begin to leak into the ___________________________________ compartment.

WORD ATTACK SKILLS

Combining Forms

Here are some important combining forms found in this chapter:

cardi/o	heart
my/o	muscle
sin/o	a space or channel
vas/o	vessel
end/o	inside

COMMUNICATION EXERCISE

You are advising Mrs. Perryman who has complained of pain in her legs due to varicose veins. She also has high blood pressure. (Practice the dialogue with a partner.)

Mrs. Perryman: My legs hurt—and look at these ugly varicose veins! My feet and legs hurt at the end of the day. They are swollen. And I get so tired!

Nurse:	Would you like me to work out a plan with you that might help?
Mrs. Perryman:	Oh, yes! That would be wonderful.
Nurse:	I would like you to wear these support hose—but no tight underwear or pants or garters that would cut off the circulation. If you can put the hose on in the morning while you are still in bed it would help.
Mrs. Perryman:	Why is that?
Nurse:	If you put them on before your legs swell, it helps keep the circulation flowing. When your legs hang off the edge of the bed they swell with the blood flowing to them.
Mrs. Perryman:	That makes sense.
Nurse:	When you are sitting, I would like you to keep your feet elevated if you can. Do you get much exercise?
Mrs. Perryman:	No, not very much.
Nurse:	Let's see if you can do more walking. You can begin with just 15 minutes at a time. If you could do swimming or water aerobics it would be a big help.
Mrs. Perryman:	Where could I do that?
Nurse:	The YMCA and the parks department sometimes have programs. I can check into it and let you know. Are you a smoker?
Mrs. Perryman:	No, not for years.
Nurse:	That's good, because smoking constricts the blood vessels even more. About your diet—if we can get you on a low-salt, low-fat, heart-healthy diet that will help a lot. I will show you how to read the food labels. That's it—diet, exercise, wearing support hose, and keeping your legs elevated.
Mrs. Perryman:	That sounds like a lot to do.
Nurse:	Yes, it is, but you will feel so much better—and it could even save your life! Next week when I visit, we will see if we can tell the difference in your blood pressure, too.

CHAPTER 20

Care of Patients with Coronary Artery Disease and Cardiac Surgery

evolve Go to http://evolve.elsevier.com/deWit for additional activities and exercises.

TERMINOLOGY

Directions: Define the following terms.

Angina pectoris: ***(492)***____

Coronary insufficiency: ***(488)*** ____________________________________

Drug-eluting stent: ***(498)*** _____________________________________

Myocardial infarction: ***(493)*** ___________________________________

Necrosis: ***(493)*** ____

Ischemia: ***(493)*** ____

COMPLETION

Directions: Fill in the blanks to complete the statements.

1. As the coronary vessels narrow, the patient may experience symptoms of ischemia such as ________________ and ________________________. ***(489)***
2. ____________________________________ is the major contributing factor to the formation of this fatty material that contributes to the process of atherosclerosis. ***(488)***
3. Women are more likely to experience heart attacks after reaching __________________; however, poor ____________ habits, __________________ lifestyle, and _____________ levels of stress contribute to development of cardiovascular disease earlier in life. ***(493)***
4. Any activity that increases the heart's workload increases its need for ______________. ***(489)***
5. The prognosis of the patient who suffers an acute myocardial infarction (MI) depends on the ____________________ of the artery obstructed, the location, and the ______________________ of heart tissue that is damaged. ***(493)***

6. Another treatment method for occlusion of a coronary artery other than coronary artery bypass graft is the procedure called ______________________________. ***(502)***

7. It is important to stress to the patient that she has ________________ over her rehabilitation and prognosis. ***(499)***

8. A thrombolytic agent must be administered within __________ hours of experiencing the symptoms of MI, in order to prevent or decrease damage to the heart muscle. ***(407)***

9. After receiving a heart transplant, the patient must take ________________ for life. ***(505)***

10. Two constant potential complications that the heart transplant patient must deal with are ________________ and ________________. ***(506)***

11. The doctor orders IV fluid for a postoperative patient to infuse at 125 mL/hour. The drop factor is 10 gtts/mL. What is the drip rate? ________________ ***(58)***

TABLE ACTIVITY

Cardiac Surgeries

Directions: Fill in the blocks below with the type of surgery that matches the description. The first block has been done for you.

Type of Surgery	Description
coronary artery bypass graft (CABG)	surgery bypasses the blocked artery, replacing it with sections of a vein or artery taken from another part of the patient's body
	does not require stopping the heart's activity, and therefore does not require using the heart-lung machine ***(501)***
	is invasive and similar to the procedure used for cardiac catheterization where a catheter is introduced through the femoral vessel ***(502)***
	part of the latissimus dorsi muscle is detached from its natural position and brought around to the front of the body ***(504)***
	can be accomplished with a mechanical or biological device ***(504)***
	performed for selected patients who have end-stage left ventricular failure resulting from cardiomyopathy ***(505)***

APPLICATION OF THE NURSING PROCESS

Care of a Patient with Angina Pectoris

Directions: Provide the answer to the following questions.

Scenario: Mr. Locke, age 55, is admitted to the hospital with chest pains. Over the past year, he has gradually become more fatigued and uncomfortable whenever he exerts himself. His admitting diagnosis is possible angina pectoris.

1. What other information from Mr. Locke's history could be helpful in assessing his cardiovascular status? *(493)*

   a. ________________________________

   b. ________________________________

   c. ________________________________

   d. ________________________________

2. Two nursing diagnoses on Mr. Locke's nursing care plan are Pain and Knowledge deficit. List three specific nursing interventions appropriate for each nursing diagnosis.

   Pain related to decreased coronary artery circulation: *(494)*

   a. ________________________________

   b. ________________________________

   c. ________________________________

   Knowledge deficit related to self-care: *(495)*

   a. ________________________________

   b. ________________________________

   c. ________________________________

3. Which of the following objective data indicates that Mr. Locke's level of physical activity is appropriate to his recovery?
   a. Patient asks for assistance when he becomes fatigued.
   b. Patient's heart rate and respiratory rate are stable after ambulation.
   c. Patient's activity is observed by the physical therapist.
   d. Family tells you that he is walking like he used to prior to hospitalization.

PRIORITY SETTING

Directions: Read the scenario and prioritize as appropriate.

You are working in an extended care facility. Mr. Ido is walking down the hall and reports to you that he is having angina. He has a PRN order for sublingual nitroglycerine and he asks you to assist him with the medication that is on his bedside table. *Prioritize the steps in administering the nitroglycerine.* ***(493)***

_______ a. If the pain has not eased or if BP increases, administer second tablet.

_______ b. Give one tablet, placed under the tongue, wait 5 minutes.

_______ c. Notify the physician regarding pain.

_______ d. Assist the patient to lie in bed.

_______ e. Wait 5 minutes, reassess pain.

_______ f. Obtain a baseline BP.

_______ g. Reassess pain and recheck BP.

_______ h. Administer a third tablet if pain persists.

_______ i. Recheck BP; it should have decreased.

NCLEX-PN® EXAM REVIEW

Directions: Choose the best answer(s) for the following questions.

1. The risk factors that lead to a higher incidence of atherosclerosis include which of the following? *(Select all that apply.)* ***(488-489)***
   1. High levels of high-density lipoproteins
   2. Cigarette smoking
   3. A history of hypertension and diabetes mellitus
   4. Age (> age 40), gender, and race
   5. Women on oral contraceptives or estrogen replacement therapy

2. Which of the following is the most significant in diagnosing damage to the myocardium? ***(496)***
   1. Elevated level of troponin
   2. Elevated level of creatine phosphokinase (CPK)
   3. Elevated level of creatine phosphokinase-MB (CK-MB)
   4. Elevated level of lactate dehydrogenase (LDH)

3. The patient is taking lovastatin (Mevacor) for treatment of hypercholesterolemia. The patient should have follow-up because of the potential for: ***(490)***
   1. nephrotoxcity.
   2. cardiotoxicity.
   3. hepatotoxicity.
   4. ototoxicity.

4. The patient presents in the emergency department with severe chest pain. Which of the following are likely to be prescribed during the initial emergency care? ***(497)***
   1. Morphine, oxygen, nitrates, aspirin
   2. Beta-blockers, clopidogrel (Plavix)
   3. Simvastatin (Lipitor), lorazepam (Ativan)
   4. Oxygen, dobutamine (Dobutrex)

5. Which of the following statements by the patient indicates a need for additional teaching about taking his nitroglycerine? ***(493)***
   1. "I should try to sit or lie down before I take a tablet."
   2. "If I get a headache, I should not take any more."
   3. "I can take up to three tablets before I call my doctor."
   4. "The tablets should be stored in a dark bottle."

6. A patient who has had an acute myocardial infarction may be prescribed a stool softener. The purpose of the stool softener in this case is to: ***(497)***
   1. counteract the effects of prolonged bedrest.
   2. conserve energy associated with walking to toilet.
   3. counteract the side effects of medications.
   4. decrease the risk of bradycardia associated with straining.

7. Which of the following is a contraindication for thrombolytic therapy, such as t-PA (Activase)? ***(497)***
   1. History of hypertension
   2. History of hemorrhagic stroke
   3. Symptom onset within past 12 hours
   4. Intraspinal surgery during childhood

8. The patient is admitted for an acute MI. Which of the following symptoms or findings is expected within 24 hours after the attack? ***(497)***
   1. Continuous, dull substernal chest pain
   2. A slightly elevated temperature
   3. An abnormal electrocardiogram
   4. A decline in the level of LDH

9. The nurse knows that there are several types of angina. Which of the following is considered the most urgent and in need of immediate attention? ***(492)***
   1. Exertional angina
   2. Variant angina
   3. Vasospastic angina
   4. Unstable angina

10. For a patient who is taking a statin drug, an important teaching point to include would be to: ***(490)***
    1. report muscle tenderness or pain that persists for more than a few days.
    2. increase consumption of grapefruit juice to supply K^+.
    3. have follow-up appointments to monitor platelet count.
    4. discontinue medication when the target weight goal is met.

11. One of the major goals of cardiac rehabilitation is to: ***(499-500)***
    1. assist the patient to return to previous level of functioning.
    2. ensure that the patient can perform activities of daily living.
    3. increase activity based on individual progress and needs.
    4. teach the patient how to resume sexual relations.

12. There are several patients on a busy cardiac rehabilitation unit who need assistance. Which task would be appropriate to assign to the nursing assistant? ***(4)***
    1. Find out why a depressed patient is not doing his physical therapy.
    2. Answer a family member's question about how to contact a local support group.
    3. Escort a patient who has been discharged home to his wife's car.
    4. Listen to a patient who is complaining about the bad hospital food.

CRITICAL THINKING ACTIVITIES

Scenario A

You are at the local park for a neighborhood picnic. You notice that Mrs. Grandville, a middle-aged, obese woman, is holding her hand over her chest. She tells you that she is "having a little indigestion from the potato salad;" however, you notice that she is breathing faster than normal and she appears anxious. On further questioning, she admits to chest pressure, but she says that she will just drive herself home and rest. She declines your offer to help or your advice about going to the hospital.

1. What coping mechanism is Mrs. Grandville using to respond to the symptoms? ***(499)***

   ____

2. Explain in your own words how the use of this coping mechanism affects her decision-making.

   ____

   ____

   ____

3. Write a brief dialogue that you could use with Mrs. Grandville, so that she can make an informed decision.

   ____

   ____

   ____

   ____

   ____

   ____

   ____

Scenario B

You are making home visits to Mr. Ketauna, an elderly patient who has chronic cardiomyopathy. The family reports that Mr. Ketauna is mentally active, although he is somewhat depressed, because over the past several years his quality of life has steadily been decreasing. They are considering asking the doctor if he would be a candidate for a heart transplant. You suggest that the family talk to the doctor and you decide to do some research to help clarify their concerns.

1. List at least five of the criteria for heart transplant. ***(505)***

   a. ______________________________

   b. ______________________________

   c. ______________________________

   d. ______________________________

   e. ______________________________

2. What are some of the ethical implications for the above criteria when trying to determine who will or will not receive an organ transplant?

____

____

____

____

____

____

____

____

3. In your own words, discuss some adjustments that the family and the prospective recipient would have to make while waiting on the transplant list.

____

____

____

____

____

____

____

____

STEPS TOWARD BETTER COMMUNICATION

VOCABULARY BUILDING GLOSSARY

Term	Definition
col lat'er al	(adj.) parallel, secondary
com pen' sa tor y	(adj.) making up for, counterbalancing
com'pro mise	(noun) a settlement between two sides that both agree on; (verb) 1. to make such an agreement; 2. to expose to danger by unwise action
e'ti ol'o gy	(noun) the cause, origin
ex'tra cor por'e al	(adj.) outside the body
fi'brous	(adj.) made of fibers, long thin strands of tissue
prog no'sis	(noun) an advance indication, a forecast or prospect of the probable outcome
wean, weaning (ween)	(verb) a gradual withdrawal

COMPLETION

Directions: Fill in the blanks with the appropriate word from the Glossary above to complete the statements.

1. The pathology report will help determine the ________________ of the disease.
2. ________________ plaques build up in the arteries, occluding the blood flow.
3. The ________________ for the patient depends on the size and location of the obstruction in the artery.
4. The oxygen demands from exertion may ____________________ the coronary circulation of an elderly person.
5. Patients whose bodies have a strong ____________________ mechanism may have a well-developed ________________________ circulation.
6. When the heart-lung machine is used to pump and oxygenate the blood, the procedure is called ____________________ circulation.
7. After surgery, ________________ from the ventilator is begun if oxygenation is adequate.

MATCHING

Directions: Match the abbreviation on the left with the correct meaning on the right.

1. ______	CAD	a.	Coronary care unit
2. ______	CHF	b.	Percutaneous transluminal coronary angioplasty
3. ______	CK	c.	Myocardial infarction
4. ______	CCU	d.	Coronary artery bypass graft
5. ______	ECG	e.	Congestive heart failure
6. ______	MI	f.	Acute coronary syndrome
7. ______	CVP	g.	Central venous pressure
8. ______	PAP	h.	Metabolic equivalents
9. ______	PCWP	i.	Creatine kinase
10. ______	PTCA	j.	Coronary artery disease
11. ______	CABG	k.	Pulmonary artery pressure
12. ______	IABP	l.	Pulmonary capillary wedge pressure
13. ______	ACS	m.	Intra-aortic balloon pump
14. ______	MET	n.	Electrocardiogram

COMMUNICATION EXERCISE

The following words are often used to describe the pain associated with these conditions:

angina pectoris:	dull, tightness, ache
acute myocardial infarction:	sudden, severe, crushing, burning, pressure, squeezing, knife-like (left arm more frequently indicated)

1. Can you give two reasons why people often have heart attacks while shoveling snow?

   a. ______________________________

   b. ______________________________

2. Unscramble this sentence:

   consumed Grapefruit when be not a juice should drug taking statin.

   ____

CHAPTER 21

The Neurologic System

evolve Go to http://evolve.elsevier.com/deWit for additional activities and exercises.

REVIEW OF ANATOMY AND PHYSIOLOGY

Terminology

Directions: Match the term on the left with the correct statement, function, or definition on the right. ***(511-515)***

1. _______ Pyramidal tracts
2. _______ Meninges
3. _______ Subarachnoid space
4. _______ Nerve stimulus
5. _______ Neurotransmitter
6. _______ Reflex arc
7. _______ Myelin sheath
8. _______ Synapse

a. Space between two neurons
b. Covering of nerves that insulates them
c. Physical, chemical, or electrical event that changes cell membrane and conducts as an electrical impulse along nerve pathway
d. Path traveled by a stimulus from point of stimulus through spinal cord and back to effector site
e. Protective membranes that cover the brain and help protect the spinal cord
f. Conduction pathways, beginning in the cerebral cortex and ending in the spinal cord, that control skeletal muscle movement
g. Space through which cerebrospinal fluid travels and where villi help regulate amount of circulating fluid
h. Secreted at the synapse

Matching

Directions: Match the part of the brain on the left with its function(s) on the right. (There may be more than one answer for each.) ***(516)***

1. _______ Cerebrum
2. _______ Cerebellum
3. _______ Thalamus
4. _______ Hypothalamus
5. _______ Midbrain (brain stem)
6. _______ Pons (brain stem)
7. _______ Medulla oblongata

a. Mediates visual and auditory reflexes
b. Responsible for balance
c. Controls body temperature
d. Center of thinking and consciousness
e. Relay between spinal cord and cerebrum
f. Controls appetite and water balance
g. Helps regulate respiration
h. Regulates heartbeat, respiration, and blood pressure
i. Responsible for coordination of movement
j. Links nervous system and endocrine system
k. Control center for swallowing
l. Responsible for judgment and learning

SHORT ANSWER

Changes that Occur with Aging

1. Reaction time is slowed with aging because there is a ______________________________ ______________________________. *(515)*

2. With advanced age, there is a loss of neurons and slower nerve conduction causes a decrease in the efficiency of the ______________________________. *(515)*

3. Although the ability to learn is not affected by aging, the process of learning is ______________________________. *(515)*

4. Continued intellectual function in the healthy elderly is promoted by ______________________________ ______________________________. *(515)*

5. With aging there is often a decrease in ____________________ memory, but often ____________________ is unaffected. *(515)*

COMPLETION

Nursing Management

Directions: Fill in the blanks to complete the statements.

1. A response to a stimulus may be ______________________________ or ______________________________ movement. *(525)*

2. Reflexes cause ______________________________ movements. *(519)*

3. The "neuro check" assesses neuromuscular function when the nurse asks the patient to ____________ ______________________________ ______________________________. *(523)*

4. A normal response to scraping an object across the sole of the foot will result in ____________ ____________________ of the toes. *(522)*

5. A positive Babinski reflex in someone older than 20–24 months of age is ____________________. *(522)*

6. A diagnostic test for a possible herniated lumbar disc is called a ______________________________ ______________________________. *(521)*

7. A potential side effect of the radiopaque contrast medium used for many diagnostic x-rays is ______________________________.

8. An electromyelogram tests the function of the ______________________________. *(519)*

9. When the pupil of one eye is increasing in size, it indicates____. ***(526)***

10. The acronym PERRLA stands for ____. ***(526)***

SHORT ANSWER

Directions: Answer the following questions in the spaces provided.

1. List three specific things you might notice a patient doing that could indicate poor coordination and balance, and write them as if you were documenting them on the patient's chart. ***(525)***

   a. ____

   b. ____

   c. ____

2. List four reasons why a lumbar puncture is performed. ***(519)***

   a. ____

   b. ____

   c. ____

   d. ____

3. Describe what an electroencephalogram (EEG) is and what it is *not*. ***(519)***

   ____

   ____

   ____

   ____

   ____

4. List at least four pieces of information you think would be significant during an admission assessment of a patient's neurologic status. This information would be obtained while taking the patient's health history. One example would be recent infections affecting the sinuses or face. ***(523)***

   a. ____

   b. ____

   c. ____

   d. ____

NCLEX-PN® EXAM REVIEW

Directions: Choose the best answer(s) for the following questions.

1. Causative factors of neurologic problems include: *(Select all that apply.)* ***(516)***
   1. alcohol consumption.
   2. cigarette smoking.
   3. cocaine use.
   4. hypertension.
   5. lack of exercise.
   6. pesticides.

2. Promotion of blood pressure control can help prevent brain damage from: ***(516)***
   1. medications.
   2. stroke.
   3. myocardial infarction.
   4. atherosclerosis.

3. Tests for coordination and balance check areas controlled by: ***(518)***
   1. tendons and muscles.
   2. the pons and medulla.
   3. the left cerebral hemisphere.
   4. the cerebrum and cerebellum.

4. A vital sign that can indicate increasing intracranial pressure is ______________________________. ***(523)***

5. Which one of the following signs would be the most important to report if found when a patient has had a head injury? ***(526)***
   1. Weak hand grips
   2. BP rising from 128/78 to 134/82
   3. Restless movements of the extremities
   4. One pupil larger than the other

6. When assessing the level of consciousness in a patient, the nurse should be sure to: ***(524)***
   1. always repeat questions using the same words.
   2. phrase questions so that they cannot be answered simply with a yes or no.
   3. ask different questions each time the patient is assessed.
   4. use vocabulary in the questions that is familiar to the patient.

7. When a patient has hemiplegia or quadriplegia, it is important to provide relief for pain and: ***(529)***
   1. muscle spasms.
   2. diplopia.
   3. paresthesias.
   4. vasoconstriction.

8. One of the most common nursing diagnoses for patients with a neurologic problem is: ***(832)***
   1. Impaired mobility.
   2. Self-care deficit.
   3. Impaired verbal communication.
   4. Chronic confusion.

9. Measures that help a patient with dysphagia include: *(Select all that apply.)* ***(533)***
   1. check swallowing ability before feeding.
   2. purée foods to ease swallowing.
   3. maintain an upright position for 30 minutes after eating.
   4. keep a nonstressful atmosphere at meal time.
   5. feed at a steady pace.
   6. refrain from talking while the patient is eating.

10. A high priority of nursing care for the patient who is confused is: ***(534)***
    1. enhancing mobility.
    2. providing safety.
    3. adequate nutrition.
    4. promoting sleep and rest.

CRITICAL THINKING ACTIVITIES

1. Why is positioning so important for the patient who is unconscious? ***(529)***

2. What would you teach a patient who is about to have an electromylogram (EMG)? ***(519)***

STEPS TOWARD BETTER COMMUNICATION

VOCABULARY BUILDING GLOSSARY

Term	Pronunciation	Definition
myriad	mir'i ad	many, a vast number
mechanism	mek'an ism	a method, a process by which something happens
nystagmus	nis tag'mus	rapid involuntary movement of the eyeball
widened pulse pressure		greater difference between systolic and diastolic
mnemonic	ne mon'ik	a memory device to help aid the memory and recall facts

COMPLETION

Directions: Use the correct word from the Glossary above to complete the sentence.

1. When checking the eyes, if ____________________ is found, it indicates an abnormality.

2. A ______________ of causes can affect the neurologic system and cause problems.

3. A ____________________________________ occurs when the systolic pressure goes up and the diastolic goes down.

4. A verse, or an abbreviation (e.g., PERRLA), is a good ____________________ to help recall facts or lists of things.

5. Excess carbon dioxide in the blood is one of the ____________________ that can cause intracranial pressure to rise after a head injury.

WORD ATTACK SKILLS

Prefixes

Directions: Form a word combining the correct prefix below with the word stem listed. Write the meaning of the word. Use a dictionary as necessary.

Prefix	Meaning
a-, in-, an-, im-	no, not, without, lack of
dys-, dis-, mal-	bad, difficult

Word Stem	Combined Word	Meaning
1. -orders	____________________	____________________
2. -paired	____________________	____________________
3. -voluntary	____________________	____________________
4. -noxia	____________________	____________________
5. -oriented	____________________	____________________
6. -effective	____________________	____________________
7. -orientation	____________________	____________________

Directions: Several words in this chapter have the same prefix. Write the meanings for the following words by attaching the prefix cereb- (brain), dys- (bad, difficult), or hemi- (half, partly) to the suffix listed. Use your dictionary as needed.

Suffix	Word	Meaning
1. -brum	____________________	____________________
2. -bellum	____________________	____________________
3. -bral	____________________	____________________
4. -paresis	____________________	____________________
5. -plegia	____________________	____________________
6. -phasia	____________________	____________________

COMMUNICATION EXERCISES

Dialogue Practice

Directions: Discuss with a partner.

A. With a partner, use the guidelines in Focused Assessment 21-1 in the textbook to perform an assessment. Practice asking each question. Practice charting your assessment.

B. As a second language learner, do you think the steps to help an aphasic person (self talk, parallel talk, expansion, and modeling) would help someone learning a new language? Why or why not? What happens in each of the steps?

Explanations

What would you say to a patient who asked why the doctor does a knee jerk (patellar reflex) test?

___

Orientation and Function Questions

Directions: Make a short list of questions you could ask an alert patient in order to assess his mental function.

___

___

___

CHAPTER 22

Care of Patients with Head and Spinal Cord Injuries

evolve Go to http://evolve.elsevier.com/deWit for additional activities and exercises.

COMPLETION

Head and Spinal Cord Injuries

Directions: Fill in the blanks to complete the statements.

1. When a concussion occurs, there is ____________________ and a ____________________ due to the brief disruption of consciousness. ***(540)***

2. An acceleration-deceleration injury causes __________ brain injuries. ***(541)***

3. Elderly people are more susceptible to subdural hematoma after a bump on the head because the brain tends to ________________ within the cranial vault and __________________ may be torn. ***(541)***

4. An ____________________ hematoma results after a head injury from rapid leakage of blood from the ____ which quickly elevates ____. ***(541)***

5. If clear fluid is leaking from the ear after a head injury, it should be tested to see if there is ____________________ present. ***(542)***

6. Initial measures after a head injury include securing a ____________________________ and elevating ____. ***(543)***

7. Subdural hematoma is relieved by _______________________ or _______________________. ***(543)***

8. Traumatic spinal cord injuries occur from compression, _______________________, _______________________, or tearing of the cord. ***(550)***

9. A complication of spinal cord injury from disruption in the nerve communication pathways between upper and lower motor neurons is _____________________. ***(553)***

10. Following the immediate flaccid paralysis that may occur with spinal cord injury, ____________________ often occurs. ***(553)***

11. To avoid muscle spasms in the spinal cord–injured patient, when positioning the patient avoid ____. ***(554)***

12. Autonomic dysreflexia is dangerous because it can cause sudden ______________________________ ______________________________. *(554)*

13. A common problem in spinal cord–injured patients is ____________________ reflux that predisposes to ______________________________. *(555)*

14. Paraplegia occurs when spinal cord injury occurs at the level of ______________________________. *(551)*

15. If a patient has a cervical spine injury and is in a halo traction device, you should never ______________________________ device. *(552)*

SHORT ANSWER

Intracranial Pressure

Directions: Answer the following questions in the spaces provided.

1. The classic signs of increasing intracranial pressure are ______________________________ ____________________, ____________________, ____________________and ______________________________. *(546)*

2. The earliest sign of increasing intracranial pressure is usually a change in ______________________________ ______________________________. *(546)*

3. Some necessary nursing interventions that may increase intracranial pressure in the patient suffering from a head injury are ______________________________ ______________________________. *(549)*

4. A priority concern for the nurse caring for a patient after intracranial surgery is ______________________________ ______________________________. *(543)*

5. Pathophysiologically, a head injury causes swelling and pressure against cerebral veins and arteries that interferes with the flow of blood, causing ____________________ and ____________________ of the tissues. *(545)*

6. Normal intracranial pressure is ____________________ mm Hg. *(546)*

7. Pupil changes occur with increasing intracranial pressure because ______________________________ ____________________. *(546)*

8. Positioning of the patient with increased intracranial pressure is extremely important to help __________ ______________________________ and reduce ______________________________ ______________________________. *(549)*

9. Seven indications that intracranial pressure is rising are: ***(548)***

   a. ______________________________

   b. ______________________________

   c. ______________________________

   d. ______________________________

   e. ______________________________

   f. ______________________________

   g. ______________________________

COMPLETION

Back Pain and Ruptured Intervertebral Disc

Directions: Fill in the blanks to complete the statements.

1. Health care workers are prone to back pain just from ______________________. ***(557)***
2. Back pain and disorders can be prevented by proper ______________ and the use of ______________________ and ______________________________. ***(557)***
3. In the elderly, one reason for degeneration of the spinal vertebrae is ______________________. ***(558)***
4. Chronic back pain is defined as pain that lasts for more than ______________ or occurs on a ______________________. ***(558)***
5. Signs of a herniated lumbar disk may include pain radiating down ______________ into the ______________ or ______________________________. ***(558)***
6. Signs of a herniated cervical disk may include pain in the ______________ and ______________, radiating down the arm with ______________________ and ______________________________. ***(558)***
7. Patients who are experiencing back pain should not ___________ or ___________ for long periods of time. ***(558)***
8. Surgical removal of a damaged disk may be performed by a percutaneous laser ______________. ***(559)***
9. If a spinal fusion is necessary, a ______________________ must be performed. ***(559)***
10. After spinal surgery, a priority nursing measure is to keep the spinal column in ______________ ______________________. ***(559)***

APPLICATION OF THE NURSING PROCESS

Directions: Write a brief answer to each question.

Your patient has sustained a closed head injury in an automobile accident and was admitted to the ICU. The priority nursing diagnosis on the care plan is "Risk for injury related to potential increased intracranial pressure."

1. Write two appropriate expected outcomes for this diagnosis for this patient. ***(544)***

   a. ______________________________

   b. ______________________________

2. Nursing interventions that would be carried out to help the patient achieve the expected outcomes would be: ***(544)***

   ____

   ____

   ____

3. Criteria by which you would evaluate whether the expected outcomes have been met are:

   ____

   ____

PRIORITY SETTING

You are assigned the following patients:

a. Mr. Hopper, age 23, who has a C-5 injury sustained in a diving accident and is in cervical tongs and on a Roto-Rest bed.
b. Mrs. Hernandez, age 48, who has a ruptured disk at L-5. She has just had a diskectomy this morning.
c. Ms. Chinn, age 72, who suffered a back injury and a pelvic fracture in an automobile accident. She is on bedrest and has paresthesia in her right leg and foot.

Mr. Hopper is complaining of muscle spasms and pain. Mrs. Hernandez calls complaining of nausea. Ms. Chinn calls and asks for help, explaining that she has experienced some incontinence and the bed is wet.

In which order would you attend to these patients' needs? ______________________________

NCLEX-PN® EXAM REVIEW

Directions: Choose the best answer(s) for the following questions.

1. Discharge teaching for the patient who has sustained a concussion should include instructions to: ***(546)***
   1. take the prescribed analgesic for headache every 4 hours.
   2. lie down flat at home and move around as little as possible.
   3. force fluids to prevent dehydration and infection.
   4. report immediately any severe headache or persistent vomiting.

2. Planning for the patient who has sustained a head injury would include listing which *one* of the following nursing diagnoses as the highest priority in the care plan? ***(545-546)***
   1. Sensory perception alteration related to cerebral bleeding
   2. Risk for infection related to skull fracture
   3. Incontinence related to decreased level of consciousness
   4. Risk for injury related to possible increase in intracranial pressure

3. The first priority in assessing the patient with head trauma at an accident scene is determining: ***(543)***
   1. whether spinal injury is present.
   2. the level of consciousness using the Glasgow coma scale.
   3. whether the airway is patent.
   4. whether hypotension is present.

4. Baclofen is a drug used to help prevent muscle spasms. The side effects of this drug include: *(Select all that apply.)* ***(555)***
   1. Seizure activity
   2. Diplopia
   3. Rash
   4. Nausea and vomiting
   5. Fatigue
   6. Urinary urgency

5. Mannitol is an osmotic diuretic that helps decrease intracranial pressure. Nursing interventions for the patient receiving this drug include: *(Select all that apply.)* ***(555)***
   1. monitor intake and output.
   2. observe for chest pain.
   3. monitor for increasing salivation.
   4. watch for electrolyte imbalances.
   5. check skin turgor.

6. A patient with a daughter who is engaged to be married suffered an accident that left him paraplegic. He says to his minister, "If God will let me just walk my daughter down the aisle for her wedding, I'll never complain about being in this chair again." This indicates which stage of grief or mourning? ***(554)***
   1. Shock and denial
   2. Anger
   3. Bargaining
   4. Depression
   5. Adjustment

7. Mr. Pineda suffered a closed head injury and has increased intracranial pressure. The physician has prescribed mannitol 1 g/kg IV every 6 hours. Mr. Pineda weighs 162 lbs. How many grams of mannitol would be the correct dose to be given every 6 hours? ____________ g ***(58)***

8. Which of the following is a priority nursing intervention for the patient with a spinal cord injury who is at risk of autonomic dysreflexia? ***(554)***
   1. Careful monitoring of urinary output.
   2. Preventing cold draughts of air from touching the patient.
   3. Using an abdominal binder to raise blood pressure.
   4. Providing frequent massage of the legs.

9. Autonomic dysreflexia can lead to which of the following? ***(554)***
   1. Heat stroke from loss of thermoregulation
   2. Paralytic ileus
   3. Severe muscle cramps
   4. Severe hypertension

CRITICAL THINKING ACTIVITIES

Scenario A: Mr. Schultz sustained a head injury in a bicycle accident. He was admitted to the ICU from the emergency department as his level of consciousness was decreasing. He is arousable, but very drowsy. His vital signs are BP 132/84, P 78, R 16, T. 98.8° F. Vital and neuro signs are ordered every hour. A pulse oximeter is attached and he is placed on a cardiac monitor.

1. What diagnostic tests would most likely be ordered to determine the extent of damage from his head injury? ***(542)***

His pulse pressure shows widening after 3 hours, and he is more difficult to arouse.

2. What medications would you expect he might receive? ***(555)***

His condition worsens and one pupil begins to dilate. He is placed on mechanical ventilation.

3. When suctioning his endotracheal tube, why is it especially important to oxygenate him well beforehand? ***(552)***

Scenario B: Mr. Schultz was found to have a subdural hematoma. Burr holes were performed and the hematoma evacuated. You are caring for him postoperatively. ***(554-555)***

1. What would you pay particular attention to when positioning him?

2. Why is it important to maintain a quiet, nonstimulating atmosphere for this patient?

3. Besides increasing intracranial pressure, what is the next complication against which you would direct your nursing care?

STEPS TOWARD BETTER COMMUNICATION

VOCABULARY BUILDING GLOSSARY

Term	Pronunciation	Definition
contracoup	con'tra coo'	a counter or opposite blow—the contents of the cranium hit the inside of the skull, then bounce back and hit the other side, causing a second injury or contracoup
noxious	nok'shus	unpleasant and harmful
precipitating	pre sip'i ta' ting	causing
"goose bumps"		roughness of the skin as the hairs stand erect, caused by cold or fear
"log rolling"		the method of moving or turning a patient by rolling him to one side by using a blanket beneath him to wrap and roll him so that the body moves as one unit; and the exchange of assistance to take such action

COMPLETION

Directions: Fill in the blanks with the appropriate words from the Vocabulary Building Glossary above.

1. Bleeding into the brain is a ______________________ factor for an increase in intracranial pressure.
2. The patient who has a spinal cord injury is repositioned on the side by ______________________ him as a single unit.
3. Mr. Eagle hit his head hard on the windshield, his head bounced backwards and he ended up with an injury on the front of the brain and a ______________________ injury on the back of the brain.
4. ______________________ odors in the room of a patient after brain surgery may cause the intracranial pressure to rise.
5. A reaction seen with autonomic dysreflexia is ______________________ on the skin.

WORD ATTACK SKILLS

Directions: Find the word stem that combines with the prefix to make the combined word. Write the meaning. Use a dictionary as needed.

Prefix	Word Stem	Combined Word	Meaning
dys-	-reflexia	dysreflexia	disordered response to stimuli
under-	-lying	underlying	at the base or bottom of, a cause
oto-	________	otorrhea	________
rhino-	________	rhinorrhea	________
contra-	________	contralateral	________
	________	contracoup	________
ipsi-	________	ipsilateral	________
hema-	________	hematoma	________
hemo-	________	hemodynamic	________
hypo-	________	hypothermia	________
	________	hypoxia	________
hyper-	________	hyperextension	________
	________	hyperreflexia	________
un-	________	uninterrupted	________
poly-	________	polyuria	________
vaso-	________	vasoconstriction	________
	________	vasodilation	________
im-	________	immobility	________
in-	________	innervation	________
	________	inability	________
over-	________	overdistended	________
re-	________	rehabilitation	________

COMMUNICATION EXERCISE

Dialogue Practice

Write out what you might say to the mother of a 16-year-old boy, who suffered a head injury, to reassure her and involve her in the plan to help her son. Cover why she shouldn't try to keep him awake (sleep is helpful for healing, but he will be aroused periodically to check the level of consciousness.) Explain to her how she can help with passive range of motion exercises and with keeping his hands in good anatomical position.

Documentation

Document what you told her below:

____

____

____

____

CULTURAL POINTS

Many cultures have taboos about discussing sexual matters with outsiders or with someone of the opposite sex who isn't a spouse. Even in cultures open about sex, people may be hesitant to talk about their personal situations and concerns. As a nurse, you will need to be able to interact with patients about sexual problems. The patient with a spinal cord injury who is paraplegic will surely have sexual concerns. After reading the section in your text about this, think about how you would communicate with the patient about such concerns. Ask a classmate to interact with you so that you can practice what you would say.

CHAPTER 23

Care of Patients with Disorders of the Brain

evolve Go to http://evolve.elsevier.com/deWit for additional activities and exercises.

COMPLETION

Seizure Disorders and Epilepsy

Directions: Fill in the blanks to complete each statement.

1. Seizures are classified as ______________________ or ______________________. ***(564)***
2. During a grand mal seizure, the person usually loses ____________________________ and ____________________ tone. ***(564)***
3. A common side effect of the hydantoin anticonvulsant drugs is ________________________________ ____________________________. ***(565)***
4. The goal of anticonvulsant therapy is to control the seizures by using the ______________ amount of the drug with the ____________________ side effects. ***(567)***
5. Absence or petit mal seizures usually last for _______________________________ and the person remains ______________________. ***(564)***
6. IV phenytoin must be mixed with ______________________________ only. ***(566)***

SHORT ANSWER

Directions: Complete the following statements.

1. Other than epilepsy, seizures can be caused by: ***(563)*** ______________________________________ ______________________________________ ______________________________________.
2. Seizures are the result of: ***(563)***______________________________________.
3. Automatisms are: ***(564)*** ______________________________________.
4. The manifestations of epilepsy depend on: ***(564)***______________________________________ ______________________________________.

5. Status epilepticus is dangerous because: ***(565)*** ____

____.

6. The home treatment of status epilepticus is: ***(566)***______________________________________.

MATCHING

Cerebrovascular Accident

Directions: Match the term in the first column with the brief definition in the second column. ***(572)***

1. _______	Aphasia	a.	Loss of ability to form vocal sounds
2. _______	Dysphasia	b.	Unsteadiness or lack of coordination
3. _______	Aphonia	c.	Inability to recognize an object by sight, touch, or hearing
4. _______	Hemiplegia	d.	Reduced sensation on one side
5. _______	Atrophy	e.	Difficulty speaking
6. _______	Ataxia	f.	Impairment of or difficult speech
7. _______	Hemiparesthesia	g.	Paralysis of arm and leg on one side
8. _______	Diplopia	h.	Double vision
9. _______	Dysarthria	i.	Muscle wasting
10. _______	Agnosia	j.	Loss of ability to communicate by either spoken or written word

COMPLETION

Directions: Fill in the blanks to complete the sentence.

1. Transient ischemic attacks differ from cerebrovascular accidents in that there is no ____________________ ____. ***(567-568)***

2. Individuals most at risk for stroke include those with ______________________________, a history of ______________________________ and ______________________________. ***(568)***

3. A priority concern for the nurse caring for a patient after intracranial surgery is ____________________ ____. ***(574)***

4. The symptoms of a stroke caused by thrombosis occur ______________________________, whereas those caused by embolus occur ______________________________. ***(572)***

5. An individual who experiences a cerebrovascular accident (CVA) in the right hemisphere of the brain often has paresis or paralysis on the ______________ side. ***(572)***

6. The results of lumbar puncture in a patient who has had a subarachnoid hemorrhage will show ____________________________ in the cerebrospinal fluid. ***(569)***

7. Nursing interventions for the patient with a cerebral aneurysm include keeping the patient as ______________________________________ as possible. ***(575)***

8. An embolus causing a stroke often arises from the ______________ in a patient who has ______________________________. *(571)*

9. Structures that can cause an intercerebral hemorrhage are a(n) ______________________ and a(n) ____. *(569)*

10. A subarachnoid hemorrhage often causes ______________________ of neurologic ______________ and loss of ______________________________. *(569)*

COMPLETION

Brain Tumor

Directions: Fill in the blanks with the correct words to complete the statement.

1. Three characteristic signs of a brain tumor are ______________________________, ______________________, and ____. *(580)*

2. An infratentorial brain tumor often causes a loss of ______________________ and ______________________________. *(580)*

3. Most symptoms of brain tumor are related to ______________________________________. *(580)*

4. Diagnostic studies to verify presence of a brain tumor are ______________, ______________, and ______________________________. *(581)*

5. Two complications of a brain tumor are ______________________ and ______________ ______________________. *(582)*

Infections and Inflammatory Disorders of the Nervous System

Directions: Fill in the blank(s) with the correct words to complete the sentence.

1. Meningitis is an ______________________ of the ______________________ covering the ______________ and ______________________. *(582)*

2. Bacterial meningitis frequently follows an ______________________________ infection. *(582)*

3. Classic signs of meningitis are ____ ____. *(582)*

4. A ______________________ rash on the chest and extremities accompanies ______________ meningitis. *(582-583)*

5. Meningitis is confirmed by a ______________________, where CSF pressure is ______________ and glucose is ______________________. *(583)*

6. For the patient with meningitis, it is important to watch for ______________________, as well as neurologic deficits and seizures. *(583)*

7. The signs and symptoms of viral meningitis are ______________________, ______________, ______________________, and ____________________________. *(584)*

8. The course of viral meningitis is usually ______________________________. *(584)*

9. Encephalitis is spread by vectors such as ________________________ and ______________. *(585)*

10. Nonvector-transmitted encephalitis is an ______________________________ disorder. *(584)*

APPLICATION OF THE NURSING PROCESS

Directions: List three nursing activities that would be included in the nursing care plan of a patient with each of the following nursing diagnoses.

1. Impaired verbal communication related to cerebrovascular accident *(572)*

   a. ____

   b. ____

   c. ____

2. Self-care deficit related to hemiplegia (patient is a 62-year-old male) *(578)*

   a. ____

   b. ____

   c. ____

3. An expected outcome for "Self-care deficit related to hemiplegia" might be: *(578)*

   ____

4. A long-term expected outcome for the nursing diagnosis of "Impaired verbal communication related to cerebrovascular accident" would be:

   ____

5. Evaluation criteria for the expected outcome in #4 would be: ______________________

   ____

PRIORITY SETTING

A patient who has been diagnosed with a thrombotic cerebrovascular accident was admitted yesterday and is assigned to you. The patient has left-sided hemiplegia, particularly of the arm. According to the orders and care plan, you are to carry out the following. It is now 7:30 AM. Breakfast is served at 8:00 AM. Indicate in what order you would carry out or check the following:

_______ a. Neurologic check q 2 hr.

_______ b. Vital signs q 4 hr.

_______ c. IV of 0.9% NS at 50 mL/hr.

_______ d. Blood glucose via glucometer AC and HS

_______ e. Urine sample to lab for urinalysis

_______ f. Monitor for seizure activity

_______ g. Up in chair three times a day with assistance

_______ h. Assist with bath

NCLEX-PN® REVIEW

Directions: Choose the best answer(s) to each of the following or supply the missing words to complete the statement.

1. During a seizure, it is important for the nurse to observe: ***(566)***
   1. the type of aura the patient experiences.
   2. where movement occurs and how it progresses.
   3. the quality and rate of respirations during the seizure.
   4. the position of the patient's arms and legs during the seizure.

2. During a grand mal seizure, you could expect the patient to experience: *(Select all that apply.)* ***(564)***
   1. loss of muscle tone.
   2. tonic-clonic movements.
   3. automatisms.
   4. absence for a few seconds.
   5. possible urinary incontinence.
   6. unilateral movements of limbs.

3. The teaching plan for the patient with epilepsy should include: *(Select all that apply.)* ***(567)***
   1. refrain from drinking alcohol.
   2. wear a Medic-Alert bracelet or necklace.
   3. do not go anyplace by yourself.
   4. don't become overly tired.
   5. eat bananas to replace potassium loss.
   6. swim only with a partner.

4. A neurologic occurrence where the patient has sudden weakness or numbness on one side of the body that lasts a short time is called a ______________________________. ***(568)***

5. Hydrocephalus is a complication after an intercerebral bleed because: ***(582)***
   1. blood in the cerebral ventricular system interferes with the resorption of CSF.
   2. excessive amounts of CSF are produced after an intercerebral bleed.
   3. excessive hormone production increases the production of CSF.
   4. the ventricles become blocked by blood clots.

6. A CVA occurring on the right side of the brain may cause motor problems: ***(572)***
   1. on the left side of the body.
   2. on the right side of the body.
   3. on both sides of the body.
   4. only in the lower extremities.

7. One of the best things for the self-esteem of the neurologically impaired person is: *(579)*
   1. to establish small, accomplishable goals.
   2. time to adapt to body changes.
   3. a way to be a productive member of society.
   4. contact with friends and family.

8. A distinction of migraine headaches is that they often begin with: *(586)*
   1. a headache at the base of the skull radiating upward.
   2. pain in the forehead area that worsens with movement.
   3. sudden, diffuse, excruciating pain in the head.
   4. visual disturbances such as scotoma.

9. An effective treatment to stop a migraine headache for many people is to: *(586)*
   1. place an ice bag on the throbbing area of the head.
   2. lie down in an odor-free, darkened room with the eyes closed.
   3. sit very still in an upright position with the eyes closed.
   4. apply heat packs to the forehead and neck.

10. A patient experiencing status epilepticus is receiving phenytoin IV. He is to receive 18 mg/kg over 24 hours. He weighs 162 lbs. The total amount he should receive is ___________ . If he is to receive this medication mixed with 500 mL of 0.9% NaCl every 8 hours, each 500 mL IV should contain _________ mg of phenytoin. *(58)*

CRITICAL THINKING ACTIVITIES

Scenario A: Mrs. Margarita Rosario has been found to have an aneurysm in the brain. She has had headaches for many years, but they have become much worse lately. She also has type II diabetes and hypertension for which she takes several medications. She has been admitted to your unit.

1. How might this aneurysm be treated? *(573-574)*

2. If the aneurysm begins to leak, what symptoms might Mrs. Rosario have? *(574)*

3. What would you expect the treatment of this patient to be? *(574)*

4. What is your priority nursing responsibility? *(575)*

Scenario B: Mr. Tompkins, age 76, suffered a CVA with right hemiplegia. He is in the recovery stage and has been admitted to the rehabilitation institute. He is achieving some feeling in his right arm and leg, but is still unable to walk or use his arm effectively.

1. What particular deficits might this type of CVA have caused that will affect his everyday living? *(575)*

2. What therapies would you expect him to undergo at the rehabilitation institute? ***(579)***

3. What would you do when he has crying spells? ***(578)***

4. What medications would you expect to be administering related to the CVA? ***(571)***

STEPS TOWARD BETTER COMMUNICATION

VOCABULARY BUILDING GLOSSARY

Term	Pronunciation	Definition
seizure	see' zur	sudden attack or occurrence of a disease; convulsion; caused by abnormal electrical activity in the brain
spasm	spa' zim	strong involuntary contractions
untoward [effects]	un tord'	inconvenient, awkward, unexpected
groggy	grog' ee	weak and unsteady, possibly confused (may come from "grog," an alcoholic drink)
intractable [seizures]	in trak' ta bel	unmanageable, hard to control
susceptible	su sep' ti bel	likely to be affected by
debilitating	de bil' ih ta ting	making weak, or feeble; losing energy and ability
ischemia	is ke' mia	deficiency of blood, or obstruction
aura	or' a	atmosphere surrounding something; a radiation of light

COMPLETION

Directions: Fill in each blank with the appropriate word from the Glossary above.

1. When the patient woke up, he seemed a little ____________________ and wasn't ready to eat his breakfast.
2. The child's legs seemed to be in __________________________ and she couldn't straighten them.
3. A person who is poorly nourished is more ______________________ to disease.
4. The man was found on the floor having an apparent ______________________.
5. The severe seizures are ______________________ and need to be better controlled.
6. The man was discouraged because his stoke was so ______________________.

7. The woman usually was warned that a migraine was coming on by the ___________ she saw beforehand.

8. The family was surprised by the _________________________ effects of their father's illness.

COMMUNICATION EXERCISE

Explanations

A. Directions: Can you put these symptoms in lay terms so that the patient's family can understand them?

"Homonymous hemianopsia, hemiplegia or hemiparesis, agnosia, apraxia, aphasia, and dysphagia are some of the problems caused by a CVA."

____

____

____

____

____

____

____

B. Directions: Explain the difference between a shunt and a stent.

____

____

PRONUNCIATION SKILLS

Directions: Practice pronouncing these words aloud.

Symptomatology	Sym to ma tol'o gy
Electroencephalogram	E lec tro' en ceph'a lo gram
Homonymous hemianopsia	Ho mon'i mous hem'i ah nop'si a
Cytomegalovirus encephalitis	Cy to meg'a lo vir'us en ceph'a li'tis

MATCHING

Directions: Write the correct meaning after each word.

1. Idiopathic	____________	no known cause
2. Neoplasm	____________	narrowing of the blood vessels
3. Flaccid	____________	tumor
4. Vasoconstriction	____________	both sides
5. Bilateral	____________	limp, hanging loose, weak, soft

COMMUNICATION EXERCISE

Directions: Write a short dialogue or monologue of what you would say to the patient or family in each of these cases. Practice it with another student.

Provide encouragement for a stroke patient with left-sided hemiparesis who is learning how to walk again. Show patience and encouragement. What would you say if the patient becomes frustrated and angry? Write out some ideas of how you would provide encouragement and how you would handle the anger.

____

____

____

____

CHAPTER 24

Care of Patients with Degenerative Neurologic Disorders

evolve Go to http://evolve.elsevier.com/deWit for additional activities and exercises.

COMPLETION

Degenerative Neurologic Disorders

Directions: Fill in the blanks to complete the statements.

1. Parkinson's disease affects the part of the brain that controls ____________________ and ____________________. *(592)*

2. Parkinson's disease leads to a deficiency of ____________________ in the brain. ***(693)***

3. Four drugs that help control tremor, rigidity, and drooling are ____________________, ____________________, ____________________, and ____________________. ***(595)***

4. Signs and symptoms of multiple sclerosis depend on the extent to which inflammation and scarring of the ____________________ have occurred. ***(598)***

5. Multiple sclerosis is a disease of the central nervous system, and its symptoms are caused by ____________________ of the nerve fibers. ***(598)***

6. When caring for a patient with confusion, it is important for the nurse not to ____________________ items around in the patient's room.

7. The progression of Alzheimer's disease results in the patient requiring ____________________ ____________________. ***(602)***

8. Amyotrophic lateral sclerosis is a ____________________ neuromuscular disease characterized by degeneration of the ____________________ in the anterior horns of the ____________________ and the lower cranial nerves. ***(602)***

9. Guillain-Barré syndrome sometimes occurs after ____________________ immunization. ***(603)***

10. Pathologic changes that occur with Guillain-Barré syndrome are ______________________________,
______________________________, ______________________________, and ______________________________. ***(603)***

11. When the lower brainstem becomes involved in Guillain-Barré, the ______________________________ are affected. ***(603)***

12. Guillain-Barré syndrome is characterized by the appearance of an ______________________________
______________________________. ***(603)***

13. The patient with Guillain-Barré suffers paresthesias, muscular aches and cramps, and
______________________________. ***(603)***

14. Diagnosis of Guillain-Barré is by history, physical, ______________________, ______________________,
and __________________ conduction studies. ***(603-604)***

15. Huntington's disease is genetically transmitted and is characterized by ______________________________
______________________________. ***(605)***

16. Huntington's disease causes deterioration in ______________________________ capacity and
______________________________ disturbances. ***(605)***

17. Common observable symptoms of myasthenia gravis include ______________________ of the eyelids,
______________________________, and difficulty chewing and swallowing. ***(605)***

18. The purpose of plasma exchange as a treatment of myasthenia gravis is to mechanically remove
____. ***(608)***

19. One method of assisting the patient who is having difficulty with short-term memory and recognition of items in the environment is to place ____
____.

TABLE ACTIVITY

Directions: Complete the following table comparing three neurologic diseases: Parkinson's disease, multiple sclerosis, and myasthenia gravis.

	Parkinson's Disease *(592-598)*	**Multiple Sclerosis** *(596-602)*	**Myasthenia Gravis** *(605-607)*
Definition			
Clinical manifestations			
Cause			
Diagnostic measures			
Medical management			
Special nursing concerns and patient problems			

PRIORITY SETTING

You are assigned to a variety of patients who have several medications to be administered at 8:00 AM. Breakfast is served at 8:00 AM. You plan to start dispensing the medications ordered for 8:00 AM at about 7:45 AM in order to get them all administered on time. Consider the nursing implications of the diagnoses and the drugs to be administered. Decide on the order of priority in which you will give each patient's medications and indicate the numerical order in the blanks provided.

The patients and medications are:

______ a. Mrs. Hubers, diagnosis of type 2 diabetes and pneumonia. She is to receive Diabinese and Biaxin.

______ b. Mr. Hunter, diagnosis hypertension and heart failure. He is to receive digoxin, furosemide, and losartan.

______ c. Ms. Johnson, diagnosis myasthenia gravis. She is to receive Mestinon.

______ d. Mr. Takura, diagnosis Parkinson's disease. He is to receive Sinemet, Cogentin, and Metamucil.*

*What special nursing implication regarding the administration of Metamucil should be considered? ______________________________

NCLEX-PN® EXAM REVIEW

Directions: Choose the best answer(s) for the following questions or fill in the blank with the correct answer.

1. Signs and symptoms of Parkinson's disease include: *(Select all that apply.)* ***(593)***
   1. tremor.
   2. head jerking.
   3. drooping eyelids.
   4. bradykinesia.
   5. rigidity.
   6. muscle atrophy.

2. The patient with Parkinson's disease often has difficulty with: ***(593)***
   1. maintaining sitting or standing posture.
   2. balance and movement.
   3. coordination and speech.
   4. respiration and rapid pulse.

3. Patients taking levodopa to control Parkinson's disease often have side effects including: ***(594)***
   1. orthostatic hypotension.
   2. gastrointestinal bleeding.
   3. muscle aches.
   4. headache.

4. The patient who is admitted with weakness of a leg, blurred vision, and spasticity of muscles, and a positive Lhermitte's sign most likely will be diagnosed with: ***(599)***
   1. Parkinson's disease.
   2. multiple sclerosis.
   3. myasthenia gravis.
   4. amyotrophic lateral sclerosis.

5. An important factor in planning nursing care for the patient with multiple sclerosis is to remember that the patient: ***(600)***
   1. fatigues very easily and has the most strength in the afternoon.
   2. will have periods of both remission and exacerbation of the disease.
   3. responds best in a very warm environment.
   4. needs increased calories in the diet.

6. Baclofen is used for multiple sclerosis patients to: ***(601)***
   1. decrease urinary incontinence.
   2. decrease inflammation.
   3. decrease spasticity.
   4. control pain.

7. A nursing intervention for safety of the patient with Guillain-Barré syndrome is to: ***(604)***
   1. keep intubation equipment and an Ambu bag at the bedside.
   2. keep the head of the patient's bed elevated 15–30 degrees at all times.
   3. have the patient perform range of motion exercises at least three times a day.
   4. keep the room darkened and the environment quiet to prevent agitation of the patient.

8. Postpolio syndrome, which occurs in people who previously had polio, is characterized by: ***(605)***
   1. new onset of weakness, pain, and fatigue.
   2. paralysis of the previously affected limbs.
   3. headaches and muscle aching in the affected limbs.
   4. weakness in the extremities with spasm.

9. The first clinical manifestation of amyotrophic lateral sclerosis is usually: ***(603)***
   1. difficulty breathing.
   2. bilateral tremors.
   3. ascending paralysis.
   4. weakness of voluntary muscles.

10. Huntington's disease is genetically transmitted and usually causes death after signs appear within ____________ years. ***(605)***

CRITICAL THINKING ACTIVITIES

Scenario A: Joleen Jensen, age 23, has just been diagnosed with multiple sclerosis. Her doctor thinks she has the relapsing-remitting type. She is a graduate student at the university. She has been having trouble with her vision.

1. What can she expect with this type of multiple sclerosis? ***(598-599)***

2. How would you help her decide what to do about her vision problems as they are interfering with her studying? ***(600)***

3. Her physician has talked with her about using beta-interferon to help control her disease. What could you tell her about this medication? ***(600)***

Scenario B: Antonio Katsigris, age 46, has recently been diagnosed with myasthenia gravis. He is not familiar with the disease and has many questions.

1. What could you tell him about the disease? ***(605)***

2. What are the biggest dangers with this disease? ***(605-606)***

3. What would you tell him about the usual treatment for the disease? ***(606)***

STEPS TOWARD BETTER COMMUNICATION

VOCABULARY BUILDING GLOSSARY

Term	Pronunciation	Definition
collaborate	co lab'o rate	to work together
ascending	a send' ing	going upward
dyspepsia	dis pep'si a	indigestion
plateau	plat oh'	a level place after an increase; a fairly level area of high ground
drooling		water or saliva coming out of the mouth, usually due to lack of muscle control

COMPLETION

Directions: Complete the following sentences with one of the Glossary words above.

1. ____________________ the stairway takes much more energy than coming down.
2. The nursing staff and the physical therapists agreed to ____________________ on solving the problem.
3. Because of his stroke, his facial muscles were paralyzed and Mr. Branson had difficulty preventing himself from ________________________.
4. The patient's rehabilitation efforts seemed to reach a ____________________ that it was difficult to get beyond.
5. Mrs. Johnson's ______________________ made her irritable after meals.

GRAMMAR POINTS

Collaborate is the base verb meaning to work together, **collaborator** is a noun (one of the people who does the working together), **collaboration** is a noun referring to the action of working together, **collaborative** is an adjective describing the kind of action.

Drool is the base verb; **drooler,** a noun, would be a person (not commonly used); **drooling** would be the noun describing the action (from the participle).

COMMUNICATION EXERCISES

a. Dialogue Practice

? ***Think critically about...*** A patient comes into the clinic complaining about hand tremors and "stiffness" of the joints that started recently, excessive sweating, and some urinary incontinence. You notice that her gait is abnormal. What would be a priority question you would ask her as you start history-taking?

Use the above as the basis for a dialogue. With a partner, practice asking the questions in Focused Assessment 24-1 for the Patient with Parkinson's Symptoms in the textbook.

b. Explanations

With a partner, practice explaining to a patient with myasthenia gravis why wearing a Medic-Alert emblem/bracelet is a good idea.

CULTURAL POINTS

Directions: For discussion in a group:

People with the disorders described in this chapter have a number of physical manifestations relating to their illness (tremors, lack of muscle control, strange gaits, tics, etc.). How do you think this affects their going out in public? What about their feelings about going out in public? How are they received by the people they meet or who observe them? What nursing problems could this cause?

If there are people in your class from other cultures, ask how these people would be treated in their culture. Are there differences among the cultures?

What might you as medical personnel be able to do to help the situation?

CHAPTER 25

The Sensory System: Eye and Ear

Go to http://evolve.elsevier.com/deWit for additional activities and exercises.

PART 1 – THE EYE

REVIEW OF ANATOMY AND PHYSIOLOGY

Terminology

Directions: Match the term on the left with the correct definition, function, or statement on the right. ***(611-614)***

1. ______	Pupil	a.	Protect eye against debris in air.
2. ______	Choroid	b.	Sits between lens and retina and contains vitreous humor.
3. ______	Iris	c.	Allow for focusing of light on lens and retina.
4. ______	Anterior chamber	d.	Contain an enzyme that kills bacteria.
5. ______	Posterior chamber	e.	Between the lens and the cornea.
6. ______	Eyelashes	f.	Eversion of the lower lid that may occur with aging.
7. ______	Eyelids	g.	Secrete aqueous humor.
8. ______	Tears	h.	Central opening allowing light into interior.
9. ______	Suspensory ligaments	i.	Located between sclera and retina; contains brown pigment.
10. ______	Ectropion	j.	Help trap foreign particles, keeping them out of the eye.
		k.	Colored portion of the eye.

Labeling

Directions: Label the following structures on the diagram of the eye. ***(612)***

sclera
pupil
Schlemm's canal
ciliary process
cornea
conjunctiva
anterior chamber
choroid
lens
optic disk
posterior chamber
iris
optic nerve
retina
vitreous body

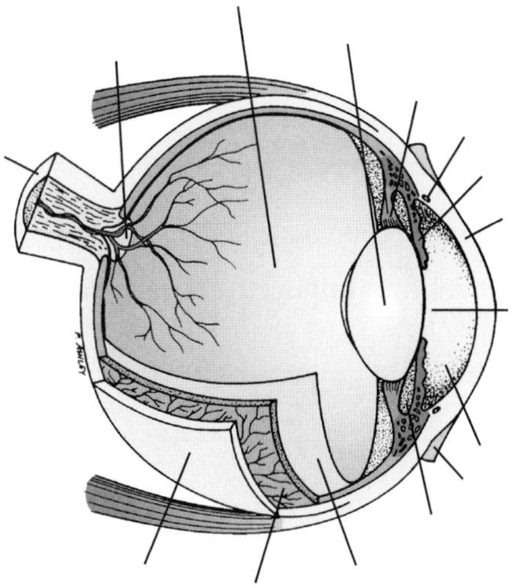

COMPLETION

Prevention of Eye Disease and Diagnostic Tests

Directions: Fill in the blanks with the correct words to complete the statements.

1. Everyone over the age of 40 should have an eye examination every ______________________. ***(616)***
2. When using machinery that might cause debris to fly into the eye, ______________________________ should be worn. ***(615)***
3. Diabetes mellitus and hypertension are the two major causes of ______________________. ***(620)***
4. ______________________________________ is the diagnostic test used to evaluate blood vessel abnormalities in the eye. ***(618)***
5. With aging, the ability of the ________________ to dilate decreases, causing difficulty for the older person in going from a ______________________ into a ____________________________. ***(613)***

APPLICATION OF THE NURSING PROCESS

Directions: Write a brief answer to each question.

1. List the five danger signals of eye disease that should be looked for upon assessment of each person. ***(616)***
   a. ______________________________
   b. ______________________________
   c. ______________________________
   d. ______________________________
   e. ______________________________
2. List five guidelines for assisting a blind person. ***(622-623)***
   a. ______________________________
   b. ______________________________
   c. ______________________________
   d. ______________________________
   e. ______________________________
3. What are four important steps in administering eye drops? ***(622)***
   a. ______________________________
   b. ______________________________
   c. ______________________________
   d. ______________________________

NCLEX-PN® EXAM REVIEW

Directions: Choose the best answer(s) for each of the following questions.

1. When assessing for visual acuity, which of the following steps are appropriate? *(Select all that apply.)* ***(618)***
   1. Position the chart 20 feet from the patient.
   2. Express the result of the test for each eye as a whole number.
   3. Occlude one eye at a time, testing the unoccluded eye.
   4. Indicate the line at which the person should begin reading.
   5. Express the result of the test as a fraction.

2. Subtle signs of decreasing vision found upon history-taking are: ***(620)***
   1. becoming less interested in a hobby such as sewing.
   2. developing a bruise on the shin from the open door to the dishwasher.
   3. seeing better when using prescribed glasses.
   4. wanting a light on in the room when watching television.

3. When examining a patient for a visual problem, an indication that a problem is present is: ***(617)***
   1. pupils that are quite small.
   2. blinking several times during the exam.
   3. leaning forward slightly when looking at the examiner.
   4. squinting when asked to read a few sentences from a card.

4. When setting up a dinner tray for a visually impaired person, you would: ***(623)***
   1. place the person's hands on each side of the plate.
   2. describe where each type of food is located using the "clock" method.
   3. allow the person to cut up the meat.
   4. make certain there are no shadows in the room.

5. A part of community teaching that is not necessary for the prevention of eye problems is: ***(623)***
   1. wearing a hat when outdoors.
   2. wearing sunglasses that block UVA and UVB rays when outdoors.
   3. using eyedrops when returning inside from being in the sun.
   4. eating a diet rich in fruits and vegetables that contain antioxidants.

CRITICAL THINKING ACTIVITES

1. Develop a teaching plan on protecting vision for a community or school group. ***(623)***

2. Explain the Amsler Grid test to your elderly relatives and/or neighbors and perform an assessment for macular degeneration using the grid. ***(619)***

PART II – THE EAR

REVIEW OF ANATOMY AND PHYSIOLOGY

Labeling

Directions: Label the diagram of the ear with the following parts. ***(625)***

pinna
semicircular canals
auditory meatus
cochlea
eustachian tube
malleus
vestibular nerve CN VIII branch
incus
cochlear nerve CN VII
stapes
tympanic membrane
vestibule
facial nerve

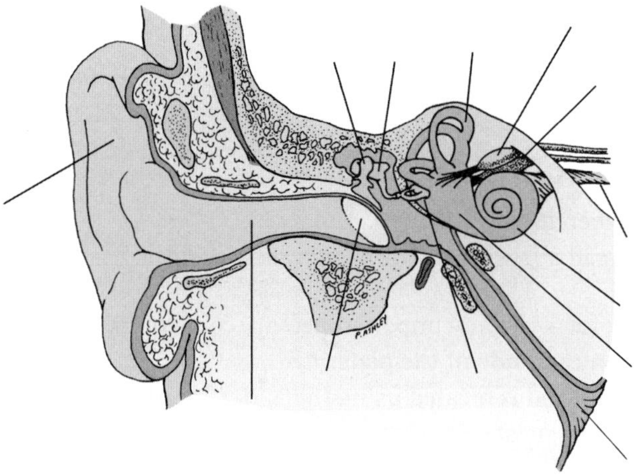

SHORT ANSWER

Prevention of Hearing Loss

Directions: Write a brief answer for each question.

1. What are three things a nurse might do to contribute to the prevention of hearing loss? ***(624)***

 a. ______________________________

 b. ______________________________

 c. ______________________________

2. What are four signs of hearing loss? ***(630)***

 a. ______________________________

 b. ______________________________

 c. ______________________________

 d. ______________________________

3. What are five common medications that are potentially ototoxic and may cause hearing loss? *(627)*

   a. ______________________________

   b. ______________________________

   c. ______________________________

   d. ______________________________

TABLE ACTIVITY

Conductive Versus Sensorineural Hearing Loss

Directions: Complete the following table comparing conductive and sensorineural hearing loss. ***(624)***

Characteristic	Conductive	Sensorineural
Location of dysfunction		
Common causes		
Treatment		

COMPLETION

The Ear and Hearing Loss

Directions: Fill in the blanks with the correct words to complete the statements.

1. The ear is examined by use of the ______________________________. *(628)*

2. A simple hearing test is the ________________________ test. *(628)*

3. A test for status of equilibrium is the ________________ test. ***(628)***

4. When ear drops are administered, they should first be ________________________ or they may cause discomfort or dizziness. ***(632)***

5. When ear drops are instilled, the patient should remain in the lateral position for ________________ minutes. ***(632)***

6. When communicating with a hearing-impaired person, it is best to position yourself ____________________ of the person. ***(632)***

7. When working with a patient who has a hearing aid, the nurse should make certain that the aid ____. ***(632)***

8. Many people do not know that hearing aids from a reputable dealer usually have a ________________ ________________________________. ***(632)***

9. People who are deaf may ________________ themselves because of embarrassment and frustration over difficulty in communicating. ***(624)***

10. Exposure to environmental loud noise causes a ________________________ hearing loss that is often not correctable. ***(626)***

NCLEX-PN® EXAM REVIEW

Directions: Choose the best answer(s) for each of the following questions.

1. When assessing a patient who complains of a mild hearing loss, the nurse should *first*: ***(628)***
   1. schedule an audiogram.
   2. inspect the ear canal for cerumen.
   3. inquire about past episodes of upper respiratory infection.
   4. lavage the ear canal for clearer vision of the eardrum.

2. When explaining the tests that a patient with hearing loss will undergo, the nurse would tell the patient that the test for a possible tumor of the eighth cranial (acoustic nerve) is: ***(629)***
   1. electronystagmography.
   2. the Tine test.
   3. the Rinne test.
   4. an audiogram.

3. When the nurse works with a patient who has a slight to moderate hearing deficit, she should: *(Select all that apply.)* ***(632)***
   1. write everything down for him.
   2. face him and gain his attention before speaking.
   3. speak very loudly and slowly.
   4. be certain that his hearing aid is on if he wears one.

4. Decreases in hearing often occur with aging because of: *(Select all that apply.)* ***(626)***
   1. vascular changes from diabetes.
   2. loss of elasticity of the tympanic membrane.
   3. nerve cell atrophy in the ear and brain.
   4. arteriosclerosis and decreased blood flow.

5. Which action when working with someone with a hearing deficit is *not* necessary? *(Select all that apply.)* *(632)*
   1. Speak slowly and clearly.
   2. Validate understanding by getting feedback.
   3. Reinforce instructions with printed sheets.
   4. Use correct vocal tones to fit the patient.

CRITICAL THINKING ACTIVITIES

1. Formulate a teaching plan for college students on how to protect hearing.

2. Plan how you would handle the situation if you go to a concert, dance, or other place that has music that is playing too loudly.

STEPS TOWARD BETTER COMMUNICATION

VOCABULARY BUILDING GLOSSARY

Term	Pronunciation	Definition
acuity	ah ku' ĭ tee	clearness, sharpness
enun'ciate	ee nun' cee āt	to speak clearly
opaque	o pāk'	light cannot go through it
pitch	pich	degree of highness or lowness of a sound
take it for granted		to not think about something, especially a gift or normal behavior, such as sight, food, or family; to assume it will always be there

COMPLETION

Directions: Fill in the blanks with the correct words from the Vocabulary Building Glossary to complete the statements.

1. The patient could hear low sounds but had difficulty hearing sounds with a high _____________.

2. A cataract makes the lens of the eye ____________________.

3. After age 70, Joe noticed that the __________________________ of his hearing had decreased.

4. When a patient has a hearing loss, it is important that the nurse ______________________________ words.

5. After age 40, many people develop decreased visual __________________________ and need glasses.

6. When hearing loss occurs, it is often the high _____________________ that are most difficult to hear.

VOCABULARY EXERCISE

Review of Terms and Combining Forms

opthalm/o	eye
ot/o	ear
aural	relating to the ear
superior	above
inferior	below
lateral	toward the side
medial	central, in the middle

PRONUNCIATION SKILLS

Vestib'ulococh'lear (ves tib' u lo kok' lee ar)

Eusta'chian (u sta' che an)

ABBREVIATIONS

OD	right eye
OS	left eye
OU	both eyes

[One way to remember this is to think that right eye (OD) comes first in the alphabet; left eye (OS) comes second in the alphabet, and both eyes (OU) comes last.]

Directions: Practice pronouncing the above words and abbreviations with a peer. Have your partner write down the words or abbreviations as you say them. Check the list for accurate enunciation.

COMMUNICATION EXERCISE

With a peer, practice assessment by using Focused Assessment 25-1 and Focused Assessment 25-2 in the textbook to take a history. Ask your partner questions to help clarify points that require more explanation.

CHAPTER 26

Care of Patients with Disorders of the Eyes and Ears

evolve Go to http://evolve.elsevier.com/deWit for additional activities and exercises.

PART 1 – THE EYE

COMPLETION

Eye Disorders

Directions: Fill in the blanks with the correct words to complete the statements

1. Seeking prompt attention for a corneal abrasion helps prevent ______________________________. ***(640)***

2. The treatment for severe corneal scarring is ____ termed a ______________________________. ***(640)***

3. If a chemical splashes into the eye, the eye should be treated with ________________________________ for at least ____________________ with __________________________ or __________________________. ***(641)***

4. If a foreign body is stuck on the surface of the eye, the best thing to do is __________________________ ______________ and to ____. ***(641)***

5. A cataract causes a blurring of vision because the ________________ becomes ______________________ ________________________________. ***(642)***

6. Cataract surgery is performed when the loss of vision ____ ________________________________ the person's life. ***(642)***

7. Glaucoma is often ______________________ until damage to vision has occurred from ______________ ________________________________ and pressure on the ___________________________________. ***(644)***

8. The characteristic sign of closed angle glaucoma is ____ ____________________________. ***(645)***

9. Drugs used in the treatment of glaucoma act to ____ of ____ or decrease ______________________________. ***(645)***

10. Uncontrolled glaucoma causes ______________________________. ***(648)***

11. The sudden occurrence of flashes of colored light is a sign of ______________________________. ***(650)***

12. Retinopathy is often a disorder that occurs in patients with diabetes mellitus and is either from ____________________ of blood vessels or ____________ of blood vessels with ________________. ***(650)***

13. Early symptoms of macular degeneration are inability to see ______________________________ of ________________ and ________________. ***(653)***

14. The patient who has just had eye surgery should be positioned with the head ________________ and should not lie on the ______________________ side. ***(655)***

15. When administering preoperative mydriatic eye drops you should wait _________ minutes between the instillation of one drop and the other. ***(654)***

APPLICATION OF THE NURSING PROCESS

Directions: Write a brief answer to each question.

1. List five nursing diagnoses frequently encountered for patients with disorders of the eye.

   a. ____

   b. ____

   c. ____

   d. ____

   e. ____

2. Give four assessment findings that may indicate the presence of a cataract. ***(642)***

   a. ____

   b. ____

   c. ____

   c. ____

3. Your clinical patient is scheduled for same-day surgery in the ambulatory surgery unit. Eye drops are ordered to be instilled three times at 15-minute intervals. The patient has just been admitted to the unit. An IV is to be started, a gown put on by the patient, the preoperative checklist is to be completed, and the patient is to be ready for surgery in 60 minutes. In what order of priority should these actions take place?

SHORT ANSWER

Retinal Detachment and Eye Surgery

Directions: Read the clinical situation and write brief answers to the questions that follow.

Situation: Mr. Cox, age 82, is scheduled for a scleral buckle for a retinal detachment. He will be hospitalized at least overnight.

1. Considering the procedure Mr. Cox is undergoing, what should be included in his teaching plan to prepare him for the early postoperative period? *(652)*

   a.

   b.

   c.

   d.

   e.

2. What safety precautions should be taken during Mr. Cox's hospital stay? *(654)*

   a.

   b.

   c.

   d.

3. Name three instructions that should be included in Mr. Cox's discharge teaching specific to the type of surgery he had. ***(650)***

   a. ______________________________

   ____

   b. ______________________________

   ____

   c. ______________________________

   ____

4. List five goals or expected outcomes for nursing interventions in the postoperative care of all patients who have had surgery of the eye.

   a. ______________________________

   b. ______________________________

   c. ______________________________

   d. ______________________________

   e. ______________________________

COMPLETION

Eye Medications

Directions: Fill in the blanks with the correct words to complete the statements. ***(647)***

1. Pilocarpine is a ______________ medication that works by ______________ the pupil.
2. Patients who use pilocarpine should not __________ at __________.
3. Acetazolamide (Diamox) is a commonly used medication. It works by decreasing the __________ of ______________.
4. Atropine eye drops are used to __________ the eyes and to ______________ the muscles of accommodation.
5. Atropine is used during ______________ in order to visualize the ______________ of the eye.
6. When gentamicin (Garamycin) eye drops are prescribed, the patient should be taught to also use a ______________ and __________ each time the face is washed to prevent reinfection.
7. Pred Forte is a ______________ eye drop used to decrease ______________ and ______________.
8. Fluorescein sodium drops are used to __________ the cornea and if a corneal scratch is present, it will show up as ______________.

NCLEX-PN® EXAM REVIEW

Directions: Choose the best answer(s) for each of the following questions.

1. Mrs. Messina is scheduled for a cataract extraction with intraocular lens implant of the right eye. Assessment of Mrs. Messina during preoperative care would include: *(Select all that apply.)* ***(642)***
   1. food likes and dislikes for dietary selections.
   2. degree of retained vision and history of previous hospitalizations.
   3. ability to instill eye drops and administer self-care.
   4. ability to understand and follow directions postoperatively.

2. Planning for safety needs for a patient with a right cataract extraction and intraocular lens implant in the immediate postoperative period would include: *(Select all that apply.)* ***(643-644)***
   1. placing the call light cord and console on her left side.
   2. unplugging the television so that she is not tempted to watch it.
   3. keeping her in bed for 12 hours.
   4. medicating quickly if she becomes nauseous from anesthesia.

3. The *most* important goal for the cataract patient with lens implant in the early postoperative period is: ***(644)***
   1. no evidence of nausea or vomiting.
   2. control of pain and discomfort.
   3. prevention of intraocular hemorrhage.
   4. stabilization of vital signs within 4 hours.

4. The *most* important nursing intervention in the recovery period before discharge from the day surgery unit to ensure success of eye surgery is: ***(644)***
   1. medicating for pain before it becomes severe.
   2. answering the call light promptly.
   3. assisting the patient to walk to the bathroom.
   4. positioning the patient per orders.

5. Evaluation of measures to prevent complications of the cataract procedure include: *(Select all that apply.)* ***(644)***
   1. checking the degree of eye pain.
   2. checking security of the eye dressing.
   3. assessing the amount of nausea.
   4. checking the amount of redness of the operative eye.

6. The therapeutic response expected of a mydriatic eye medication is: ***(647)***
   1. dilation of the pupil.
   2. constriction of the pupil.
   3. decrease of intraocular pressure.
   4. decreased production of aqueous humor.

7. Mr. Schultz has come to the emergency department with severe eye pain. He is diagnosed with closed angle glaucoma. The physician orders IV Diamox 150 mg in 200 mL of D_5W to be given over 15 minutes. The vial of the drug contains 500 mg in 2 mL. How many mL would be added to the D_5W for this infusion? ____________

PART II – THE EAR

COMPLETION

Ear Disorders

Directions: Fill in the blanks with the correct words to complete the statements.

1. When a patient first arises after ear surgery, he is likely to be ______________________, and should be assisted with ambulation. ***(661)***

2. Symptoms of labyrinthitis are loss of hearing in the affected ear, severe dizziness with nausea and vomiting, and ______________________________________. ***(657)***

3. A tympanoplasty involves surgical reconstruction of the ______________________________________ and ____________________________ to restore middle ear function. ***(657)***

4. Besides difficulty in hearing, ear problems and deafness are often accompanied by ___________________________, which can cause considerable fatigue in the person.

5. Meniere's disease causes ________________________________, ______________________, and _______________________________. ***(658)***

6. Hereditary deafness is usually due to changes in the _____________________ of the ear and causes a ___________________________ hearing loss. ***(658-659)***

7. Conductive hearing loss can often be helped by a ________________________ or corrected with ____. ***(659)***

NCLEX-PN® EXAM REVIEW

Directions: Choose the best answer(s) for each of the following questions.

1. When planning care for the patient admitted with a severe episode of Meniere's disease, the nurse's priority goal for the patient is to: ***(658)***
   1. restore hearing to previous levels.
   2. control pain with analgesia.
   3. resolve infection within 5 days.
   4. ensure that no fall will be sustained during hospitalization.

2. The nurse would expect to implement which of the following orders for the patient with Meniere's disease? ***(658)***
   1. Keflin 250 mg q 6 hours IV
   2. Lasix 20 mg three times a day
   3. Morphine 4 mg IM q 4 hours PRN pain
   4. Compazine 25 mg IM q 3–4 hours PRN nausea and vomiting

3. The teaching plan for the discharged patient who has Meniere's disease would probably include instructions about: ***(658)***
   1. the side effects and dosage schedule for Antivert.
   2. adding extra sources of vitamins C and A to the diet.
   3. working to decrease stress in daily life.
   4. controlling allergy symptoms.
   5. avoiding the use of earphones for listening to music.

4. When evaluating the success of the teaching program on diet for the patient with Meniere's disease, the nurse would assess for avoidance of foods high in: ***(658)***
   1. sugar.
   2. fat.
   3. potassium.
   4. sodium.

5. The patient who has had a stapedectomy should be instructed to: ***(661)***
   1. keep the head elevated when in bed.
   2. sneeze and cough with the mouth closed.
   3. apply the ear protector for sleep.
   4. sleep with the affected ear up.

6. When teaching the elderly patient about care of his hearing aid, you would include which of the following actions? *(Select all that apply.)* ***(632)***
   1. Keep the battery in the hearing aid.
   2. Clean the ear mold regularly with alcohol.
   3. Never put the hearing aid in water.
   4. Open the battery cover when the hearing aid is not in the ear.

7. Meclizine (Antivert) is a drug that is used for patients with Meniere's disease. This drug is used to reduce dizziness and is: ***(658)***
   1. an anticholinergic.
   2. a corticosteroid.
   3. an antihypertensive.
   4. a beta-blocker.

8. Ms. Smith just had a stapedectomy. She has an IV of $D_5\frac{1}{2}$ NS hanging and there are 760 mL left in the bag. It is prescribed to run at 100 mL/hour. The IV tubing delivers 10 drops per mL. You should set the drip rate at __________ gtts/min. ***(58)***

SHORT ANSWER

Tinnitus and Hearing Loss

Directions: Write a brief answer to each question.

1. What are four medical or nursing interventions that might be helpful to the patient with vertigo? ***(668)***

   a. ______________________________

   b. ______________________________

   c. ______________________________

   d. ______________________________

2. What are four possible causes of tinnitus? ***(651-652)***

   a. ______________________________

   b. ______________________________

   c. ______________________________

   d. ______________________________

3. Can you list four suggestions you might make to help a person deal with chronic tinnitus? ***(658)***

   a. ______________________________

   b. ______________________________

   c. ______________________________

   d. ______________________________

4. Name two types of therapy that might be useful in the rehabilitation of a person with a hearing loss. ***(659)***

   a. ______________________________

   b. ______________________________

CRITICAL THINKING ACTIVITIES

Case Study: Otosclerosis

A 62-year-old female is at the ear, nose, and throat clinic regarding her hearing loss which is getting worse. She has had a progressive loss of hearing since her late 40s. She wears bilateral hearing aids. She can hear better in her left ear than her right ear. Her mother had hearing loss from her 40s on as well. Her evaluation has determined that she has otosclerosis. Treatment options are discussed and she has made a decision to have a stapedectomy of the right ear. ***(658-659)***

1. Why is it significant that her mother had early hearing loss?

2. What diagnostic tests would you expect she underwent during the evaluation?

3. Why is the stapedectomy to be done on the right ear rather than the left ear?

4. What preoperative teaching would you do? What would you cover?

Postoperatively, she is nauseous and states that she is quite dizzy when she tries to sit upright. She has meclizine, Percocet, and compazine ordered. ***(661)***

5. Which medication would you administer for the nausea? Which for the dizziness?

6. What safety interventions should you implement?

When the external ear dressing is removed, the patient states she can't hear a thing out of the left ear and becomes upset and tearful.

7. What is the probable cause of her inability to hear in that ear now? What could you say to her at this time that might calm her down?

STEPS TOWARD BETTER COMMUNICATION

VOCABULARY BUILDING GLOSSARY

Term	Pronunciation	Definition
am'plified	am' plah fīd	increased, made louder or bigger
ap'titude	ap' tĭ tūd	good ability
bear in mind		remember; think about
catch all	kech' awl	containing a wide variety of different things
phenom'enon	fah nom' ah non	an unusual or interesting fact or occurrence
prompt	prom' t	quick; on time

COMPLETION

Directions: Fill in the blanks with the correct words from the Vocabulary Building Glossary to complete the statements.

1. Joan has a special ________________________ for nursing.
2. Seeing flashing lights after a retinal detachment is an odd ________________________________.
3. The nurse should always ____ that asepsis is always important in caring for patients with an eye or ear surgery.
4. ________________________ music at concerts may be damaging to the ear and cause a loss of hearing.
5. The term *hearing loss* is a ____________________________ for several different types of physiologic problems.
6. An ear infection should receive ______________________ medical attention.

GRAMMAR POINTS

Review of Terms and Combining Forms

kerat/o	cornea
phot/o	light
optic, opt/o	vision
os, oste/o	bone
tax/o	order, coordination
toxic, tox/o	poison
opia	vision
humor	any fluid or semifluid in the body

PRONUNCIATION SKILLS

Sup' purative (sup' u rah tiv)
Trabec' uloplasty (trah bek' u lo plas tee)
Labyrinthi' tis (lab ĭ rin thi' tis)

ABBREVIATIONS

ARMD	age-related macular degeneration
IGF	insulin-like growth factor
LVES	low-vision enhancement system

Practice pronouncing the above words and abbreviations with a peer. Have your partner write down the words or abbreviations as you say them. Check the list for accurate enunciation.

With a peer, practice assessment by using Focused Assessment 25-2 and Focused Assessment 25-3 in the textbook to take a history and gather physical data. Ask your partner questions to help clarify points that require more explanation.

CHAPTER 27

The Gastrointestinal System

evolve Go to http://evolve.elsevier.com/deWit for additional activities and exercises.

REVIEW OF ANATOMY AND PHYSIOLOGY

Terminology

*Directions: Match the term on the left with the appropriate statement on the right. (**666-667**)*

1. ______	Teeth	a.	Populate large intestine and help break down waste products
2. ______	Esophagus	b.	Break down food into small pieces that can be acted upon by enzymes
3. ______	Chyme	c.	Stimulated by ingestion of food; initiates elimination
4. ______	Small intestine	d.	Carries food from pharynx to stomach
5. ______	Intestinal villi	e.	Decreased secretion of hydrochloric acid in stomach
6. ______	Sigmoid	f.	Absorb food particles into bloodstream
7. ______	Bacteria	g.	Stores fecal material until elimination is initiated
8. ______	Rectum	h.	Under voluntary control
9. ______	Gastrocolic reflex	i.	Composed of food particles, mucus, hydrochloric acid, intrinsic factor, pepsinogen, and gastrin
10. ______	Age-related change	j.	Portion of colon located on left side of abdominal cavity
11. ______	External anal sphincter	k.	Bile and pancreatic enzymes added to chyme here

TABLE ACTIVITY

Causes and Prevention of Digestive Disorders

Directions: Complete the following table by giving the pathology and preventive measures for various causative factors in the development of digestive disorders. ***(668)***

Causative Factors	Pathology (What Occurs)	Preventive Measures
Psychologic and emotional stress and tension		
Mechanical and chemical irritants		
Infectious agents: bacteria, virus, parasites		

APPLICATION OF THE NURSING PROCESS

Directions: Provide a brief answer to each of the following questions.

1. Your patient is scheduled for a diagnostic workup related to epigastric pain. What information about the patient's health history and that of her family would be helpful? ***(676)***

   a. ______________________________

   b. ______________________________

   c. ______________________________

   d. ______________________________

   e. ______________________________

2. The patient is scheduled for an esophagogastroduodenoscopy (EGD). How would you explain this procedure to her? What special care would she need before and after the procedure? *(672)*

   a. Procedure: ______________________________

   b. Care before EGD: ______________________________

   c. Care after EGD: ______________________________

3. When examining the abdomen, you would perform the steps in a particular order. What order should the examination be performed? *(676-677)*

   ____

4. Why is checking the color of the urine a part of the gastrointestinal assessment? *(677)* ______________________________

5. What is the purpose of performing percussion of the abdomen? *(677)* ______________________________

6. What data found upon assessment would indicate that fats are not being digested properly? *(677)* ______________________________

7. What assessment data might indicate that bile is not reaching the intestine? *(677)* ______________________________

8. Why is it important to determine what medications and supplements a patient is taking when there is a problem in the gastrointestinal system? *(677)*

   ____

9. When a patient is experiencing nausea and vomiting, what would be an appropriate nursing diagnosis? *(678)*

____

10. When the nursing diagnosis is Constipation related to idiopathic origin, what would be an appropriate expected outcome? *(678)*

____

____

11. List three specific nursing interventions for the patient who suffers from constipation. *(678)*

a. ______________________________

b. ______________________________

c. ______________________________

12. How would you evaluate whether the above interventions were effective? *(678)*

____

____

____

PRIORITY SETTING

Directions: You are assigned to a newly admitted patient who is suffering from abdominal pain and vomiting. You need to perform the following actions. Place them in the order of priority in which you would perform them by numbering them using 1 as the first action.

_____ a. Collect a urine specimen.

_____ b. Percuss the abdomen.

_____ c. Give the patient an emesis basin and tissues.

_____ d. Auscultate for bowel sounds.

_____ e. Weigh the patient.

_____ f. Instruct the patient about intake and output recording.

_____ g. Have the patient change into a gown.

_____ h. Palpate the abdomen.

_____ i. Record a health history.

_____ j. Auscultate the lungs and heart.

NCLEX-PN® EXAM REVIEW

Directions: Choose the best answer(s) for the following questions.

1. The doctor schedules a patient for a colonoscopy. In preparing him for this procedure, you explain that: *(672)*
   1. he will be heavily sedated and not remember much of the procedure.
   2. the procedure takes only about 6 minutes.
   3. he may have a clear liquid breakfast before the procedure.
   4. he can go back to work as soon as the procedure is over.

2. Risk factors for the development of gallbladder disease include: *(Select all that apply.)* ***(668)***
   1. repeated viral infections.
   2. obesity.
   3. Crohn's disease.
   4. working with heavy metals.
   5. diabetes mellitus.
   6. rapid weight loss.

3. Which of the following actions help to prevent liver disease? *(Select all that apply.)* ***(668)***
   1. Keeping weight within normal limits.
   2. Avoiding excessive alcohol intake.
   3. Eating food containing vitamin A.
   4. Using appropriate precautions when using garden pesticides.
   5. Avoiding contraction of hepatitis B or C.
   6. Providing adequate ventilation when using toxic household cleaners.

4. One action that can decrease the risk of pancreatic cancer is to: ***(670)***
   1. eat a well-balanced diet.
   2. obtain 30 minutes of exercise at least 3 times a week.
   3. refrain from drinking any alcohol.
   4. refrain from smoking cigarettes.

5. When patients undergo diagnostic tests of the gastrointestinal system, elderly patients in particular must be closely watched for: ***(674)***
   1. dehydration and electrolyte imbalance.
   2. nausea and vomiting.
   3. diarrhea.
   4. constipation from contrast media.

6. Hyperactive bowel sounds in one quadrant and not in any other plus nausea and vomiting may indicate: *(677)*
   1. pancreatitis.
   2. cholecystitis.
   3. gastrointestinal bleeding.
   4. intestinal obstruction.

7. Your patient is receiving an IV of D_5½NS 1000 mL ordered to run at 150 mL/hr. The IV tubing delivers 15 drops per mL. You would set the IV to run at ____________ gtts/min. ***(58)***

8. Your patient is to have a liver biopsy. You would teach her which of the following? *(Select all that apply.)* ***(673)***
   1. Nothing is allowed by mouth for 4–8 hours prior to the procedure.
   2. Local or general anesthesia will be used.
   3. Patient will be positioned on the right lateral side for the procedure.
   4. The procedure takes about an hour.
   5. It will be necessary to lie on the right side for 1–2 hours postprocedure.
   6. Heavy lifting or strenuous activities are to be avoided for 1–2 weeks.

CRITICAL THINKING ACTIVITIES

A 78-year-old is admitted with nausea, vomiting, diarrhea, and dehydration. An IV of D_5RL is started at 125 mL per hour. The patient also has hypertension and osteoarthritis of the knees. The vomiting has stopped, but the patient is still somewhat nauseous.

1. Considering the nausea and vomiting, what measures would you take to help rehydrate the patient? ***(678)***

2. Considering the diagnosis of hypertension, what fluids would you need to use with caution in this patient?

3. What nursing measures would you institute because of the diarrhea? ***(678)***

STEPS TOWARD BETTER COMMUNICATION

VOCABULARY BUILDING GLOSSARY

Term	Pronunciation	Definition
absorption (noun)	ab sorp' tion	the uptake of a substance into or across tissues
alleviate; alleviating (verb)	a lee'vi ate	to lessen, to make less severe
assimilation (noun)	as sim i la' tion	the transformation of food into tissue
atrophy (verb)	a' tro fee	to dry up, become withered, waste away

COMPLETION

Directions: Fill in the blanks with the correct words from the Vocabulary Building Glossary to complete the statements.

1. Taste buds may ____________________ as a person ages.
2. Every attempt is made to ____________________ pain.
3. What organ is described as having a "head" and a "tail"? ____________________________

MATCHING

Directions: Match the abbreviation or word on the left with the correct term on the right.

1. ______	BUN	a.	Upper gastrointestinal
2. ______	BE	b.	Gastrointestinal
3. ______	RUQ	c.	Left lower quadrant
4. ______	UGI	d.	Barium enema
5. ______	LLQ	e.	Blood urea nitrogen
6. ______	GI	f.	Right upper quadrant
7. ______	Mastication	g.	Converting nutrients to energy
8. ______	Peristalsis	h.	Chewing
9. ______	Metabolism	i.	Rhythmic squeezing action

COMMUNICATION EXERCISE

Scrambled Sentences

Directions: Arrange the words in the correct order to make a sentence.

1. avoided Heavy weeks. are or to be 1–2 activities for lifting for strenuous

   ____

2. be anesthetic or will general used. local A

   ____

3. history have digestive Do a family of problems? you

   ____

CULTURAL POINT

Certain diseases have a genetic predisposition. This means people may tend to inherit that disease from their parents. Because of this, people of certain races or ethnic groups may be more liable to get a particular disease. This is one reason that taking a family medical history is so important. If you are working in an area with a particular ethnic population (Jewish, Native American, Asian, etc.) be sure to inform yourself and be on the lookout for the related symptoms of diseases that are genetically predisposed to that group. Working with the groups for education and prevention is also recommended.

CHAPTER 28

Care of Patients with Disorders of the Upper Gastointestinal System

evolve Go to http://evolve.elsevier.com/deWit for additional activities and exercises.

REVIEW OF ANATOMY AND PHYSIOLOGY

COMPLETION

Upper Gastrointestinal Disorders

Directions: Fill in the blanks to complete the statements.

1. Obesity causes about ________________________ deaths in the U. S. each year. ***(684)***
2. A surgical procedure for obesity that can be done laparoscopically is ______________________________ ______________________________. ***(686)***
3. In North America, an emphasis on a slim body has been an influence that has contributed to the development of ____ in young women. ***(687-688)***
4. Excessive drinking of alcohol and excessive smoking can contribute to the mouth disorder ________________________. ***(688)***
5. If it is suspected that a patient may have dysphagia, it is best to give ___________________________ before feeding foods. ***(688-689)***
6. A risk factor for cancer of the esophagus is gastric ________________ and the development of ____. ***(690)***
7. A hiatal hernia is a defect in the wall of the __________________________. ***(690)***
8. About 90% of patients who have GERD have a ___________________________. ***(690)***
9. The main cause of gastritis is ____. ***(694)***
10. The habit of taking large doses of unbuffered aspirin can cause __________________________ or ____. ***(695)***
11. An objective sign of gastrointestinal (GI) bleeding is ____________________________. ***(696)***
12. Large amounts of blood in the GI tract cause ________________________. ***(696)***
13. Subjective symptoms of GI ulcer include ____ ____. ***(696)***

14. Decreased blood pressure and increased pulse do not occur in the patient with a GI bleed until he has lost more than ________________ of his blood. *(696)*
15. When GI bleeding occurs, the hemoglobin and hematocrit readings do not show a drop before ________ hours. *(696)*
16. The IV solution usually ordered when a patient is experiencing a GI bleed is ________________ ________________. *(691)*
17. The danger associated with GI bleeding is possible ________________ and ________________. *(698)*
18. Dumping syndrome sometimes occurs after the patient has had a ________________ ________________. *(702)*
19. Symptoms of dumping syndrome include ________________, ________________, ________________, and ________________. *(702)*

SHORT ANSWER

Ulcer Disease

Directions: Read the clinical situation and answer the questions that follow.

Situation: Mrs. Galt, age 41, works two jobs to help support herself and her children. Recently, she has been skipping meals to save time and money. In the past few months, she has had frequent bouts of heartburn, has lost 15 pounds, and occasionally vomits up blood-streaked, partially digested food. She was seen by a physician at her neighborhood clinic who told her she may be developing a peptic ulcer and that she should eat more regularly and take an antacid when she has heartburn.

1. A peptic ulcer is ________________. *(695)*
2. Although she is suffering from anxiety about her home situation, Mrs. Galt's ulcer is not diagnosed as a stress ulcer. How does a stress ulcer differ from a peptic ulcer? *(695)*

____

____

Mrs. Galt continues to have epigastric pain and becomes too sick to work. She is admitted to the hospital for a diagnostic workup and treatment.

3. What information about Mrs. Galt's health history and that of her relatives would be helpful in establishing a diagnosis of peptic ulcer? *(695)*

   a. ________________________________

   b. ________________________________

   c. ________________________________

   d. ________________________________

   e. ________________________________

4. What daily pattern of pain would you expect Mrs. Galt to describe when asked about her pain? ***(696)***

____

____

5. What type of diagnostic test would most likely be performed first? ***(696)***

____

6. What are the three major complications of peptic ulcer? ***(698)***

a. ____

b. ____

c. ____

7. Her physician prescribes esomeprazole (Nexium) for Mrs. Galt. List the three results that are expected from this drug. ***(697)***

a. ____

b. ____

c. ____

8. Mrs. Galt is also told to take an antacid four times a day, to avoid foods that disagree with her, and to return to the outpatient clinic in 3 months for follow-up. What information do you think Mrs. Galt will need to take care of herself properly, recover from her illness, and return to work? ***(698)***

a. ____

b. ____

c. ____

d. ____

e. ____

9. Some patients are not able to respond to medical management and must have surgery. List four surgical procedures that might be performed to treat gastric and duodenal ulcers. ***(699)***

a. ____

b. ____

c. ____

d. ____

APPLICATION OF THE NURSING PROCESS

Directions: Provide the answer to the following questions.

Mr. Timmons has cancer of the stomach. He has been vomiting and unable to eat and was admitted to the hospital yesterday. He has lost 7 lbs. in the last week. He was started on TPN yesterday afternoon.

1. Which of the following nursing diagnoses would be appropriate for this problem?
   a. Altered nutrition, less than body requirements r/t vomiting and inability to keep food in the stomach
   b. Readiness for enhanced fluid balance r/t nausea and vomiting
   c. Deficient fluid volume related to vomiting
   d. Risk for deficient fluid volume related to vomiting

2. Can you write an expected outcome for the correct nursing diagnosis for Mr. Timmons' problem?

   ____

3. List three interventions appropriate for Mr. Timmons related to the administration of the TPN. ***(704-705)***

   a. ______________________________

   b. ______________________________

   c. ______________________________

4. What are comfort interventions often used for the patient who is vomiting? ***(694)***

   ____

   ____

   ____

5. What evaluation criteria would be needed to determine whether the interventions are effective and the expected outcome is being met? ***(694)***

   ____

   ____

PRIORITY SETTING

You are caring for the following patients: Ms. Schultz, an elderly lady with gastroenteritis and dehydration; Mr. Hooper, a 45-year-old working man with a bleeding peptic ulcer, Ms. Peterson, a 48-year-old woman who is second day postoperative after an abdominal surgical procedure for weight control. Indicate in which order you would attend to the following needs of these patients. It is presently 7:45 AM.

______ a. Ms. Schultz urgently needs to go to the bathroom.
______ b. Mr. Hooper has just vomited again and has called for his nurse.
______ c. Ms. Peterson is calling for more pain medication.
______ d. Ms. Peterson needs assistance with her bath.
______ e. Mr. Hooper is scheduled for a gastroscopy at 9:30 amand needs to be prepared.
______ f. Ms. Schultz has not yet been assessed for this shift.

NCLEX-PN® EXAM REVIEW

Directions: Choose the best answer(s) for the following questions.

1. Obesity is a growing problem. Some factors are controllable, some are not. Which of the following contribute to obesity? *(Select all that apply.)* ***(684)***
   1. A high protein, moderate fat diet
   2. Vitamin and supplement intake
   3. A diet high in calories and fat
   4. Family genetic make-up
   5. Large dinner plates and growing portion sizes
   6. Prepackaged foods and "fast food"

2. Complications of obesity include: *(Select all that apply.)* ***(685)***
   1. hypertension.
   2. diabetes mellitus.
   3. multiple sclerosis.
   4. asthma.
   5. cholelithiasis.
   6. coronary artery disease.
   7. arthritis of the knees.

3. A person is considered obese if he or she weighs more than ____________ percent above ideal weight for height and body type. *(Fill in the blank.)* ***(685)***
   1. 10%
   2. 30%
   3. 5%
   4. 20%

4. One treatment for dysphagia is to use a therapy directed at: ***(688)***
   1. puréeing all foods.
   2. increasing swallowing muscle strength.
   3. controlling breathing while swallowing.
   4. keeping the head tilted back when swallowing.

5. The surgical procedure of hemiglossectomy is performed for the treatment of: ***(689)***
   1. esophageal cancer.
   2. hiatal hernia.
   3. cancer of the mouth area.
   4. stomach cancer.

6. Esophagogastroduodenoscopy with biopsy is used for the definitive diagnosis of: ***(672)***
   1. hiatal hernia.
   2. cancer of the tongue.
   3. bulemia.
   4. esophageal cancer.

7. Your patient who has had gastric surgery has a nasogastric tube attached to suction. The drainage container had 250 mL in it at the beginning of the shift. You have irrigated the tube twice with 30 mL of sterile water. At the end of the shift there is 420 mL of drainage in the container. The NG output for the shift is _________ mL.

8. Proton pump inhibitors such as rabeprazole (Aciphex) work by: ***(697)***
   1. increasing HCl secretion in the stomach.
   2. neutralizing stomach acid.
   3. both neutralizing and suppressing stomach acid.
   4. suppressing the secretion of stomach acid.

9. A nursing implication for esomeprazole (Nexium) is to: ***(697)***
   1. administer the drug only with food.
   2. not to administer the drug with digoxin (Lanoxin).
   3. administer the drug along with an antacid.
   4. do not administer the drug along with orange or grapefruit juice.

10. When caring for a patient with nasogastric suction, you would test the drainage for blood if you found: ***(705)***
    1. copious greenish drainage in the container.
    2. coffee ground-like material in the tubing.
    3. complaints of continued nausea by the patient.
    4. a rising blood pressure and pulse rate.

CRITICAL THINKING ACTIVITIES

Scenario A: Mr. Sims comes to the ambulatory clinic because he is having severe heartburn (GERD). He was diagnosed with a hiatal hernia a year ago. You are assigned to take his history and will do the teaching reinforcement that he needs.

1. What questions would you ask him? ***(690-691)***

2. Describe the specific teaching you would do for this patient. ***(691)***

Scenario B: Ms. Harper is second day post-gastrointestinal surgery and has an NG tube attached to suction. There is little drainage in the suction container after 4 hours. ***(705)***

1. What would you do *first?*

2. What other interventions would you perform?

STEPS TOWARD BETTER COMMUNICATION

VOCABULARY BUILDING GLOSSARY

Term	Pronunciation	Definition
regurgitation	ree gurj ah ta' shun	bringing food from the stomach back to the mouth; repeating something without thinking about it
swoosh		rushing sound of air moving quickly
dumping	dump'ing	dropping a mass suddenly
intrinsic factor	intrin'sic fac'tor	glycoprotein necessary for the absorption of vitamin B_{12} from the gastrointestinal system
manifested	man'ifested	showing symptoms of something
adverse	ad'verse	negative, unfavorable
adhere	ad heer'	to follow, to stick to
abound	ah bownd'	exist in great numbers; to be multiple
despite	des pit'	in spite of; not prevented by

COMPLETION

Directions: Fill in the blanks with the appropriate words from the Vocabulary Building Glossary to complete the statements.

1. Sometimes after a subtotal gastrectomy and vagotomy, ______________________ syndrome occurs.
2. Recurrent stomach pain, nausea, and ____________________________ may be signs of peptic ulcer.
3. One way to check the placement of a nasogastric tube before a feeding is by placing a stethoscope over the gastric region, inserting air into the tube, and listening for a ____________________.
4. Patients who lack __________________________________ tend to develop pernicious anemia.
5. People trying to lose weight often have problems trying to _________________ to their diet.
6. People who regularly take antacids ____________________ in our society.

MATCHING

Directions: Match the abbreviation on the left with the correct term on the right.

1. ______	TCDB	a.	milliliter
2. ______	NG	b.	hemoglobin
3. ______	NSAIDs	c.	turn, cough, deep breathe
4. ______	mL	d.	nasogastric
5. ______	Hb or Hgb	e.	nonsteroidal antiinflammatory drugs

PRONUNCIATION SKILLS

Directions: Take turns practicing with a peer pronouncing these words to increase your ability to speak English clearly.

gas'troesophage'al (gas' tro ee sof ah jee' al)	pertaining to the stomach and esophagus
hy'poglyce'mic (hi' po gli see' mik)	having low serum glucose
mal'occlu'sion (mal' ah cloo' zhun)	top and bottom teeth do not come together properly
meta'bolism (mah tab' ah lizm)	process of the building up and breaking down tissue

The pronunciation of the letters **"ai"** in the two words constraint and contraindicated are different. In the first word, they make the long **"a"** sound because they are in the same syllable and are pronounced together (as in pain and complain). In the second word, they are pronounced separately because they are in different syllables:

con straints (kon strants')

con tra in di ca ted (kon' trah in' di ka' ted)

CHAPTER 29

Care of Patients with Disorders of the Lower Gastrointestinal System

evolve Go to http://evolve.elsevier.com/deWit for additional activities and exercises.

SHORT ANSWER

Assessment and Pathophysiology

Directions: Provide brief answers for the following questions.

1. Describe the proper sequence for assessment of the abdomen. ***(676-678)*** ______________________

____

____

2. When assessing for a hernia, you would check the ______________ and ______________ areas, looking for ____

____. ***(710)***

3. The person who has irritable bowel syndrome may have symptoms such as: ***(711)*** ______________

____

____

4. When diverticulosis is suspected, a ______________________ is usually ordered to confirm the diagnosis. ***(671)***

5. The pathophysiologic explanation for diverticulitis is: ***(714)*** ______________________

____

____

6. Signs and symptoms of an intestinal obstruction include: ***(716)*** ______________________

____

____

7. If an elderly person develops appendicitis, the presenting signs and symptoms may differ from those in a younger adult. The older adult may present with only ______________________________

______________________. ***(719)***

8. Peritonitis may occur when the appendix ruptures. The pathophysiologic explanation is: *(720)* ________

____

____

____

9. When assessing for a malabsorption problem, you would specifically ask if the patient has noticed: *(720)*

____

____

10. Hemorrhoids may be internal or external and usually present with: *(721)* ________________

____

COMPLETION

Lower Gastrointestinal Disorders

Directions: Fill in the blank to complete the statement.

1. A medication that can cause blackish stools is ______________________. *(772)*
2. Severe malabsorption problems of the small intestine often necessitate ______________________ ______________________. *(720)*
3. Early signs and symptoms of cancer of the colon include ______________________ and ______________________. *(723)*
4. After a barium enema is performed, the barium must be removed or it can cause ______________________ or ______________________. *(671)*
5. An abdominoperineal resection requires a ______________________ colostomy. *(728)*
6. Three days before surgery on the colon, the patient may be placed on a ______________________ diet. *(730)*
7. Because of prolonged exposure of the abdominal cavity during surgery and the loss of body fluids, patients who have colon surgery must be closely watched for signs of ______________________. *(730)*
8. If a hernia becomes incarcerated, it can cause ______________________ of the protruding part. *(710)*
9. Instead of surgery, hemorrhoids can sometimes be removed by ______________________ or ______________________. *(721)*
10. A diet high in ______________________ is thought to contribute to the formation of cancer of the colon. *(723)*

LABELING

Ostomies

Directions: Write the correct names of the procedures depicted in the three drawings below. ***(729)***

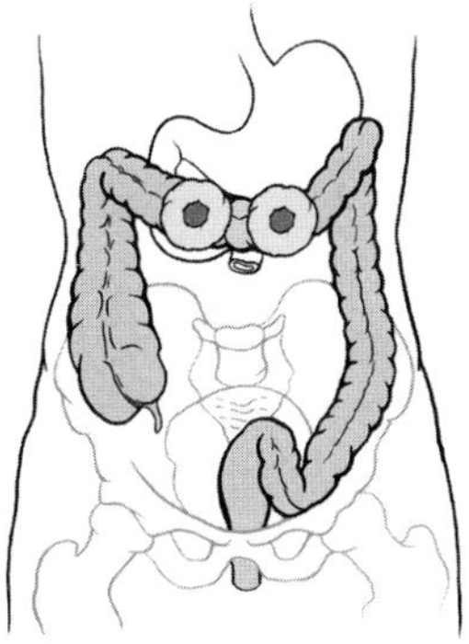

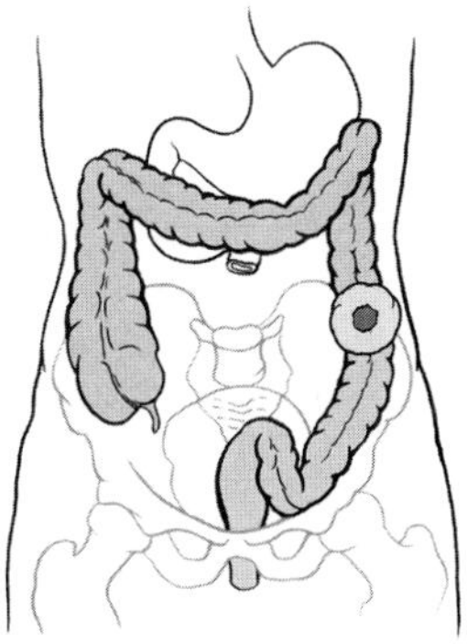

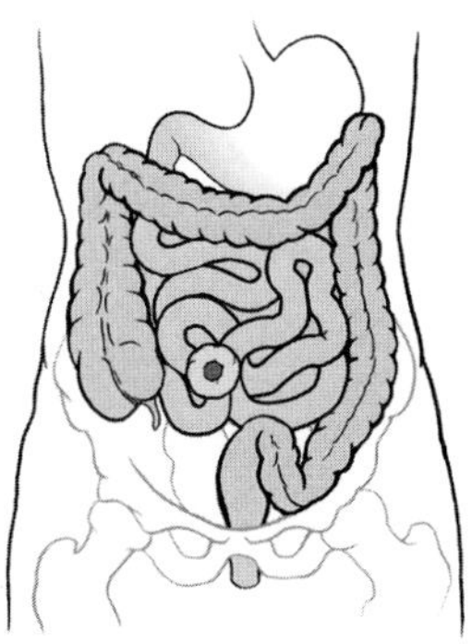

1. ____________________
   ____

2. ____________________

3. ____________________

COMPLETION

Directions: Fill in the blanks to complete the statements.

1. The discharge from an ascending colostomy is normally ____________________. ***(727-729)***
2. A potential problem for the patient with a sigmoid colostomy is ____________________. ***(727-729)***
3. A double-barrelled colostomy is ____________________. ***(727-729)***
4. The discharge from an ileostomy is ____________________. ***(727-729)***
5. An ileostomy is often performed on the patient who has ____________________. ***(727-729)***
6. A continent ileostomy is drained by ____________________. ***(727-729)***
7. The problem with a sigmoid conduit is that ____________________ often occurs. ***(727-729)***
8. The postoperative nursing care plan of a patient with an ileostomy should include monitoring the patient for signs of ____________________ and ____________________. ***(727-729)***
9. Normal coloration for a new stoma is ____________________. ***(727-729)***
10. A noticeable blanching or lightening of color in a stoma may indicate ____________________ ____________________. ***(731-733)***
11. A purplish hue to the stoma may indicate ____________________ ____________________. ***(731-733)***

12. Stomach cramping and a significant drop in the amount of material being discharged from an ileostomy could indicate ____. *(731-733)*
13. When a patient has prolapse of a stoma, the nurse should ____
____. *(731-733)*
14. Stenosis of the stoma can usually be corrected by ____
____. *(731-733)*

SHORT ANSWER

Directions: Write a short answer for each of the following questions.

1. What are two major principles that should be followed to protect the skin around the stoma from irritation and breakdown? *(734)*

   a. ____

   b. ____

2. What is the major reason for irrigating a colostomy? *(734)* ____

   ____

3. What three nursing interventions may help prevent cramping, nausea, and dizziness during a colostomy irrigation? *(734)*

   a. ____

   b. ____

   c. ____

4. What three nursing interventions may help a patient prevent or overcome repeated expulsion of gas from the colostomy? *(736)*

   a. ____

   b. ____

   c. ____

5. What three nursing interventions may help a patient prevent or overcome obstruction of the ileostomy? *(736)*

   a. ____

   b. ____

   c. ____

6. List four nursing interventions that might be helpful in assisting the patient to adjust psychologically to

an ostomy. *(735)*

a. ___

b. ___

c. ___

d. ___

COMPLETION

Medications

Directions: Fill in the answers to the following questions. ***(712-713)***

1. List two important points the nurse should teach the patient who has diphenoxylate hydrochloride (Lomotil) prescribed.

   a. ___

   b. ___

2. What is a contraindication to using a stool softener? ___

3. Name a major problem with the use of contact laxatives. ___

4. Give an important nursing implication for administering a histamine receptor antagonist to a patient who is also taking an antacid.

   ___

5. How should a patient who has an antispasmodic prescribed be taught to take it? ___

6. What should the diabetic patient taking an oral hypoglycemic drug and sulfasalazine be specifically told to prevent a problem?

   ___

PRIORITY SETTING

You are assigned the following patients: Ms. K., a newly admitted female, 68 years old, with probable intestinal obstruction. Mr. P., a 46-year-old male 1 day postoperative for a ruptured appendix and peritonitis. Ms. T., a 72-year-old female with diverticulitis and dehydration. Ms. S., a 56-year-old female patient with Crohn's disease on total parenteral nutrition (TPN). You have just received shift report for the previous shift. Place the following tasks and needs in the order in which you would attend to them.

______ a. Ms. T. is calling for pain medication.
______ b. Assessment (data collection) for Ms. T.
______ c. Wound irrigation and dressing change for Mr. P.
______ d. Assessment (data collection) for Mr. P.
______ e. Ms. K. is vomiting and calling for help.
______ f. Assessment (data collection) for Ms. K.
______ g. Assessment (data collection) of Ms. S. including blood sugar determination.

NCLEX-PN® EXAM REVIEW

Directions: Choose or supply the best answer(s) for the following questions.

1. The cause of irritable bowel syndrome is unknown, but several things seems to trigger episodes, including: *(Select all that apply.) (711)*
   1. consumption of milk products.
   2. overeating of sweets.
   3. consumption of caffeine.
   4. extra-stressful situations.
   5. alcohol consumption.
   6. food intolerances or allergies.

2. A female, age 26, has been diagnosed with ulcerative colitis. She is hospitalized prior to intestinal surgery. When gathering data on this patient, you would expect to obtain a history of: *(717)*
   1. alternating bowel pattern of diarrhea and constipation.
   2. intolerance to milk and milk products.
   3. episodes of bloody, mucoid diarrhea.
   4. relatives with a history of the disorder.

3. In planning care for a patient with ulcerative colitis, you would determine appropriate interventions for the nursing diagnoses of: *(Select all that apply.) (718)*
   1. Nutrition, less than body requirements.
   2. Ineffective coping.
   3. Constipation.
   4. Insomnia.
   5. Sedentary lifestyle.
   6. Diarrhea.

4. An important nursing intervention for the patient with ulcerative colitis is to: *(718)*
   1. restrict all substances containing caffeine.
   2. force fluids to prevent dehydration.
   3. teach relaxation exercises to decrease stress.
   4. guaiac test all stools for the presence of blood.

5. Evaluation data that would indicate that therapy for intestinal inflammation is effective would be: *(Select all that apply.)*
   1. a decrease in the number of diarrheal stools.
   2. an increase in appetite and food consumption.
   3. an increase in hemoglobin and hematocrit.
   4. an increase in weight and energy.
   5. decrease in temperature.
   6. decreased need for pain medication.

6. Treatment of ulcerative colitis sometimes involves resting the bowel. In this event, the patient is placed on __________. *(718)*
   1. long-term intravenous fluids
   2. a bland diet for several weeks
   3. a low-residue diet for 3 weeks
   4. total parenteral nutrition

7. When a patient is receiving TPN, the nurse incorporates which safety factor into the plan of care? *(704-705)*
   1. Never speeding up the TPN solution if it falls behind schedule.
   2. Carefully monitoring and assessing intake and output.
   3. Changing the peripheral IV site every 48 hours.
   4. Monitoring for signs of hypoglycemia during each nursing shift.

8. A male patient, age 67, has lost 8 lbs. over the past 6 months and has experienced diarrhea. When he goes to the doctor for a checkup, he is asked to have tests for the presence of blood in his stool. The tests are positive. His doctor recommends further tests to see if he has colon cancer. Which *one* of the following statements about cancer of the colon is true? *(623)*
   1. Cancer of the colon occurs more in females than males.
   2. Nutrients that seem to protect against it are folic acid and iron.
   3. It is curable if caught in the early stages.
   4. Intestinal obstruction may be the first sign.

9. A sign of colon cancer that a patient might experience is: *(623)*
   1. nausea.
   2. excessive gas.
   3. pain after eating.
   4. black stool.

10. The colonoscopy shows a small, apparently localized tumor in the upper sigmoid colon. The treatment of choice for this tumor would be: *(723)*
    1. radiation and then chemotherapy for 3 months.
    2. hemicolectomy with colostomy.
    3. abdominoperineal resection.
    4. hemicolectomy.

11. The patient has an order to "force fluids." The intake and output records indicate the following for this shift:

	Intake	Output
0730		650 mL
0800	250 mL	
0900	220 mL	
1000	175 mL	420 mL
1100	225 mL	
1200	110 mL	
1300	455 mL	
1400	180 mL	675 mL
1500	220 mL	

The intake and output for the shift are: I = __________ O = __________

12. A patient with diverticulitis and dehydration is receiving intravenous fluid. The order reads D_5NS 1000 mL at 150 mL/hr. The available IV tubing delivers 10 gtts/mL. The IV should run at ____________ gtts/min. *(58)*

CRITICAL THINKING ACTIVITIES

Scenario: Ms. Rubens has had inflammatory bowel disease for the past 5 years. Her specific diagnosis is Crohn's disease. She is tired of feeling ill all the time, the diarrhea episodes, and inability to work full-time. The infliximab (Remicade) infusions don't seem to help much any more. She is presently anemic, has lost 10 lbs. in the past few months, and is seeking treatment that will help her have an improved lifestyle. She enters the hospital for hyperalimentation with TPN.

1. When you come onto your shift and are assigned this patient, which laboratory values would you check in the medical record? *(718)*

2. How do the signs and symptoms of Crohn's disease differ from those of ulcerative colitis? *(717)*

3. Why is surgery not a first choice for patients with Crohn's disease? *(718)*

4. What type of drug is infliximab? What are its major side effects? *(713)*

STEPS TOWARD BETTER COMMUNICATION

VOCABULARY BUILDING GLOSSARY

Term	Pronunciation	Definition
adhere	ad heer'	negative, unfavorable
adverse	ad'verse	negative, unfavorable
manifested	man'ifested	showing symptoms of something
mush		a soft, wet mass; consistency of cooked cereal
constraints	kon stran'ts	limitations
"worry wort"		person who worries about everything
offend'ing	ah fend' ing	causing a problem
gur'gle	ger' gul	sound of water or liquid bubbling (as in boiling or moving over stones)
bout	bowt	a short, difficult period
empathy	em' pa thee	understanding another person's feelings
effluent	ef' floo ent	material discharged or flowing out
blanching	blanch' ing	turning white or light-colored

COMPLETION

Directions: Fill in the blanks with the appropriate words from the Vocabulary Building Glossary to complete the statements.

1. The patient's stool was the consistency of ________________.
2. Because the patient worried about every little thing, she was called a ______________________________.
3. The ____________________ from a new ileostomy must be carefully measured.
4. The patient was having trouble with his ileostomy because he did not ____________________ to the dietary guidelines.
5. Ostomy patients do worry about ______________________ those around them with bad odors.
6. The patient's intestinal disease was ________________________ by frequent bouts of bloody diarrhea.
7. While auscultating bowel sounds, the nurse heard a ________________ in the left upper quadrant.
8. The nurse checked the reddened area on the patient's buttocks for ______________________ when she turned him to determine if a pressure ulcer was developing.
9. The patient who ignores signs of colon cancer may have an ______________________ outcome.
10. The patient with diverticulitis was experiencing another __________ of severe abdominal pain.
11. The nurse must try to develop _________________ for patients who are experiencing a tremendous body image change due to an ostomy.

MATCHING

Directions: Match the abbreviation on the left with the correct term on the right.

1. ______	BM	a.	Inflammatory bowel disease
2. ______	IBS	b.	Bowel movement
3. ______	IBD	c.	Total parenteral nutrition
4. ______	TPN	d.	Irritable bowel syndrome

PRONUNCIATION SKILLS

Directions: Take turns practicing with a peer pronouncing these words to increase your ability to speak English.

def'ecate (def' ah kāt)	eliminate stool
incon'tinence (in kon' tah nens)	no control over passage of urine or of stool
piloni'dal (pī lo nīdal)	having a core of hair
sa'crococcyg'eal (sa' kro kok sij' ee al)	pertaining to the sacrum and coccyx

CULTURAL POINT

There are a variety of common terms that patients may use for digestive functions. Proper medical terms are listed below in dark print; the other terms are not medical terms and are impolite, but you should understand the meaning when you hear them.

bowel movement (BM), **defecate**, **stool**, **feces**, shit, crap, excreta, poop

gas, flatus, flatulence, pass gas, pass wind, fart, poop

diarrhea, the runs, the trots

CHAPTER 30

Care of Patients with Disorders of the Gallbladder, Liver, and Pancreas

evolve Go to http://evolve.elsevier.com/deWit for additional activities and exercises.

COMPLETION

Gallbladder Disease

Directions: Fill in the blanks to complete the statements.

1. The most frequent cause of cholecystitis is ________________________________. *(740)*
2. The symptoms of cholecystitis are usually most noticeable after the patient has ____________________ ________________________. *(741)*
3. The surgical procedure most often performed for treatment of cholelithiasis is ____________________ ______________________. *(742)*
4. Four types of people most at risk for developing cholelithiasis are those who: *(740)*
   a. ____
   b. ____
   c. ____
   d. ____
5. In addition to routine care, one of the most important aspects of the postoperative care of a patient who has had a cholecystectomy is ____ ____________________________________. *(743-744)*

Diseases of the Liver and Pancreas

Directions: Fill in the blanks to complete the statements.

1. The percentage of cases of cirrhosis related to alcoholism is between ______ and ______. *(751)*
2. Frequently, the first symptoms noted by a patient with cirrhosis are those that occur when the patient has ________________, __________________________, or ____________________________________. *(752)*
3. Ascites is the result of a condition in which there is __________________________ of the portal circulation. *(757)*

4. Medical treatment of ascites includes restriction of ________________ and ________________ and administration of ________________. *(753)*

5. The insertion of a large needle into the peritoneal cavity to remove ascitic fluid is called a ________________ ________________. *(753)*

6. A LaVeen shunt involves directing excess fluid in the peritoneal cavity from the ________________ ________________ to the ________________. *(753)*

7. Neurologic changes that occur as a result of liver failure constitute a condition called ________________ ________________. *(757)*

8. Neurologic changes that occur as a result of liver failure are characterized by ________________, ________________, ________________, and ________________. *(757)*

9. The neurologic symptoms described above are due to excess ________________ in the blood, which eventually reaches the brain cells and damages them. *(757)*

10. In an effort to minimize brain damage, a patient with neurologic symptoms due to advanced cirrhosis may be placed on a diet that is limited in ________________. *(754)*

11. The most deadly of all complications of cirrhosis of the liver is ________________ ________________. *(754)*

12. Both hepatitis B and cirrhosis increase the risk of ________________. *(758)*

13. Treatment for cancer of the liver is ________________ and ________________. *(753)*

14. If the tumor is confined to the liver, ________________ is an option. *(758)*

15. After a liver transplant, the patient must take ________________ and ________________ for life to prevent rejection of the liver. *(757)*

16. Signs of transplant rejection are fever, increasing jaundice, ________________, ________________, and changes in stool and urine color. *(758)*

17. The majority of cases of pancreatitis are caused by ________________, ________________, and ________________. *(758)*

18. Describe the typical pain from pancreatitis. (759) ________________

____

19. If the patient has pancreatitis, the laboratory tests will reveal an elevated: ________________ ________________. *(758)*

20. List four measures for treatment of pancreatitis. *(759)*

    a. ______________________________

    b. ______________________________

    c. ______________________________

    d. ______________________________

21. When powdered pancreatic enzymes are given with food, the powder should be mixed in ______________________________; it should not be allowed to remain on the ______________ because it will cause ______________. *(760)*

22. Cancer of the pancreas is twice as frequent among ______________. *(760)*

23. The main symptoms of pancreatic cancer are ______________________ and ______________________. *(761)*

NCLEX-PN® EXAM REVIEW

Directions: Choose the best answer(s) for the following questions.

1. The nurse is caring for a patient who is known to be a infected with hepatitis A. Which of the following infection control precautions should the nurse implement? *(Select all that apply.)* *(745)*
   1. Wear a mask when entering the patient's room.
   2. Wear a gown when delivering the patient's meal tray.
   3. Wear a gown and gloves when bathing the patient.
   4. Wear latex gloves when emptying the bedpan after a bowel movement.

2. Which of the following laboratory test results should you be closely monitoring when caring for a patient with pancreatitis? *(Select all that apply.)* *(759)*
   1. CBC
   2. AST and ALT
   3. Lipase
   4. Amylase

3. The nurse is caring for several patients. The postcholecystectomy patient is requesting assistance with ambulation. The patient with pancreatitis is wanting medication for nausea. The cirrhosis patient has just noticed considerable blood in his stool. The patient with possible cancer of the liver is complaining of pain. Which patient should the nurse attend to *first?*
   1. The postcholecystectomy patient
   2. The patient with cirrhosis of the liver
   3. The patient with pancreatitis
   4. The patient with possible cancer of the liver

4. Which of the following medications is used to decrease ammonia levels in the patient with liver failure? *(747)*
   1. Vasopressin (Pitressin)
   2. Esomeprazole (Nexium)
   3. Furosemide (Lasix)
   4. Lactulose (Cephulac)

5. Hepatitis virus are transmitted by various routes. Which virus is transmitted by the gastrointestinal route? ***(744)***
   1. Hepatitis A
   2. Hepatitis B
   3. Hepatitis C
   4. Hepatitis D

6. If a patient presents with pain radiating to the back at the level of the shoulder blade, which problem often displays that symptom? ***(741)***
   1. Cholelithiasis
   2. Cirrhosis of the liver
   3. Pancreatitis
   4. Cancer of the pancreas

7. Jaundice occurs when: ***(746)***
   1. too much bile flows into the intestine.
   2. the pancreas is not producing sufficient digestive enzymes.
   3. cirrhosis has caused the liver to stop producing clotting agents for the blood.
   4. bile flow out of the liver is blocked and bile pigment is entering the bloodstream.

8. Ascites occurs in advanced cirrhosis due to: ***(752)***
   1. fluid buildup related to sodium retention.
   2. obstruction to the flow of blood through the portal circulatory system.
   3. secreted enzymes autodigesting tissue causing inflammation.
   4. obstruction of bile ducts causing backup of fluid.

9. The *highest* priority of nursing care for the patient with pancreatitis would be: ***(759)***
   1. providing supplemental enzymes for digestion of food.
   2. providing skin care to relieve pruritus.
   3. medicating for nausea whenever needed.
   4. providing adequate pain control.

10. Important nursing actions for the patient with symptoms of hepatitis are: *(Select all that apply.)* ***(746)***
    1. encourage as much rest as possible.
    2. encourage a high-protein diet.
    3. offer six small meals a day to counteract anorexia.
    4. reinforce teaching of hand hygiene.

CRITICAL THINKING ACTIVITIES

Directions: Read the clinical scenario below and answer the questions that follow.

Scenario: Mr. Poe, age 29, is admitted to the hospital with possible viral hepatitis. He was in an automobile accident 6 weeks ago and had received two units of blood. One week ago, he returned from a vacation at the seashore where he had eaten a significant amount of shellfish. Within the past few days, he has felt very weak and tired and finally went to his doctor, who hospitalized him.

1. What would you look for in Mr. Poe's health history that would be helpful to the health care provider in diagnosing his illness? ***(746)***

   a. ____________________

   b. ____________________

   c. ____________________

   d. ____________________

2. List subjective and objective data that would indicate inflammation or damage to Mr. Poe's liver. ***(746)***

   Subjective data: ____________________

   Objective data: ____________________

Within a few days of admission, Mr. Poe began to exhibit signs of severe jaundice. His diagnosis was type B viral hepatitis with liver damage.

3. List specific nursing actions that can be taken to help Mr. Poe with each of the following problems.

   a. Abdominal pain: ***(750)*** ____________________

   b. Bleeding tendency: ***(750)*** ____________________

   c. Nausea, vomiting, and anorexia: ***(750)*** ____________________

4. What special precautions to prevent the spread of infection would you expect to be necessary in the care of Mr. Poe? ***(751)***

5. An IV infusion is ordered for Mr. Poe. The order reads D_5W 1000 mL at 100 mL/hr. The tubing set delivers 15 drops per mL. How many drops per minute should the IV run to infuse within the allotted time? ______________________________ *(58)*

6. What might be given to individuals who were in close contact with Mr. Poe to provide them with passive immunity against type B hepatitis? *(746)*

____

____

7. If Mr. Poe were to become a carrier of type B hepatitis, he would be at high risk for developing what conditions? *(751)*

   a. ______________________________

   b. ______________________________

   c. ______________________________

8. What should Mr. Poe know in order to avoid future liver damage from hepatotoxins? *(749)*

____

____

____

STEPS TOWARD BETTER COMMUNICATION

VOCABULARY BUILDING GLOSSARY

Term	Pronunciation	Definition
accessory	ek ses' ah ree	additional, supplemental
geared	geer' d	aimed, intended for, adapted for a particular situation
prevalent	prev'alent	common, often occurs, widespread
dammed up		stopped by a blockage

COMPLETION

Directions: Fill in each blank with the appropriate word from the Vocabulary Building Glossary.

1. Hepatitis is quite ____________________ among travelers.

2. The gallstone ______________________________ the common duct, causing a backup of bile in the gallbladder and liver.

3. Much of the care of the patient with hepatitis A is ________________ toward preventing the spread of infection.

4. The pancreas is an ______________________________ organ of the digestive system.

PRONUNCIATION SKILLS

These words are somewhat difficult to pronounce:

cholelith'iasis (ko le li thī' ah sis)
cholan'giopan'creatog'raphy (ko lan' jee o pan' cree ah tog' rah fee)
phagocyte (far' go sī t)
phagocytic (far' go sit' ic)

Directions: Practice pronouncing the above words with a peer partner.

Short "i" Sound

Short i (ĭ) is the sound of the letter **"i"** in the words it, is, infect, minute, and liver. It is usually written with the letter "i," but sometimes with the letter "y."

Directions: Draw a line under the letters in the following words that have the sound of short "i." Then practice pronouncing the words out loud.

liver, filter, topic, digestive, insulin, lipid, sluggish, lipase, nutrition, cirrhosis, irritation, toxins, cholelithiasis, fluid deficit, bilirubin, pitressin infusion, carcinogenic, phagocytic

WORD ATTACK SKILLS

Combining Forms

These combining forms are used frequently in Chapter 30:

chol/e	bile
lith/o	stone
-iasis	condition
-angi/o	vessel
pancreat/o	pancreas
-graphy	recording

Directions: Using vertical lines, break each word into its word elements (parts) and give the meaning of the word.

1. cholelithiasis: ______________________________

2. cholangiopancreatography: ______________________________

GRAMMAR POINTS

When asking questions during assessment about things that happened in the past over a period of time, it is often necessary to use the verb construction *have* plus the past participle form of the verb (the present perfect tense). *Examples:*

Have you had any pain?
Have you had any injuries?
Have you had any problems with . . .?
Have you used cleaning agents containing carbon tetrachloride?
How long have you taken this medication?
Have you taken any other drugs?
Have you been exposed to pesticides or toxins?
Have you been exposed to hepatitis?
Have you been tired lately?
How long have you been drinking?

This is different from talking about something that happened in the past and was completed. These statements use the simple past form of the verb. *Examples:*

Did you see the doctor recently?

I saw him last week.

When did you have the accident?

I had it last year in February.

CHAPTER 31

The Musculoskeletal System

Go to http://evolve.elsevier.com/deWit for additional activities and exercises.

REVIEW OF ANATOMY AND PHYSIOLOGY

COMPLETION

Changes Occurring with Aging

Directions: Complete the following statements.

1. As we age, bone density decreases because of ______________________________ ______________________________. *(767)*
2. Kyphosis in the elderly is because of ______________________________ ______________________________. *(767)*
3. The bones of the elderly break more easily because they are ____________________ and ____________________. *(767)*
4. Stiffness and crepitation in the joints is a result of joint ____________________ and erosion from ____________________. *(767)*
5. Muscle movement is slowed in the elderly due to ____________________ and becoming ____________________. *(767)*
6. Nighttime muscle cramping in the elderly is increased because of ____________________ and accumulation of ____________________. *(767)*
7. As bone mass decreases with aging, ____________________ may occur and ____________________ become more common. *(767)*

SHORT ANSWER

Causes and Prevention of Musculoskeletal Disorders

Directions: Provide short answers to complete the following statements.

1. Trauma contributes to musculoskeletal disorders by ______________________________ ______________________________. *(765)*

2. Poor nutrition can contribute to musculoskeletal problems because there may be ____________________ ____. *(768)*

3. Malignant tumors can contribute to musculoskeletal disorders is two ways: ***(765)***

   a. ______________________________

   b. ______________________________

4. Five measures that can help prevent musculoskeletal disorders are: ***(768)***

   a. ______________________________

   b. ______________________________

   c. ______________________________

   d. ______________________________

   e. ______________________________

MATCHING

Diagnostic Tests

Directions: Match the procedure on the left with the most appropriate phrase on the right.

1. ______	Bone scan *(769)*	a.	Measurement of range of motion of a joint
2. ______	Arthroscopy *(770)*	b.	Apply ice or cold packs, support joint with pillows
3. ______	Arthrocentesis *(771)*	c.	Grading ranges from 0 (paralysis) to 5 (normal)
4. ______	Synovial analysis *(771)*	d.	After procedure, watch for signs of infection, hemarthrosis, swelling, and injury to joint or loss of feeling
5. ______	Culture *(771)*	e.	Normal findings are clear, viscid fluid containing no or very few blood cells
6. ______	Goniometry *(772)*	f.	After procedure, monitor site of venipuncture for signs of inflammation and hematoma
7. ______	Muscle strength *(771)*	g.	Examination of bone tissue to identify infecting organism

APPLICATION OF THE NURSING PROCESS

Directions: Answer the questions that follow.

1. List three significant findings the nurse might record when taking a history during assessment of a patient with a disorder of the musculoskeletal system. *(773)*

   a. ______________________________

   b. ______________________________

   c. ______________________________

2. List three observations that are significant in assessing musculoskeletal state. *(773)*

   a. ______________________________

   b. ______________________________

   c. ______________________________

3. Three nursing diagnoses concerning physical aspects that would probably be found on the care plan for the patient who has severe rheumatoid arthritis affecting the hands, knees, and hips are: *(773-775)*

   a. ______________________________

   b. ______________________________

   c. ______________________________

4. Expected outcomes for the above nursing diagnoses might be: *(773-775)*

   a. ______________________________

   b. ______________________________

   c. ______________________________

COMPLETION

Directions: Fill in the blanks to complete the statements

1. A primary goal when positioning orthopedic patients is to prevent ______________________________. *(778)*

2. After turning and repositioning a patient, the nurse should check to see if he is in good ______________________________. *(778)*

3. When making the bed of a patient who must be lifted and turned frequently, the nurse should place a ______________________________ on the bed. *(774)*

4. Joint mobility is maintained by regularly performing ______________________________ exercises. *(778)*

5. A patient who is immobilized for a long period of time loses ______________________________ from his bones.

6. Lengthy immobilization tends to cause muscle ______________________________. *(777)*

7. Rehabilitation of the orthopedic patient begins ______________________________.

8. If ankylosis of a joint is unavoidable, the joint is braced so that the extremity will have ______________________________. *(778)*

9. Flexion and extension exercises work to preserve ______________________________ and to promote ______________________________. *(777)*

10. ______________________________ exercise is helpful in preventing osteoporosis. *(768)*

PRIORITY SETTING

Directions: You are assigned to ambulate a 72-year-old female patient who is recovering after a pelvic fracture. She had been on bedrest and is still somewhat weak. Place the actions you would take into the order in which you would carry them out. She uses a cane to ambulate.

_____ a. Plan how far you will go with her as she will have to come back as well.

_____ b. Have her stand still to dispel any dizziness.

_____ c. Check the orders.

_____ d. Assist to sit in the chair.

_____ e. Assess her ability to move, stand, and ambulate.

_____ f. Attach the gait belt to her.

_____ g. Assist to the side of the bed.

_____ h. Identify the patient.

_____ i. Ambulate back to the room.

_____ j. Perform hand hygiene.

_____ k. Hand her the cane.

_____ l. Assist to stand.

_____ m. Ambulate the correct distance.

_____ n. Assist to sit on the side of the bed.

NCLEX-PN® EXAM REVIEW

Directions: Choose the best answer(s) to the following questions.

1. Magnetic resonance imaging is used to help diagnose a variety of musculoskeletal problems. Which of the following instructions would you give the patient who is to undergo an MRI? *(Select all that apply.)* ***(770)***
    1. A consent must be signed for this procedure.
    2. You must remove all metal from your body.
    3. You will be given a contrast media to drink.
    4. You will need to remain perfectly still for 15–60 minutes.
    5. If you are claustrophobic, you may ask for a sedative beforehand.

2. When assessing whether crutches have been fitted to the patient properly, you know that when walking with them, the: *(Select all that apply.)* ***(780)***
    1. axillary bar should be two finger-breadths below the axilla.
    2. elbow should be flexed at a 45-degree angle.
    3. elbow should be flexed at a 30-degree angle.
    4. the crutches should be about 16 inches shorter than the patient's height.

3. Although the following are all good sources of calcium, calcium is not absorbed readily from: ***(768)***
    1. green leafy vegetables.
    2. canned sardines.
    3. cheese and yogurt.
    4. milk.

4. When teaching a patient to do quadriceps and gluteal muscle exercises, you would instruct to do them how many times an hour while awake? _______________ *(779)*

5. When checking the joints during a focused assessment, you should: *(Select all that apply.)* ***(773)***
   1. palpate them for tenderness.
   2. position them to full extension and flexion.
   3. inspect them for swelling or deformity.
   4. assess for warmth over the joint.
   5. determine range of motion without pain.

6. Proper exercise and positioning of joints for an immobile patient is extremely important because a contracture can begin to occur within as little as: ***(777)***
   1. 6–8 weeks.
   2. 10 days.
   3. 2 weeks.
   4. 3–7 days.

7. When a walker is used for ambulation, it is important that it be appropriate height for the patient. Most walkers have adjustable legs. When walking with it, the walker height is correct when the patient's elbow is: ***(779)***
   1. locked to sustain the weight of the upper body.
   2. bent at 15–30 degrees.
   3. at a 45-degree angle to swing the walker forward.
   4. just slightly bent.

8. Because the patient is immobilized, the physician has ordered Lovenox, low–molecular-weight heparin injections. The order reads: enoxaparin sodium 60 mg Subcut. per day in 2 divided doses. On hand is enoxaparin sodium 30 mg/mL. How much medication would you draw up for each injection? _____________ mL ***(58)***

CRITICAL THINKING ACTIVITIES

1. If you need to make the bed for a patient in traction, what steps would you take to accomplish the task?

Scenario A: You are to teach a patient about proper and safe use of crutches. The patient cannot bear weight on the left leg. ***(780)***

1. Describe how you would teach the patient to go up and down stairs.

2. What safety measures would you teach?

Scenario B: You are assigned a patient who has rheumatoid arthritis who is recovering from an appendectomy. You need to have the patient exercise her joints. *(778)*

1. How would you prepare the patient to do the exercises?

2. What would you do to prevent excessive pain during the exercise sessions?

STEPS TOWARD BETTER COMMUNICATION

VOCABULARY BUILDING GLOSSARY

Term	Pronunciation	Definition
deficit	def' ah sit	not enough, insufficient, less than required
distal		farthest away from, remote
dowager	dow' ah jer	an older woman, usually with money and property
initiate	in i'shee āt	to start, begin
flaccid	flas' id	limp, soft
trigger	trig' ger	initiate, cause to begin

COMPLETION

Directions: Fill in the blanks with the correct words from the Vocabulary Building Glossary to complete the statements.

1. When an injury has occurred to an extremity, the nurse checks the pulse ______________ to the area of trauma.
2. An abnormal finding on a musculoskeletal assessment would be ______________ muscles in the right lower extremity.
3. Accidentally brushing against the weights of a traction device may ________________ pain for the patient.
4. Osteoarthritis often causes a ________________ in joint motion.
5. Sometimes the nurse must ________________ action to obtain heat or cold treatments for a patient who needs them.
6. The bent-forward position of the elderly lady showed that she had a ________________ hump.

COMMUNICATION EXERCISE

Directions: Here are some examples of what to say if a patient were to ask you the following questions.

1. What is the difference between a tendon and a ligament?

   Ligaments hold the joint together. Tendons anchor muscle to bone.

2. What is the purpose of cartilage?

   Cartilage provides a cushion between the bones of the joint.

3. What is the difference between a sprain and a strain?

   A sprain involves stretching or tearing of ligaments around a joint. A strain involves pulling and tearing of a muscle or a tendon or both.

WORD ATTACK SKILLS

Directions: Study the word parts and answer the related questions.

1. ankyl/o crooked or bent

   Can you think of a joint whose name came from this word element? ________________

2. ab- from
   ad- to
   re- gain
   -sorb to attract or retain substances

   Directions: Write the meanings of the following words:

   a. Absorb: ____

   b. Adsorb: ____

   c. Resorb: ____

3. -esthesi/o

   If *anesthesia* means without pain and *paresthesia* means having numbness or tingling, what does *para-* mean? ______________________

Pronunciation

Directions: Practice pronouncing the following words with a peer.

throm'bophlebit'is (throm' bo flee bī' tus)
ankylo'sis (ang' kee lo' sis)
kypho'sis (ki fo' sis)

Also practice pronouncing the terms given in Focused Assessment 31-1 of the textbook.

Descriptive Terms

Directions: Here are some terms commonly used to describe findings of physical assessment:

Posture: erect, slumped, rounded-shouldered, straight

Gait: normal, rolling, heel-toe, toe-heel, ataxic, ambling, slow, rapid, bouncy

Range of motion: full, limited, diminished, little

Spine: normal curve, S-shaped, abnormally curved, tender, rounded

Joints: normal, reddened, swollen, painful, deformed, immovable, contracted, freely movable

Skeletal muscles: good tone, well-developed, underdeveloped, tense, hard, soft, poor tone, atrophic, painful

COMMUNICATION EXERCISE

Assessment Questions: History-Taking

Using Focused Assessment 31-2 in the textbook, practice asking and answering the questions with a peer. Answer either from your own experience or with imaginary answers. When you are the "patient," do not look in the book. Your responsibility is to listen and ask for repetition and clarification when you do not understand.

CHAPTER 32

Care of Patients with Musculoskeletal and Connective Tissue Disorders

evolve Go to http://evolve.elsevier.com/deWit for additional activities and exercises.

COMPLETION

Musculoskeletal and Connective Tissue Disorders

Directions: Fill in the blanks to complete the statements.

1. In addition to joint swelling, the patient with rheumatoid arthritis often has considerable ________________ and ________________. ***(797)***
2. Rest, exercise, analgesics, and ________________ are the main treatments for osteoarthritis. ***(795)***
3. After hip replacement, it is extremely important that the affected leg be kept ________________. ***(800)***
4. For traction to be effective, the weights must be kept ________________. ***(793)***
5. The most common cause of osteomyelitis is ________________. ***(794)***
6. The muscles most commonly afflicted with muscle strain are the ________________, ________________, and ________________ muscles. ***(784)***
7. A sprain may be treated with ________________, ________________, ________________, and ________________. ***(784)***
8. Russell's traction is often used for preoperative immobilization of the patient who has a fracture of the ________________. ***(789)***
9. Signs of fat embolism in a patient who has a fracture of a long bone are ________________ and ________________. ***(794)***
10. One intervention to decrease pain for the patient suffering muscle spasms is to apply ________________ for ________________ of each hour while awake. ***(784)***
11. In addition to increasing calcium intake, one of the best ways for women to prevent osteoporosis is to perform ________________. ***(807)***
12. The most common cause of below-the-knee amputation is ________________. ***(810)***
13. The two most common problems during the postoperative period for an amputation are ________________ and________________. ***(810)***

14. The stump of a lower extremity should be elevated postoperatively for at least ______________________ ______________________. *(810)*

15. The hip should not be positioned in a flexed position of more than ______ degrees after amputation of the lower leg. *(810-811)*

SHORT ANSWER

Arthritis

Directions: Answer the following questions about arthritis in the spaces provided.

1. List four questions the nurse might ask when assessing the status of a patient with arthritis. ***(795-797, 804)***

   a. ____

   b. ____

   c. ____

   d. ____

2. What are some objective data the nurse might collect when assessing a patient with arthritis? ***(795-797)***

   a. ____

   b. ____

   c. ____

3. List some important facts that should be included when teaching a patient with arthritis about rest and exercise. ***(795, 797)***

   a. ____

   b. ____

   c. ____

   d. ____

   e. ____

LABELING

Fractures and Immobilization

Directions: Review the drawings below and identify each of the following types of fractures: comminuted, compound, greenstick, longitudinal, oblique, simple, spiral, and transverse. ***(786)***

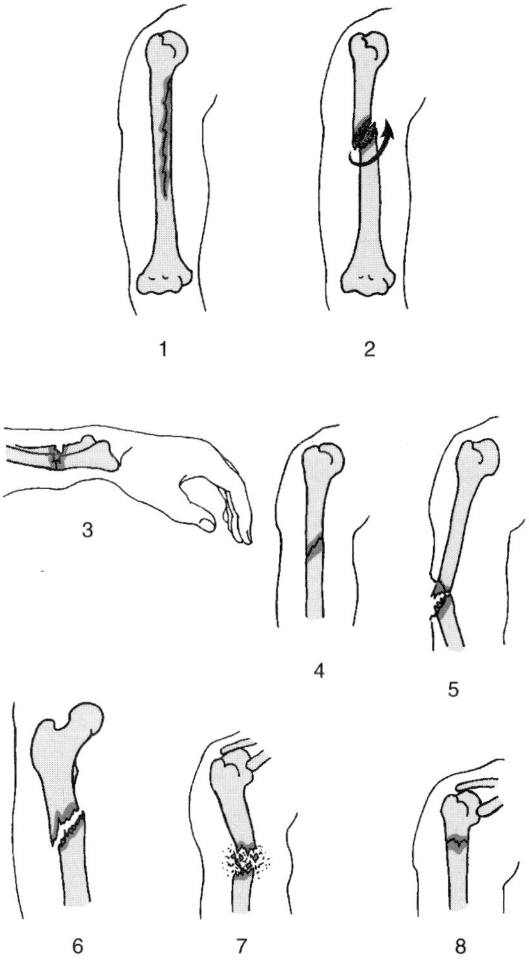

1. ______________________
2. ______________________
3. ______________________
4. ______________________
5. ______________________
6. ______________________
7. ______________________
8. ______________________

COMPLETION

Directions: Answer the following questions in the spaces provided.

1. If a patient has a synthetic cast applied and is then sent home, what will he need to know to take care of himself and the cast? ***(788, 792)***

   a. ______________________

   b. ______________________

   c. ______________________

2. Mr. King, age 29, suffered a compound comminuted fracture of the femur in an automobile accident. The fracture was treated surgically by open reduction and internal fixation, after which a cast was applied. If Mr. King's physician had chosen traction rather than a cast to immobilize the fractured femur, he probably would have used balanced suspension of the affected leg and perhaps inserted pins for skeletal traction. List five observations Mr. King would then require. *(790-791)*

   a. ______________________________

   b. ______________________________

   c. ______________________________

   d. ______________________________

   e. ______________________________

3. Explain what happens when a bone heals and why it is important to establish and maintain a sturdy union of broken bone fragments. *(787)*

   ____

   ____

   ____

   ____

   ____

APPLICATION OF THE NURSING PROCESS

Matching

Directions: Match the problem on the left with the appropriate nursing assessment or intervention on the right.

1. ______	Swelling and increased pressure within a fascial compartment *(790)*	a. Patient complains of grating sensation and unrelenting pain, especially with motion.
2. ______	Inadequate immobilization *(794)*	b. Notify the physician promptly; this is symptomatic of fat embolism. The condition could be fatal.
3. ______	Migration of a traction pin *(794)*	c. Presents as dull pain that becomes progressively worse, fever, purulent drainage, foul odor. Initiate wound and skin precautions.
4. ______	Infection of a pin site or fracture site *(794)*	d. Assess for pain at site of insertion and tenting at pin site.
5. ______	Tachypnea, disorientation, crackles and wheezing, and rash with lesions that do not blanch with pressure *(794)*	e. Do a two-point discrimination test and capillary refill time test.

Short Answer

Directions: Provide a short answer to the following questions or provide the information requested.

1. The following nursing diagnoses might be on the nursing care plan for the patient who has had a joint replacement. For each nursing diagnosis, write an expected outcome. ***(802-803)***

   a. Impaired mobility related to surgical procedure on knee.

   ____

   b. Risk for ineffective tissue perfusion related to potential for thrombus formation.

   ____

   c. Pain related to surgical procedure and rehabilitation exercises.

   ____

2. Interventions to assist in improving mobility would include: ***(804-805)*** ______________________________

   ____

   ____

3. Interventions to help prevent thrombus formation for this patient would include: ***(803)***

   a. ______________________________

   b. ______________________________

   c. ______________________________

   d. ______________________________

4. Other interventions besides analgesic administration to assist the patient with pain could include: ***(804-805)***

   ____

   ____

   ____

5. You would evaluate whether the expected outcomes are being met by gathering data regarding: ***(803)***

   ____

   ____

6. If the expected outcomes are not being met, you would: ***(804)*** ______________________________

   ____

PRIORITY SETTING

You are assigned the following patients:

a. Mr. Holmes who has just had a right knee replacement and is using a CPM machine.
b. Ms. Tuttle who has been admitted for final tests before a left hip replacement.
c. Mr. Conners who was in a motorcycle accident and has multiple injuries including a broken leg that is immobilized with balanced traction.
d. Ms. Simpson who is 2 days postoperative for an amputation of her left foot. She is diabetic.

1. Indicate the priority order in which you would do your beginning of shift rounds. ____________________
2. Which patient requires the most thorough assessment at first visit? ___________
3. All the call lights are on later in the morning. Mr. Holmes is asking for pain medication. Ms. Tuttle needs assistance to the bathroom. Mr. Connors says he doesn't feel well and sounds anxious. Ms. Simpson says her left foot is itching and would someone please help her. Which patient would you attend to first? ___________ Why?

NCLEX-PN® EXAM REVIEW

Directions: Choose the best answer(s) for the following:

1. Mrs. C. is in her first postoperative day after a total hip replacement as treatment for degenerative arthritis. In which of the following positions must Mrs. C.'s operated limb be kept at all times? ***(800)***
   1. Adduction
   2. Externally rotated
   3. Internally rotated
   4. Abduction

2. A complication common in the immobilized hip fracture patient for which you should regularly assess is: ***(801)***
   1. atelectasis or pneumonia.
   2. urinary tract infection.
   3. deep vein thrombosis.
   4. contracture of the opposite hip.

3. When the patient with the new hip is being prepared for discharge, you should give which of the following instructions to avoid dislocation of the prosthesis? *(Select all that apply.)* ***(801)***
   1. Sit on straight chairs only.
   2. Use a raised toilet seat.
   3. Do not lie on your back in bed.
   4. Use a pillow between your knees when lying down.
   5. Do not cross your legs at the knee or ankle.
   6. Be careful not to bend at the hip more than 90 degrees.

4. When a patient is to be turned by "log-rolling," you turn him by: ***(556)***
   1. placing his arms across his chest, keeping his spine and neck in good alignment, and rolling him over as one unit.
   2. bending his knees up toward his chest, putting his opposite arm across his chest, and tipping him up on his side.
   3. having him scoot to the side of the bed, reach to the opposite side rail, and pull himself over onto his side.
   4. using a roller device to pull him to the side of the bed and tip him up onto his side.

5. An assessment finding that you should immediately report to the surgeon about a patient who has just had spinal surgery is: ***(544)***
   1. blood on the dressing.
   2. complaints of headache.
   3. clear drainage on the dressing.
   4. nausea and vomiting.

6. Mr. H. fractured his right femur 3 days ago. Today he is complaining of difficulty breathing, his temperature is elevated, his pulse is rapid, and he has a petechial rash on his chest. The nurse recognizes that this represents probable ______________________________. ***(794)***

7. Whenever a patient has sustained a musculoskeletal injury, it is most important that you assess the patient's distal extremities for: ***(786)***
   1. proper position and elevation.
   2. paresthesia, numbness, and decreased pulses.
   3. signs of deep vein thrombosis.
   4. edema, swelling, and soft tissue injury.

8. The patient who returns to the floor after an reduction and internal fixation of the right hip has an IV running. The order for the next IV reads: D_5NS 1000 mL at 150 mL/hr. The IV tubing has a drop factor of 10 gtts/mL. The IV should be set to run at __________ gtts/min. ***(58)***

9. Rheumatoid arthritis patients who are receiving Enbrel or other biologic response modifiers must be watched for complications such as: *(Select all that apply.)* ***(798)***
   1. hearing loss.
   2. serious infection.
   3. severe edema.
   4. blood dyscrasias.
   5. signs of demylination.
   6. skin eruptions.

10. Disease-modifying antirheumatic drugs prevent joint and cartilage destruction by: ***(798)***
    1. suppressing the immune system.
    2. stimulating cortisol production.
    3. providing collagen to the joints.
    4. blocking pain transmission

CRITICAL THINKING ACTIVITIES

1. Your neighbor says she has an odd spot on her calf and asks you to look at it. She has a red spot that seems to have a reddish ring around it. What questions would you ask her?

2. Your older brother calls complaining of excruciating pain in his left big toe and asking for advice. What would you say to him?

3. What would you teach a patient about measures to prevent gout attacks?

STEPS TOWARD BETTER COMMUNICATON

VOCABULARY BUILDING GLOSSARY

Term	Pronunciation	Definition
knit	nit	to grow together in small bits; to make clothing (sweaters) by connecting loops of yarn with long needles
impede'	im peed'	to slow, or get in the way of
imped'iment	im ped' ah ment	something that blocks or gets in the way of action
debris'	dah bree'	pieces left of something broken

COMPLETION

Directions: Fill in the blanks with the correct words from the Vocabulary Building Glossary to complete the statements.

1. Swelling under a cast may ________________________ blood flow.
2. Before a compound fracture is set, the surgeon cleans out any ______________ in the wound.
3. A splint often causes less ___________________________ to moving about than a cast.
4. If properly immobilized, the bone disrupted by a fracture will _____________.

GRAMMAR POINTS

Giving Instructions

The words you use when talking to a patient are very important to their understanding of what things are important and necessary for them to do. Here are some terms with the meanings they will have for the patient:

You can/you may indicate that the action is *optional.*

You should/you will indicate that the action is *recommended.*

Notice that the same term in the negative is usually stronger than the positive:

You can't/you shouldn't/you may not indicate the action is *required.*

You have to/you must/you mustn't/never indicate the action is *absolutely necessary.*

Here are some examples of each category.

Optional:

You can exercise your knee joint as many times a day as you can as long as it doesn't cause swelling.

You may apply ice packs to your back for the pain for 20 minutes of each hour.

If you like, **you can** use a heating pad for the discomfort.

Recommended:

Range of motion exercises **should** be done three or four times a day.

You should keep a pillow wedged between your legs when you lie on your side after hip surgery.

You shouldn't cross your legs after hip surgery.

Required:

Don't poke anything down into the cast.

Be sure to keep your leg cast dry.

You may not smoke or have caffeine for 8 hours before the test.

You can't let the traction weights set down on the bed.

Absolutely necessary:

You have to keep your weight off your foot for at least 3 weeks.

You must lie perfectly still for the bone scan.

You mustn't have any metal on your body for the MRI test.

Never remove these screws.

Assume you are giving instructions to a patient with a new leg cast. Use some of the phrases above to give one instruction from each category.

1. Optional:____

2. Recommended:____

3. Required:____

4. Absolutely necessary: ____

Other types of instruction statements:

Expectation or possibility statements:

Should can also mean *expectation* (The discomfort **should** be minimal) or *possibility* (If there **should** be any pain, you can take aspirin). It is also used to make a request more polite (I **should** think it would be good for you to exercise more often).

Consequence statements:

Consequence statements have the form of **If you . . ., then . . .**

If you get up and move around, **then** you will heal faster.

If you use heat treatments before you exercise, **then** your joint will not be as stiff.

If you get your cast wet, **then** it will have to be replaced.

CHAPTER 33

The Urinary System

evolve Go to http://evolve.elsevier.com/deWit for additional activities and exercises.

REVIEW OF ANATOMY AND PHYSIOLOGY

Labeling

Anatomy of the Kidney

Directions: Label the following structures on the diagram of the kidney. ***(817)***

renal artery
renal vein
fibrous capsule
renal pyramid
calyx
renal pelvis
renal papilla
medulla
cortex
renal column
ureter

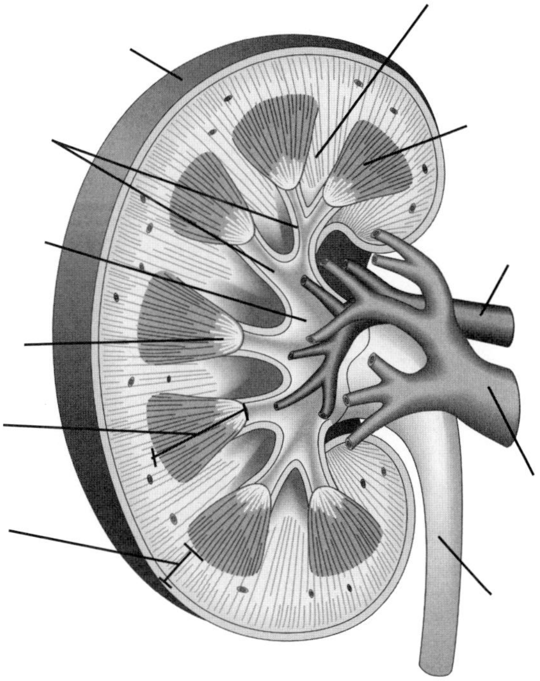

SHORT ANSWER

Assessing the Urinary System

Directions: Read the clinical scenario and answer the questions that follow.

Scenario: You are caring for several patients who have actual or are at risk for urinary disorders. In your daily assessment of these patients, you should look for specific kinds of data.

1. List five kinds of information that are of special interest when a patient has a urinary disorder. ***(825-827)***

   a. ______________________________

   b. ______________________________

   c. ______________________________

   d. ______________________________

   e. ______________________________

2. List five specific physical assessments that should be done on a patient with a urinary disorder. ***(821)***

   a. ______________________________

   b. ______________________________

   c. ______________________________

   d. ______________________________

   e. ______________________________

3. List four significant variations in the color of urine and two possible causes of each. ***(826)***

   a. Color change: ______________________________

      Possible causes: ______________________________

      ____

   b. Color change: ______________________________

      Possible causes: ______________________________

      ____

   c. Color change: ______________________________

      Possible causes: ______________________________

      ____

   d. Color change: ______________________________

      Possible causes: ______________________________

      ____

MATCHING

Diagnostic Testing

Directions: Match the diagnostic test (or test result) on the left with the most appropriate nursing action or assessment finding on the right.

1. ______ RBCs and WBCs in urine ***(822)***
2. ______ Hematuria ***(826)***
3. ______ Urine pH below 4.5 ***(822)***
4. ______ Creatinine clearance ***(822)***
5. ______ Ureteral and renal biopsy ***(825)***
6. ______ Urine culture ***(822)***
7. ______ Specific gravity below 1.010 and urine osmolality below 100 Osm/kg ***(822)***

a. Pink-tinged urine after test; increase fluid intake to minimize discomfort
b. Assess patient for signs of acidosis
c. Dilute urine
d. Instruct patient in steps to follow to collect a clean-catch midstream urine specimen
e. Assess patient for other signs of urinary tract infection
f. Try to determine at what point during urination blood first appears
g. Obtain a 24-hour urine specimen and one blood sample during test

COMPLETION

Urinary Disorders

Directions: Fill in the blanks to complete the statements.

1. An absence of urine is called ____________________, which rarely occurs, but may be associated with acute renal failure. ***(825)***
2. If your patient is having oliguria, the urinary output should be measured and recorded every ________________________. ***(828)***
3. In ____________________________, there is an abnormally high and dilute urinary output. ***(825)***
4. Urination that occurs during the night is known as________________________. ***(826)***
5. ___________________________ is voiding more often than every 2 hours because of inflammation, decreased bladder capacity, psychological disorders, or increased fluid intake. ***(826)***
6. ________________________ is a delay in starting the stream of urine which may be related to partial obstruction. ***(826)***
7. To check for ________________________________, have the patient void and then catheterize him to determine amount of urine left in the bladder. ***(826)***
8. If you suspect that the patient is having ____________________________, gently palpate the bladder for fullness. ***(826)***
9. You should encourage people to seek prompt treatment of ____________________________________ tract problems. ***(820)***

10. Emptying the bladder regularly prevents ____________________ and eliminates toxic substances. *(819)*

11. To help prevent urinary system disorders, the nurse out in the community should assist ________________ patients and ________________ patients to achieve good control of their chronic health conditions. *(819)*

12. Long-term care residents and home care patients are continuously monitored for signs of urinary tract ________________________. *(825)*

13. For critically ill patients, it may be necessary to measure urinary output every __________. *(828)*

APPLICATION OF THE NURSING PROCESS

Caring for a Patient with Urinary Incontinence

Directions: Read the scenario and provide the answers to the following questions.

Scenario: Mr. Yakada is an elderly gentleman who was recently admitted to an extended care facility. He has chronic urinary incontinence and currently he has an indwelling catheter. The family would like to have the catheter removed as soon as possible.

1. What factors could potentially contribute to Mr. Yakada's incontinence? ***(829-830)***
   a. Health conditions: ____
   ____
   ____
   b. Medications: ____
   ____

2. List three things to assess when a patient has an indwelling catheter. ***(829)***
   a. ____
   b. ____
   c. ____

3. Write an expected outcome for the nursing diagnosis: Risk for infection related to indwelling catheter.
   ____
   ____

4. List five nursing interventions to prevent infection for a patient with an indwelling catheter. ***(829)***
   a. ____
   b. ____
   c. ____
   d. ____
   e. ____

5. The physician writes an order to encourage fluids without restriction. At the end of the shift the I & O sheet indicates that Mr. Yakada had 8 ounces of water at 8:00 AM, 300 mL of juice for breakfast, 12 ounces of coffee for lunch, 10 ounces of milk for dinner and 800 mL is gone from his 1000 mL bedside water pitcher. How many mL total do you record for intake for this shift? ______________ mL

6. List five alternatives (nonsurgical) to an indwelling catheter for patients such as Mr. Yakada. ***(830-831)***

   a. ______________________________

   b. ______________________________

   c. ______________________________

   d. ______________________________

   e. ______________________________

7. Which of the following urinalysis results indicate that the expected outcome (free from infection) is being met? ***(822)***
   a. Color: amber yellow
   b. Odor: aromatic
   c. Specific gravity: 1.030
   d. White blood cells: 0–4 (per low power field)

PRIORITY SETTING

Directions: Read the scenario and prioritize the nursing actions as appropriate.

Scenario A: You are caring for Mrs. Popovitch on a rehabilitation unit. She has been doing well and is frequently ambulating off the unit with her family. She tells you that she is having urinary frequency, but currently denies any other symptoms.

1. What is your priority action?
   a. Measure and record urinary output every hour.
   b. Check to see if fluid intake is higher than usual.
   c. Obtain an order for a urinalysis.
   d. Notify the physician or RN.

Scenario B: You are working with a new nursing assistant who disconnects the catheter from the drainage bag tubing, "in order to collect a fresh urine specimen."

1. What is your priority action?
   a. Report the incident to the nurse manager.
   b. Allow her to continue and later talk to her in private.
   c. Do everything that assists her to maintain asepsis.
   d. Immediately stop her and do the procedure yourself.

NCLEX-PN® EXAM REVIEW

Directions: Choose the correct answer(s) for the following questions.

1. The patient reports having a color change in the urine. What question should the nurse ask first, in order to collect more information about this symptom? ***(826)***
   1. "Do you have any history of kidney problems?"
   2. "What color is the urine?"
   3. "Are you having any pain with urination?"
   4. "When did you first notice this?"

2. The patient is diagnosed with urinary retention. Which characteristic is least likely to be associated with this disorder? ***(832)***
   1. Dribbling of urine or passing only the overflow.
   2. Inability to void after removal of an indwelling catheter.
   3. Residual urine of greater than 100 mL.
   4. Passing urine when laughing, sneezing, or coughing.

3. A major cause of end-stage kidney disease is: ***(819)***
   1. hypertension.
   2. hyperthyroidism.
   3. prostate enlargement.
   4. kidney stones.

4. The patient is scheduled to have an intravenous pyelogram. Which of the following laboratory results should be reported to the radiologist before the patient has the procedure? ***(823)***
   1. An elevated WBC
   2. An elevated BUN
   3. A decreased RBC
   4. Urinalysis positive for nitrates

5. The nurse is explaining the procedure for a cystoscopy. After the procedure, the patient should expect which of following? ***(824)***
   1. NPO status for several hours after the procedure
   2. Burning, frequency, and pink-tinged urine
   3. Bedrest with bathroom privileges for 24 hours
   4. Indwelling catheter in place to measure output

6. The patient has returned from diagnostic testing. The physician's orders indicate to check vital signs, popliteal and pedal pulses q 15 min for the first hour, then q 2 hours x 2. This postprocedure care is appropriate for which of the following tests? ***(824)***
   1. Radionuclide renal scan
   2. Renal ultrasound
   3. Renal angiography
   4. Renal biopsy

CRITICAL THINKING ACTIVITIES

Scenario: You are caring for Mr. Whipple who is scheduled for a renal biopsy. He is very apprehensive. This is his first biopsy, and he admits that he does not know anything about it; however, he fears the worse about the procedure and the results.

1. List two purposes of a renal biopsy. ***(824)***

   a. ______________________________

   b. ______________________________

2. Write a very brief explanation of how the procedure is done and what Mr. Whipple will experience. ***(824)***

   ____

   ____

   ____

   ____

3. What two interventions could you used to help Mr. Whipple decrease his anxiety? ***(827-828)***

   a. ______________________________

   b. ______________________________

4. What is the most serious immediate postprocedure complication of a renal biopsy? ***(825)***
   a. Vomiting related to anesthesia
   b. Frank bleeding and hemorrhage
   c. Infection and inflammation
   d. Decreased urinary output

5. Mr. Whipple expresses fear and anxiety while waiting for the results. "I just can't stand this waiting. Call the doctor right now, or I am leaving the hospital!" What is the best response?
   a. "It's too dangerous for you to leave. You just had the procedure."
   b. "I'll call the doctor, if you agree to calm down and wait."
   c. "You can leave if you want to, it is your right to do as you wish."
   d. "I see that you are anxious. Let me check on the status of the report."

STEPS TOWARD BETTER COMMUNICATION

VOCABULARY BUILDING GLOSSARY

Term	**Definition**
hy poth' e size	to suggest an answer that explains a group of phenomena
pa' tent	open, unobstructed
pa' ten cy	the condition of being open

PRONUNCIATION SKILLS

Directions: Pronounce the following words.

Lithotripsy (lith'o trip' sy)	crushing stones in an organ such as the kidney
Plasmapheresis (plas'ma pher e'sis)	removal of plasma from withdrawn blood and retransfusion in a different form into the donor
Oliguria (ol i gu' ri a)	diminished urine secretion in relation to fluid intake
Polyuria (pol i u'ri a)	excessive secretion of urine
Suprapubic (su' pra pu' bic)	above the pubes
Extracorporeal (ex' tra cor po're al)	situated or occurring outside the body

COMPLETION

Directions: Fill in the blank with the correct word from the Vocabulary Building Glossary and Pronunciation Skills.

1. Make sure the tube is ________________ before you use it.
2. We ____________________ that the infection is bacterial, but we will need to check it.
3. The physician will perform a ________________ on the patient with stones.

WORD ATTACK SKILLS

Directions: Write the meaning of the word element.

1. Olig(o)-: ____
2. Poly-: ____
3. Supra-: ____
4. Extra-: ____
5. Hypo-: ____

COMMUNICATION EXERCISE

1. With a peer, practice performing a urologic assessment and history-taking. Use the Focused Assessment 33-1 Assessment: Guide to Urological Assessment in the textbook. Each partner should listen for clear pronunciation and may ask for an explanation of a word or procedure.
2. Write a dialogue you could use to ask questions about drug history.

GRAMMAR POINTS

When you are trying to establish a history from a patient, it is very important to use the correct past or present tense. You want to clearly determine what has happened in the past, such as what medications he/she has taken, as opposed to what medications are being used now.

Examples:

Have you had frequency of urination in the past?

Do you have frequency of urination now?

CULTURAL POINTS

There are many commonly used terms for urination, many which are nonmedical and were learned in childhood but are still used by adults. You may need to know these when talking with your patients. For example, I need to urinate, void, pee, make pee-pee, go pee, make water, take a leak, use the urinal, go to the toilet, etc. With your classmates, make a list of as many medical and nonmedical terms you can think of.

CHAPTER 34

Care of Patients with Disorders of the Urinary System

evolve Go to http://evolve.elsevier.com/deWit for additional activities and exercises.

COMPLETION

Directions: Fill in the blanks to complete the statements.

azotemia
thrill
dysuria
nocturia
nephrectomy

1. When a patient is in early renal failure, he has ______________________. ***(854)***

2. The patient complaining of burning is experiencing the symptom called ______________________ ______________. ***(840)***

3. You assess an arteriovenous shunt by feeling for a ____________________________ over the shunt. ***(858)***

4. Having to get up at night more than once to urinate is called ______________________________. ***(826)***

5. The patient with cancer of the kidney often undergoes a __________________________ procedure. ***(843)***

SHORT ANSWER

Cancers of the Urinary System

Directions: Provide answers for the following questions.

1. Often the only sign of cancer of the bladder is ______________________. ***(848)***

2. What are four risk factors for cancer of the bladder? ***(848)***

   a. ____

   b. ____

   c. ____

   d. ____

3. What are three diagnostic tests that are used to confirm bladder cancer? ***(848)***

   a. ______________________________

   b. ______________________________

   c. ______________________________

4. How does photodynamic therapy for bladder cancer work? ***(848)***______________________________

   ____

   ____

5. A sign of kidney cancer is hematuria. Other symptoms that may occur are ____________________, ____________________, ____________________, ____________________, and ____________________. ***(848)***

6. The primary treatment for cancer of the kidney is ____________________ before metastasis has occurred. ***(848)***

Urinary Diversion

Directions: Read the scenario and provide the answers to the following questions.

Scenario: You are caring for several patients who have urinary diversions. You recognize that while there are various surgical procedures that the physician may perform, there are some commonalities in the nursing care such as I & O and ostomy care.

1. An ileal conduit provides for evacuation of ____________________. ***(848)***

2. A cutaneous ureterostomy produces ____________________ urine. ***(848)***

3. The problem with a sigmoid conduit is that ____________________ frequently occurs.

4. The immediate postoperative nursing care plan of a patient with diversion of urinary flow should include the following nursing actions: ***(850)***

   a. Measurement of: ______________________________

   b. Observation of:______________________________

5. Write a short-term goal for the nursing diagnosis: Body image disturbance related to ostomy.

   ____

   ____

   ____

6. List three common causes of periostomal skin problems *other than* seepage of urinary waste around the stoma. ***(850)***

a. ____________________

b. ____________________

c. ____________________

7. List five nursing interventions that could help a patient prevent or overcome odor from an ureterostomy. ***(850)***

   a. ____________________

   b. ____________________

   c. ____________________

   d. ____________________

   e. ____________________

LABELING

Different Types of Urinary Diversions

Directions: Label the drawings below with the correct name of the procedure depicted, using the following list. ***(849)***

ureterosigmoidostomy (sigmoid conduit)
ileal reservoir (Kock's pouch)
cutaneous ureterostomy
ileal conduit

____

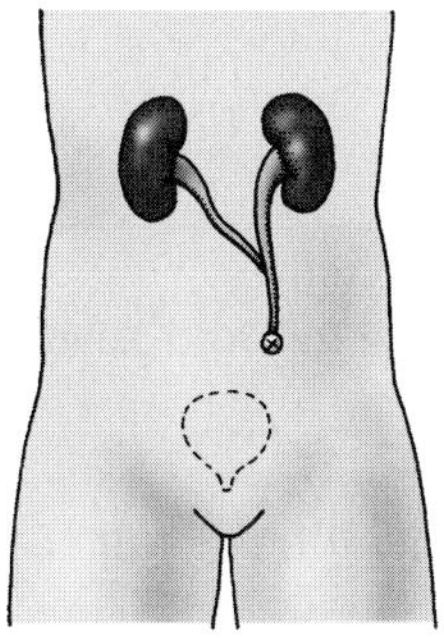

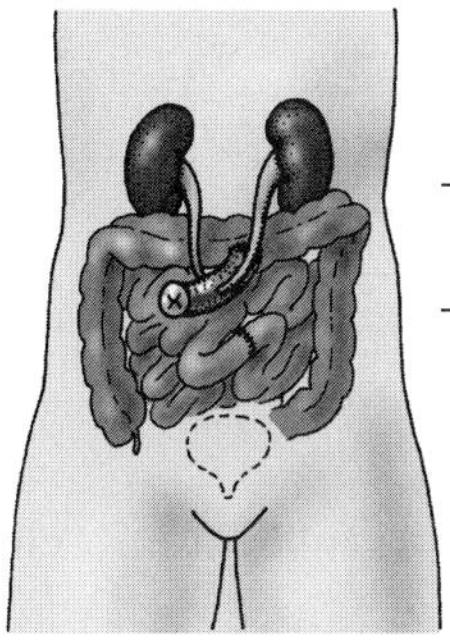

____

____

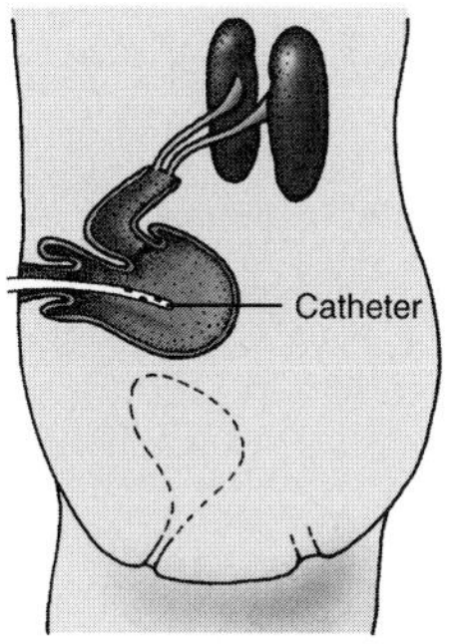

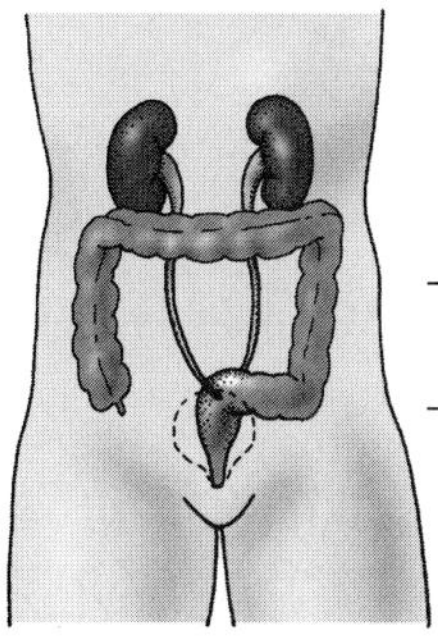

____

APPLICATION OF THE NURSING PROCESS

Caring for a Patient with a Kidney Stone

Directions: Read the scenario and provide the answers to the following questions.

Scenario: You are working in a clinic and Mr. Depp arrives in acute distress and complains of severe left lower back pain. He is restless and pacing and unable to focus on your questions. His wife tells you that he is peeing small amounts of bloody urine.

1. List at least four risk factors for kidney stones. ***(844)***

   a. ____________________

   b. ____________________

   c. ____________________

   d. ____________________

2. Which of the following nursing diagnoses is a priority for Mr. Depp?
   a. Risk for alteration in urinary elimination related to obstruction of flow
   b. Pain related to ureteral spasm and probable movement of kidney stone
   c. Risk of urinary tract infection related to urinary stasis
   d. Communication, impaired related to discomfort

3. What are three important nursing actions in the care of a patient who is trying to pass a kidney stone? ***(846)***

   a. ____________________

   b. ____________________

   c. ____________________

4. A kidney stone that is easily seen on x-ray is one that is ____________________. ***(845)***

5. When teaching a patient at risk for stone formation how to avoid developing kidney stones, you should tell him to drink enough liquids to produce at least __________ mL of urine every 24 hours. ***(854)***

6. What are three things you should teach Mr. Depp about the lithotripsy procedure? ***(846)***

   a. ____________________

   b. ____________________

   c. ____________________

7. Which of the following statements by Mr. Depp indicates that he understands the information about lithotripsy? ***(846)***
   a. "The procedure is done on a x-ray table."
   b. "I'll have to remain very still for about 10 minutes."
   c. "I should not feel any pain or discomfort during the procedure."
   d. " If I walk around as soon as I am able it will help to flush stones."

PRIORITY SETTING

Directions: Read the scenario and prioritize as appropriate.

Scenario: Mr. Wyaksit is postoperative from a kidney transplant and was transferred 5 days ago from the ICU to the general medical-surgical unit. He appeared to be recovering quickly and was independently ambulating. Last night, he tripped and fell to the floor, but appeared uninjured and told the nurse, "no damage done." This morning he is reluctant to get out of bed. Which set of assessment findings is the most critical?

a. Pulse 130/min, BP 90/60, Hct 30%
b. Fever 102° F, redness at the incision site
c. Urinary output of 25 mL/hr, rising BUN
d. Pain over the iliac fossa transplant area

NCLEX-PN® EXAM REVIEW

Directions: Choose the correct answer(s) for the following questions.

1. When the normal flow of urine is obstructed, urine can back up into the urinary tract and fill the kidney pelvis. This is called: *(843)*
   1. pyelonephritis.
   2. Staghorn calculus.
   3. hydronephrosis.
   4. renal stenosis.

2. The patient is diagnosed with a bladder infection. Which characteristic is least likely associated with this disorder? *(838)*
   1. Burning upon urination
   2. Foul-smelling urine
   3. Decreased urinary output
   4. Elevated temperature

3. Hemodialysis is performed for the end-stage kidney disease patient. Data that indicate effectiveness would be: *(857)*
   1. a rise in hemoglobin and hematocrit.
   2. a fall in glucose and sodium levels.
   3. a fall in potassium, creatinine, and urea levels.
   4. an increased alertness and a sense of well-being.

4. Other than taking baseline vital signs, an important nursing intervention to perform the morning of dialysis is: *(859)*
   1. keeping the patient NPO until after the dialysis.
   2. administrating 1 liter of normal saline to prevent shock.
   3. giving subcutaneous heparin to prevent blood clotting during dialysis.
   4. withholding blood pressure medications until the pressure has stabilized after dialysis.

5. When planning nursing care for the patient who has renal failure, the nurse encourages a diet that is: *(867)*
   1. high in calories but low in protein and potassium.
   2. high in protein, moderate in calories, and low in sodium.
   3. high in fat and protein but low in potassium and sodium.
   4. high in fiber, with mainly fruits and vegetables and some grains.

6. A nursing intervention for the patient who has just returned from surgery with a new arteriovenous shunt is to: ***(858)***
   1. maintain a heparin drip to prevent clotting in the shunt.
   2. release the elevated extremity and perform range of motion exercises every 2 hours.
   3. assess the shunt site for hematoma and check for bruit every 2–4 hours.
   4. assess the shunt for visual signs of clotting every 2–4 hours.

7. The nurse is looking at abnormal results of a urinalysis. Which finding is more specific to chronic glomerulonephritis, and is less likely to be present if the patient has an acute cystitis? ***(842)***
   1. Glucose
   2. Red blood cells
   3. Urinary casts
   4. White blood cells

8. Planning nursing care for the patient with cystitis who is experiencing considerable discomfort includes: ***(837)***
   1. decrease fluid intake to prevent discomfort of voiding.
   2. hot sitz baths to increase circulation and decrease discomfort.
   3. continuous intravenous fluid administration.
   4. obtain a urine specimen for culture and sensitivity.

9. Sulfamethoxaszole-trimethoprim (Bactrim) is prescribed for the patient's cystitis. When doing discharge teaching, the nurse would be sure to instruct the patient to: ***(839)***
   1. take the medication between meals to enhance absorption.
   2. take 3000–4000 mL of fluid per day to prevent crystallization.
   3. be aware that this medication might turn the urine orange or red.
   4. watch for signs of jaundice associated with liver toxicity.

10. What changes in the urinary system occur with aging that predispose elderly women to urinary frequency and infection? ***(838)***
    1. Decreased fluid intake to prevent incontinence
    2. An increased glomerular filtration rate
    3. Estrogen depletion that results in structural atrophy
    4. An increased bladder capacity due to loss of tone

11. Which signs and symptoms are associated with nephrotic syndrome? ***(842)***
    1. Proteinuria, hyperlipidemia, hypoalbuminemia, and severe edema
    2. Painful urination, frequent and urgent urination, and low back pain
    3. Burning, itching, frequency in voiding, and painful urination
    4. Unilateral flank pain that radiates into the genitalia and inner thigh

12. A patient has acute renal failure and is in the diuretic phase. With an increased output, there is a danger of: ***(852)***
    1. hyponatremia.
    2. hyperkalemia.
    3. fluid overload.
    4. catabolism.

13. A patient with chronic renal failure is receiving epoietin alpha (Epogen). The purpose of this medication is to: ***(857)***
    1. increase urinary output.
    2. bind phosphate; given with meals.
    3. prevent problems of calcium loss.
    4. treat anemia; promotes RBC formation.

14. One of the relevant nursing diagnoses in caring for a patient with renal failure is Activity intolerance related to metabolic changes. Which of the following interventions would be appropriate in helping the patient accomplish ADLs? *(855)*
    1. Tell the patient to do as much as he can first and then return later to help him finish.
    2. Instruct the nursing assistant to watch him do ADLs and report back on his progress.
    3. Instruct the nursing assistant to do everything for him unless he tells her that he can do it himself.
    4. Assess his energy level in the morning and then direct the nursing assistant to do specific tasks for him.

15. Which of the following is characteristic of stage 1 chronic renal failure? *(855)*
    1. BUN and serum creatinine levels begin to rise.
    2. Glomerular filtration rate falls and oliguria and edema occur.
    3. Urine concentration is decreased and polyuria and nocturia occur.
    4. Electrolyte and fluid imbalances are serious; wastes accumulate.

CRITICAL THINKING ACTIVITIES

Scenario: Mr. Sounds has chronic renal failure. His physician has decided that Mr. Sounds is a good candidate for peritoneal dialysis. This is a new therapy for Mr. Sounds, but he is eager to learn and cooperate.

1. Prepare a brief description of the purpose of peritoneal dialysis and the principle by which it works to help Mr. Sounds understand this new therapy. *(859-860)*

    ____

    ____

    ____

2. List five nursing actions specific to the care of Mr. Sounds for his peritoneal dialysis. *(859-860)*

    a. ______________________________

    b. ______________________________

    c. ______________________________

    d. ______________________________

    e. ______________________________

3. When administering peritoneal dialysis to Mr. Sounds, you would evaluate him each day. What is the most common complication? *(860)*
    a. Peritonitis
    b. Clotting of the catheter
    c. Hemorrhage from heparin in the solution
    d. Retention of in-flow solution within the abdomen

STEPS TOWARD BETTER COMMUNICATION

VOCABULARY BUILDING GLOSSARY

Term	Pronunciation	Definition
urgency	er' jen see	a need for immediate action, hurry
linked	link'ed	connected, joined
intermittent	in ter mit' ent	happening with stops and starts; periodic
pertinent	per' tin ent	pertaining to or related to; important to know in relation to a subject
flank		the side of the body between the ribs and ilium
void		to expel urine from the bladder; to make invalid

COMPLETION

Directions: Fill in each blank with the correct word from the Vocabulary Building Glossary.

1. A sign of kidney infection is pain in the ____________________ area.
2. The nurse asks the patient to ____________ into a specimen container for a urinalysis.
3. If the patient states that there has been blood in the urine, it is a very ____________________ piece of information.
4. The patient with cystitis experiences dysuria, but may also have urinary ____________________.
5. Smoking has been ____________ as a risk factor in cancer of the bladder.
6. The male with benign prostatic hypertrophy (BPH) may experience an ________________ stream when he urinates.

WORD ATTACK SKILLS

Combining Forms

nephr/o-	kidney
glomerul/o-	network of capillaries
ur/o-	urine, urinary tract
ren/o-	kidney
oli/olig/o-	little, few, scanty
poly-	many, much

Directions: Using slash marks, break these words into their word elements or parts. Write the meaning of each word part, then give the meaning of the word.

1. Glomerulonephritis: ____

____

____

2. Hypoalbuminemia: ______________________________

____

____

3. Nephrolithotomy: ______________________________

____

____

4. Pyelonephrolithotomy: ______________________________

____

____

5. Ureterosigmoidostomy: ______________________________

____

____

PRONUNCIATION SKILLS

Directions: Pronounce these abbreviations and write their meanings.

1. ARF: ______________________________
2. CRF: ______________________________
3. GFR: ______________________________
4. ATN: ______________________________
5. UTI: ______________________________
6. NSU: ______________________________
7. ESRD: ______________________________
8. ESWL: ______________________________
9. TURP: ______________________________
10. AV: ______________________________
11. CAPD: ______________________________

Pronunciation Pairs Exercise

Many words are pronounced the same except for the last letter that creates the final sound. It is important that this final sound be pronounced correctly so that the listener will understand the meaning of what is being said. Many of these sounds are difficult for the second language speaker to hear and pronounce.

Pronunciation

Directions: With a study partner, take turns pronouncing the word pairs listed below while the other listens without looking at the list. The listener should write down the words heard. Take turns speaking and then listening. Check to see that the words written by the listener are correct. (For extra practice, write the word pairs on small cards and mix up the order. Do the exercise frequently.)

life	live	barf	bark	duct	duck
of	up	ureter	urethra	tape	take
have	had	loop	lose	waste	wake
can	can't	lose	loose	help	health
out	ouch	tube	tooth	holds	holes
track	tract	gland	clamp	stones	stomas
putting	pudding	car	cart	lab	lap

CHAPTER 35

The Endocrine System

evolve Go to http://evolve.elsevier.com/deWit for additional activities and exercises.

COMPLETION

Directions: Fill in the blanks to complete the statements. ***(873-875)***

1. The hormone TSH is secreted by the ________________________________.
2. Synthesis of thyroid hormones requires an adequate dietary intake of ______________ and ______________________________.
3. Patients with primary hypothyroidism usually have low levels of __________ and __________________________________.
4. Parathormone acts on the renal tubules to increase the excretion of ________________ in the urine and the reabsorption of _______________.
5. Parathormone raises the serum calcium level by stimulating _____________________ and increasing calcium absorption in the ______________________________ tract.
6. A hormone produced by the adrenal cortex, which influences sodium and water balance, is ______________________________.
7. The adrenal medulla secretes _________________________ and _____________________________ _____________________.
8. The adrenal cortex secretes mainly __________________________ and ________________________ _____________________.
9. The mineralocorticoids affect the balance of ____________________________.
10. The glucocorticoids are essential for proper utilization of _________________, _________________, and ___________________________.
11. The primary glucocorticoid is _________________________________.
12. Primary actions of cortisol are to increase __________________ levels and to ___________________________ the inflammatory response.
13. Beta cells in the pancreas secrete the hormone ___________________.

TABLE ACTIVITY

Hormone Changes that Occur with Aging

Directions: Complete the table below. Add the hormones that increase, decrease, or essentially remain unchanged with aging. The first block is done for you. ***(876-877)***

Hormones that usually decrease with age	aldosterone, renin, calcitonin, and growth hormone; in the older female, estrogen and prolactin; and in the older male, testosterone
Hormones that may increase with age	
Hormones that remain unchanged or are slightly decreased	

SHORT ANSWER

Hypothyroidism

Directions: Read the clinical scenario and answer the questions that follow.

Scenario: You are working in an endocrinology clinic. Mrs. Venucha is an older woman who has been referred by her family doctor for a possible thyroid disorder. Mrs. Venchua tells you that she has been slowing down lately and has felt "mildly bloated, sluggish, and constipated." She agreed to have some diagnostic testing done, but she feels she needs some general information about the thyroid and the diagnostic testing.

1. List five effects of thyroid hormones. ***(878)***

   a. ______________________________

   b. ______________________________

   c. ______________________________

   d. ______________________________

   e. ______________________________

2. Name four serum tests that are done to evaluate thyroid function. ***(879)***

   a. ______________________________

   b. ______________________________

   c. ______________________________

   d. ______________________________

3. List four commonly used drugs that can alter the results of thyroid tests. ***(879)***

    a. ______________________________

    b. ______________________________

    c. ______________________________

    d. ______________________________

4. List at least three teaching points to include for a patient who needs a radioactive iodine uptake exam to assess thyroid function. ***(880)***

    a. ______________________________

    b. ______________________________

    c. ______________________________

5. Briefly describe how aging affects the thyroid gland and thyroid hormone levels. ***(878)***

    a. ______________________________

    ____

    b. ______________________________

    ____

    c. ______________________________

    ____

    d. ______________________________

    ____

APPLICATION OF THE NURSING PROCESS

Caring for Patients at Risk for Type 2 Diabetes

Directions: Read the scenario and provide the answers to the following questions.

Scenario: You are working in an ambulatory clinic. Mr. Bob, a middle-aged gentleman, comes in for a check-up and he reports having mild fatigue and some gradual but progressive weight gain over the past 6 months. He suspects he may have diabetes, "because my father had it."

1. List five or six questions to ask a patient who is suspected of having an endocrine disorder. ***(883)***

____

____

____

____

____

2. Write an example of an appropriate outcome for the nursing diagnosis: Imbalanced nutrition, more than body requirements, related to altered glucose metabolism. ***(883)***

____

____

3. List three general nursing interventions that will help a diabetic patient who has Imbalanced nutrition, more than body requirements to maintain a normal body weight. ***(883)***

   a. _______________

   b. _______________

   c. _______________

4. Write an example of evaluation outcome for the following goal: Patient will verbalize beginning understanding of diagnostic testing for diabetes at the end of teaching session. ***(883)***

____

____

____

____

____

____

5. Mr. Bob currently weighs 225 lbs. The doctor has suggested that he should gradually lose weight to achieve a target goal of 85 kg. Mr. Bob asks you help him with some calculations.

   a. How long will it take him to achieve the target goal if he can lose 4 pounds/month? _______________

   b. How long will it take him to achieve the target goal if he can lose 5 pounds/month? _______________

   c. How long will it take him to achieve the target goal if he can lose 8 pounds/month? _______________

PRIORITY SETTING

Directions: Read the scenario and prioritize as appropriate.

Scenario: You are the only nurse standing in the nurse's station and the unit secretary hands you computer printouts of several laboratory values.

1. Which patient needs priority attention?
   a. Mr. Jez has positive ketone bodies in the urine .
   b. Ms. Lukic has serum T_4 of 10 mg/dL.
   c. Mr. Doig has a 2-hour postprandial glucose of 150 mg/dL.
   d. Mrs. Kost has a fasting blood glucose of 20 mg/dL.

2. You recognize that one of the patients needs immediate attention; however, Mr. Jez, Mr. Doig, and Mrs. Kost have been assigned to other nurses. Of the four patients, Ms. Lukic is the only patient that has been assigned to you. What is your priority action?
   a. Check on Ms. Lukic.
   b. Find the nurse assigned to the critical patient.
   c. Inform the charge nurse about the lab values.
   d. Check on the most critical patient.

NCLEX-PN® EXAM REVIEW

Directions: Choose the correct answer(s) for the following questions.

1. Which gland is known as the "master gland" of the body? ***(873)***
   1. Adrenal gland
   2. Thyroid gland
   3. Pituitary gland
   4. Pineal gland

2. A patient is diagnosed with a thyroid disorder. The nurse anticipates that the patient is mostly likely to have problems with: ***(879)***
   1. metabolic rate.
   2. water reabsoprtion.
   3. bone fragility.
   4. increased blood glucose.

3. A hormone that inhibits gonadotropin-releasing hormone and therefore inhibits reproduction is: ***(878)***
   1. progesterone.
   2. estrogen
   3. melatonin.
   4. testosterone.

4. The patient is undergoing a hypertonic saline test to detect diabetes insipidus. One of the nursing responsibilities is to teach the patient to: ***(881)***
   1. produce a urine specimen using a clean-catch technique.
   2. produce a urine specimen in the marked container each hour.
   3. void in the early AM and discard the first urine specimen.
   4. produce a urine specimen at the end of the test period.

5. The doctor orders a dexamethasone suppression test to assist in the diagnosis of Cushing's disease. An appropriate nursing action would be to: *(880)*
   1. collect a clean-catch urine specimen.
   2. note the start and end time on the laboratory slip.
   3. check orders for drugs to be withheld.
   4. administer vasopressin SC as ordered.

6. A patient is being tested to determine the degree of diabetic control of blood sugar over the preceding 6–8 weeks. Which of the following is the correct test to make this determination? *(882)*
   1. Fasting blood glucose
   2. 2-hour postprandial blood glucose
   3. Glucose tolerance test
   4. Glycosolated hemoglobin

7. Which of the following is at greatest risk for injury related to bone fracture? *(874)*
   1. Patient with a thyroid disorder.
   2. Patient with a parathyroid disorder
   3. Patient with a pancreatic disorder
   4. Patient with a testicular disorder

8. The doctor orders laboratory tests for several serum electrolytes. Which of the following reflect the parathyroid function? *(881)*
   1. Calcium and phosphorus
   2. Sodium and magnesium
   3. Potassium and chloride
   4. Sodium and potassium

9. The patient needs several diagnostic tests to rule out endocrine disorders. Which of the following tasks would be appropriate to assign to the nursing assistant? *(4)*
   1. Note medications that the patient takes on laboratory slip.
   2. Ask the patient if he has any questions or needs anything.
   3. Instruct the patient on how to obtain a clean-catch specimen.
   4. Deliver the urine specimen to the laboratory.

CRITICAL THINKING ACTIVITIES

Scenario A: Your neighbor tells you that she is thinking about taking synthroid to lose weight because a relative has been taking synthroid that was obtained "through the Internet" and that person lost about 15 pounds very easily.

1. How would you respond to your neighbor? ______________________________

____

____

____

____

____

2. One of the functions of the thyroid hormones is to affect tissue response to epinephrine and norepinephrine. Briefly describe to your neighbor the potential effects on blood pressure and heart rate. ***(874)***

3. Discuss some of the problems that might occur as people try to save money by using the Internet as a health care resource. ***(885)***

Scenario B: Your cousin tells you that she thinks she has hypoglycemia. She wants your opinion about whether she might have diabetes. Her doctor has reassured her that she does not have diabetes, but she doesn't believe him.

1. Write a brief statement that you could use to redirect your cousin back to her doctor. ***(931-932)***

2. List at least five questions that your cousin could ask her doctor. ***(931-932)***

   a.

   b.

   c.

   d.

   e.

3. Would you feel comfortable giving her an opinion about the diabetes? Why or why not?

____

____

____

____

____

____

____

STEPS TOWARD BETTER COMMUNICATION

VOCABULARY BUILDING GLOSSARY

Term	Pronunciation	Definition
alter	al'ter	to change, to make different
aspect	as'pect	area, or part of a surface
assay	ass'ay	a test for purity
elicit	e lis'it	to gather information from someone
lability	labil'ity	instability
negative feedback	neg' a tive feed' back	a response to a message which is intended to change or stop the message
postprandial	post pran' di al	after dinner, or any other meal
render	ren'der	to cause a change
sluggish	slug'gish	slow-moving, inactive
stalk	stawk	1. (noun) a stem or support of a plant or organ. 2. (verb) to follow pursue secretly.
synthesis	syn'the sis	combining of parts to make a whole

COMPLETION

Directions: Fill in the blanks with the appropriate words from the Vocabulary Building Glossary to complete the statements.

1. The person who has hypothyroidism usually feels ________________________.

2. A patient should be instructed not to ____________________ their medication regimen without first consulting a physician.

3. When there is too much circulating cortisol in a person's system, he often displays emotional ____.

4. Pituitary problems may _______________________________ a female infertile.

5. When checking for thyroid disease, the examiner pays particular attention to the frontal ____ of the neck.

6. Fructosamine _____________________ is another test to monitor control of glucose over time.

7. The word *parathormone* is a _________________ of the two words *parathyroid* and *hormone*.

8. The patient gave ____________________ in response to the questionnaire about the new hospital menus.

9. She cut the ________________ of the flower so that it would fit the vase.

10. A nap is often the favorite _________________ "exercise" of many people.

11. A good history-taking will ________________ a lot of information from the patient.

WORD ATTACK SKILLS

hyper-	over, more
hypo-	under, less
endo-	internal
exo-	external
para-	beside, next to; near

PRONUNCIATION SKILLS

Directions: Take turns practicing with a peer pronouncing these words to increase your ability to speak English clearly.

adenohypophysis (ad noh hi po' us sis)	anterior pituitary
adrenocorticotropic (ah dree'no cor'tih ko tro'pik)	a hormone acting on the adrenal cortex
verbalization (ver'bal iz a' shun)	putting into words
antiinflammatory (an' ti in flam'ah tor y)	preventing inflammation
hypopituitary (hi' po pih tu' ih tar y)	decreased secretions from the pituitary gland

CHAPTER 36

Care of Patients with Pituitary, Thyroid, Parathyroid, and Adrenal Disorders

evolve Go to http://evolve.elsevier.com/deWit for additional activities and exercises.

COMPLETION

Directions: Fill in the blanks to complete the statements.

1. Simple goiter causes problems when it enlarges to the point of placing ______________________________ ______________________. ***(893)***
2. Simple goiter is treated by ____. ***(893-894)***
3. Graves' disease is another name given to ______________________________. ***(893)***
4. The first sign of thyroid cancer may be a _____________________ found on a routine physical examination. ***(899)***
5. The treatment for thyroid cancer is ____________________________________. ***(899)***
6. After a thyroidectomy, the complication of ____________________ sometimes occurs. ***(897)***
7. One type of patient who often has an imbalance of parathyroid hormone is one with ____. ***(900)***
8. Hypoparathyroidism can be caused by accidental ______________________ of parathyroid tissue during a thyroidectomy or ________________________ of the thyroid. ***(899)***
9. The chief symptom resulting from an acute lowering of serum calcium is ____________________________. ***(899-900)***
10. Laboratory testing for hyperparathyroidism involves evaluating serum levels of _______________________ and __________________________. ***(900)***
11. A person with Addison's disease must receive __________________________ and _______________________ ______________________. ***(902)***
12. The danger in an Addisonian crisis is severe _____________________ and possible shock. ***(902)***
13. Signs of diabetes insipidus are _________________________________ and polydipsia. ***(891-892)***
14. Patients with Cushing's syndrome may have weakness due to abnormal protein catabolism and show loss of ______________________________________. ***(905)***

15. *Iatrogenic* Cushing's syndrome can be caused by ________________ therapy. ***(905)***

16. The patient with diabetes insipidus may produce ______________ liters of urine in 24 hours. ***(890)***

17. Diabetes insipidus occurs as a result of decreased production of ____________, which regulates ____________________________ in the kidney tubules. ***(889)***

18. Diabetes insipidus is treated with ________________________________ orally, intravenously, or by nasal inhalation. ***(891)***

19. The syndrome of inappropriate antidiuretic hormone secretion causes ____________________________ of fluid. ***(891)***

20. Pheochromocytoma is a rare tumor of the ____________________________ which secretes catecholamines. ***(901)***

21. You receive an order to infuse 500 mL of normal saline over 6 hours. What is the pump setting?

____

SHORT ANSWER

Signs and Symptoms of Endocrine Disorders

Directions: Provide the answers to the following questions.

1. List at least five signs and symptoms of hypothyroidism. ***(898)***

   a. ____

   b. ____

   c. ____

   d. ____

   e. ____

2. List at least five signs and symptoms of adrenal cortical insufficiency (Addison's disease). ***(901)***

   a. ____

   b. ____

   c. ____

   d. ____

   e. ____

APPLICATION OF THE NURSING PROCESS

Care of Patients with Hyperthyroidism

Directions: Read the clinical scenario and answer the questions that follow.

Scenario: You are caring for a middle-aged woman, Mrs. Riata, who has been admitted for treatment of her hyperthyroidism. Mrs. Riata has been living with this diagnosis for a period of time; however, she has not had success with conservative therapy, so she is being admitted for a partial thyroidectomy. Although she is knowledgeable about the disease and the impending surgery, she is emotionally labile and appears exhausted.

1. The physical signs and symptoms of hyperthyroidism include: ***(893)*** ______________________________

____

____

2. Psychological or emotional symptoms of hyperthyroidism include episodes of: ***(893)*** ______________

____

____

____

3. Which of the following nursing diagnoses is likely to be included in the care plan for Mrs. Riata? ***(895-896)***
   a. Self-care deficit related to lethargy
   b. Altered nutrition, more than body requirements, related to decreased metabolic rate
   c. Self-esteem disturbance related to facial puffiness and swelling
   d. Constipation related to decreased gastrointestinal motility
   e. Anxiety related to agitation and difficulty concentrating

4. List three nursing actions that should be included in the postoperative nursing care plan of a patient after partial thyroidectomy. ***(895-896)***

   a. ____

   ____

   b. ____

   ____

   c. ____

   ____

5. Write an example of an evaluation outcome for the following patient goal. Patient will rest at least 7 hours per night and take frequent rest breaks during the day while in the hospital.

____

____

____

____

____

PRIORITY SETTING

Directions: Read the clinical scenario and prioritize nursing actions as appropriate. Also identify tasks that can be performed by various members of the health care team.

Scenario: You arrive for your shift at the hospital. Before you can even get your coat off, the day shift RN says, "Quick! Come and help me! I have a patient who is going down the tubes! You run to the room and recognize Mrs. Dredge who has hypothyroidism. The RN says, "The doctor has just diagnosed her with myxedema coma and wrote these orders. Will you help me and the nursing assistant so that we can take care of this lady quickly?" ***(898)***

1. Prioritize the top five interventions that need to be accomplished first.
2. Identify which tasks (if any) could be assigned to the nursing assistant or the unit secretary.
3. Identify which tasks (if any) should be done only by the RN.

_____ a. Assess response to external warming blanket

_____ b. O_2 at 3 L per N/C

_____ c. Vital signs q 2 hours and notify physician for BP <100/60 or > 160/90

_____ d. Blood glucose STAT

_____ e. Levothyroxine sodium now 0.5 mg IV push over 5 minutes

_____ f. IV access X 2 (Saline lock X 1)

_____ g. IV bolus 250 mL X1 over 30 minutes STAT

_____ h. Place on cardiac monitor

_____ i. Continuous pulse oximeter

_____ j. Maintenance IV D_5.45 NS 150 mL/hour

_____ k. Call for EKG now

_____ l. Give 1/2 amp D_{10} IV push for BS < 60

NCLEX-PN® EXAM REVIEW

Directions: Choose the correct answer(s) for the following questions.

1. A patient is admitted for a minor elective surgery. He also has a diagnosis of Cushing's syndrome. Which physical assessment findings are associated with Cushing's and are likely to be documented in the patient's record? ***(905)***
   1. Dry, scaly skin and brittle nails.
   2. Abnormal protrusion of the eyeballs
   3. Enlarged thyroid gland
   4. Buffalo hump and moon face

2. A patient is diagnosed with diabetes insipidus. Which finding is characteristic of this disorder? ***(890)***
   1. Excessive dilute urine
   2. An increased blood pressure
   3. Tachycardia
   4. Exertional dyspnea

3. The nurse is caring for a patient who has SIADH. Which of the following nursing interventions is appropriate for the care of this patient? ***(892)***
   1. Giving hypotonic enemas as ordered.
   2. Restricting fluids to 500–1000 mL/day as ordered.
   3. Administering somatropin via subcutaneous injection as ordered.
   4. Administering IV calcium gluconate as ordered.

4. The nurse is caring for a patient who is receiving large doses of radioactive iodine. The care plan should include which of the following precautions? ***(893-894)***
   1. No special precautions beyond standard precautions
   2. Wearing lead aprons when delivering nursing care
   3. Isolation of the patient for 8 days (half-life of drug)
   4. Having the patient wear a radiation detection badge

5. The patient is diagnosed with a rare tumor of the adrenal gland (pheochromocytoma). The nurse recognizes that the priority vital sign to monitor frequently is: ***(901)***
   1. respiratory rate.
   2. temperature.
   3. blood pressure.
   4. pulse.

6. The nurse is caring for a postoperative patient who has had a hypophysectomy. Which of the following nursing interventions would be appropriate in the care of this patient? *(Select all that apply.)* ***(888)***
   1. Keep the patient flat in bed.
   2. Note and report change in mental status.
   3. Change nasal drip pad as needed.
   4. Instruct patient to cough deeply.
   5. Assist the patient with mouth rinses.

7. The nurse is assessing a patient with simple goiter. The first sign usually noticed in this condition is: ***(893)***
   1. difficulty swallowing.
   2. difficulty breathing.
   3. enlargement in the front of the neck.
   4. abnormal protrusion of the eyeballs.

8. The nurse is administering an iodine preparation to a patient. A nursing implication of administering this drug includes: ***(893)***
   1. monitoring the vital signs, especially the blood pressure.
   2. diluting and administering through a straw to prevent staining teeth.
   3. administering the drug SQ in the abdominal area.
   4. monitoring the lab results for hyponatremia or hyperkalemia.

9. Which of the following statements by the patient indicates a need for additional teaching about the treatment plan for hyperthyroidism? ***(893-894)***
   1. "I could be treated with antithyroid drugs and ablation therapy."
   2. "Ablation therapy could possibly cause hypothyroidism."
   3. "I'll have a thyroidectomy first and then get ablation therapy."
   4. "I could get ablation therapy on an outpatient basis."

10. The nurse is administering antithyroid drugs to the patient. Which of the following dangerous adverse effects is a concern with antithyroid drugs? ***(894)***
    1. Agranulocytosis and hepatoxicity
    2. Hypoglycemia and neurotoxicity
    3. Hyponatremia and renal toxicity
    4. Seizures and ototoxicity

11. The nurse is carefully assessing a postoperative patient who had a thyroidectomy. Which of the following assessment findings is most likely to be associated with one of the potential complications of this surgery? ***(895-896)***
    1. Blindness
    2. Tetany
    3. Profound diuresis
    4. Hypertensive crisis

12. The nursing student is reinforcing dietary and medication teaching with a patient who is taking parathormone replacement therapy. Which of the following is an inappropriate piece of information to give this patient? ***(900)***
    1. You will be taking extra large doses of vitamin D.
    2. The goal of medications and diet is to increase your serum calcium level.
    3. You should eat generous amounts of milk, yogurt, and processed cheese.
    4. The medication and dietary modifications are lifelong therapies.

13. Which of the following therapies and medication is the physician likely to order for a patient who is experiencing an Addisonian crisis? ***(905)***
    1. Fluid restriction and prazosin (Minipress)
    2. IV glucose and levothyroxine sodium (Synthroid)
    3. Isotonic sodium chloride and calcitonin (Caltin)
    4. Fluid bolus and IV hydrocortisone (Solu-Cortef)

14. When planning care for a patient with hypothyroidism, the nurse would do which of the following? ***(898)***
    1. Provide extra snacks and encourage the patient to eat frequently.
    2. Place the patient in a cool room to avoid overheating.
    3. Provide extra time to avoid rushing the patient.
    4. Provide a calm, quiet atmosphere for episodes of emotional outbursts.

15. Which of the following endocrine disorders is most likely to mimic a cardiac disease? ***(893)***
    1. Hyperthyroidism
    2. Myxedema
    3. Sheehan's syndrome
    4. Diabetes insipidus

CRITICAL THINKING ACTIVITIES

Scenario: Your patient is diagnosed with pheochromocytoma. This is a rare condition that can be fatal. The patient was just admitted and the night nurse is not able to give you much information about pheochromocytoma; however, "the patient is stable and did not have any problems for me." ***(901-902)***

1. What is the most likely complication of this tumor if it is not treated? ______________________

____

2. What are the signs and symptoms that you might see with this condition? ______________________

____

____

____

3. Identify at least three actions (with rationale) that you should immediately take if this patient shows signs of a hypertensive crisis.

____

____

____

4. When you are working on the unit and encounter patient conditions that are unfamiliar to you (and maybe to the rest of the staff), how can you quickly access the necessary information that you need to care for the patient?

____

____

____

____

____

STEPS TOWARD BETTER COMMUNICATION

VOCABULARY BUILDING GLOSSARY

Term	Pronunciation	Definition
bulge	bulj	to extend outward, stick out, protrude
fidget	fid'get	to move nervously, especially the hands
hence	hens	for this reason, therefore
husky	hus'ky	low-sounding, rough; sturdy
idiopathic	id' ee o path' ik	the cause is not known
inertia	in er' shah	lack of movement, resisting change
lethargic	lah thar' jic	tired, inactive
moody	moo' dee	changing emotions frequently; often sad
slurred	slur'red	not clear, words run together
taper off	tap'er off	to gradually become smaller or less
tetany	tet' ah nee	muscle cramps or twitching
"think straight"		think clearly and normally
undue	un due'	excessive, too much
wringing	ring' ing	to twist or squeeze (hands or soft material)

COMPLETION

Directions: Fill in the blanks with the appropriate words from the Vocabulary Building Glossary to complete the statements.

1. If the parathyroid glands are accidentally removed during a thyroidectomy, the patient will experience ______________________________.
2. When cortisone is prescribed to treat a nonhormonal illness, it is important that the patient ____________________ the dosage gradually to prevent a hormone imbalance.
3. The patient with Addison's disease becomes very fatigued and may seem to be in a state of ______________________________.
4. The person who has a hormone imbalance may appear to be very ________.
5. Hypoparathyroidism can be caused by an ________________ atrophy of the glands.
6. While the patient was still groggy from the anesthetic, her words were ________________________________.
7. Cushing's disease is from an ________________ amount of cortisol circulating in the blood.
8. The nurse could tell that the patient was nervous because she kept __________________ her hands.
9. There was a big ________________ in the man's hip pocket where he kept his wallet.

10. Mr. Johnson was confused and kept saying, "I can't ____."

11. The mother told her child to sit still and not _________________________.

12. The medication left the patient feeling very ____________________ and not willing to do any exercise.

WORD ATTACK SKILLS

myx/o-	mucus
-crine, -crin/o	secrete

PRONUNCIATION SKILLS

Directions: Take turns practicing with a peer pronouncing these words to increase your ability to speak English clearly.

ac'romeg'aly (ak' ro meg' ah lee)	thickening of lips and nose, enlargement of extremities (hyperpituitarism)
ex'ophthal'mos (ek' sof thal' mos)	abnormal protrusion of the eye; eyes bulge or stand out in the face
myx'ede'ma (mik' sah dee' mah)	a condition resulting from low thyroid production
phe'ochromocytoma (fe' o kro'mo si' to ma)	a small tumor of the adrenal glands

CULTURAL POINT

Some people think that Americans, especially American women, are too concerned about their body images. Do you think this is true? If you are from a different country, is this different in your native country? What is the ideal body image there? Is there a relationship between body image and health?

____

____

____

CHAPTER 37

Care of Patients with Diabetes and Hypoglycemia

evolve Go to http://evolve.elsevier.com/deWit for additional activities and exercises.

COMPLETION

Directions: Fill in the blanks to complete the statements.

1. Diabetes mellitus is a complex group of disorders that have in common a disturbance in ____________________ and use of ____________________. ***(909)***
2. It is known that the risk of having some form of diabetes increases in proportion to the ____________________ of relatives who are affected, the ________________ of the relatives, and the severity of their disease. ***(910)***
3. Weight loss in patients with type 1 diabetes occurs partly because of the loss of ______________ and partly because in the absence of sufficient__________, the body begins to metabolize its own proteins and stored fat. ***(911)***
4. People with poor control over their diabetes are prone to infection because of decreased function of ______________ and abnormal phagocyte function. ***(911)***
5. The older diabetic is at risk of developing hypoglycemia up to ________ hours after exercising if the exercise is too strenuous. ***(914)***
6. ______________ insulin and ______________ are cloudy and milky in appearance and must be thoroughly mixed before they are administered. ***(914)***
7. When insulin is not present in adequate amounts to meet metabolic needs, the body breaks down ________________ and ______________ for energy. ***(929)***
8. An abundance of the byproducts of fat metabolism results in potent organic acids called __________________________. ***(929)***
9. The Dawn phenomenon is the reason why most people with diabetes do not tolerate __________________________ well in the morning. ***(930)***
10. Two out of three people with diabetes die prematurely from ___________ or _______________. ***(930)***
11. The long-term consequences of diabetes mellitus are chiefly the result of damage to the large and small _______________________. ***(930)***

12. Patients who have had diabetes for more than __________ years are likely to develop one or more of the complications of the disease.

13. Diabetic ____________________ occurs directly from changes in the renal blood circulation. ***(931)***

14. For diabetics, healing of wounds is often difficult because of the poor ____________________, and also because ______________________ levels of glucose in the blood provide a good medium for ____________________ growth. ***(931)***

15. Every patient on insulin should be monitored for ____________________ after insulin injections. ***(931)***

SHORT ANSWER

Type 2 Diabetes

Directions: Read the clinical scenarios and answer the questions that follow.

Scenario: Mr. Eick is an elderly widower with type 2 diabetes. He has been managing his own diabetic condition for the past 15 years; however, he recently moved in with his eldest daughter because he has been increasingly lonely and forgetful. Mr. Eick's daughter also has diabetes and has a good general knowledge of diabetes, but she asks you for some information specific to diabetes in the elderly.

1. Why is "tight control" not advised for elderly type 2 diabetic patients? ***(912)*** ______________________

____

2. Why is weight loss not a priority goal for an elderly diabetic patient? ***(913)*** ______________________

____

____

____

____

3. What are two problems concerning exercise for older diabetic patients? ***(914)*** ______________________

____

4. Which exercise activities are considered the safest for older diabetic patients? ***(914)***__________________

____

5. For older patients who are taking oral hypoglycemic agents, list two relevant facts related to aging. ***(919)***

   a. ____

   ____

   b. ____

   ____

SHORT ANSWER

Medications for Diabetes

Directions: Answer the following questions related to insulin injection preparation.

1. When regular insulin and long-acting insulin are to be mixed together for an injection, which insulin is drawn up first? ________________________ *(916)*

2. How are NPH and lente insulin "mixed" before being drawn up with the syringe? ***(916-917)*** __________

____

3. Why is insulin given only by injection rather than orally? ***(917)*** ______________________________

____

4. What is the proper way to warm chilled insulin? ***(918)*** ____________________________________

____

5. The patient is to receive 3 units of regular insulin and 11 units of NPH. After both medications are drawn up, how many total units will be in the syringe? ________________ units.

Directions: Answer the following questions related to oral hypoglycemic agents.

6. How do the sulfonylurea hypoglycemic agents work? ***(920)***__________________________________

____

7. If a patient is allergic to sulfonamide antibiotics, which group of antihypoglycemic agents could cause a similar allergic reaction? ***(920)***

____

8. What are the two most common side effects of the second-generation oral hypoglycemic agents? ***(920)***

____

____

9. How is metformin (Glucophage) thought to work? ***(920)*** ___________________________________

____

10. What does the drug acarbose (Precose) do? ***(920)*** _______________________________________

____

11. What are the side effects of the new insulin, brand named *Exubera*, short-acting insulin that can be taken before meals? ***(915)***

____

12. Why must you always check for drug interactions when a patient is taking an oral hypoglycemic? *(920-921)*

____

____

____

APPLICATION OF THE NURSING PROCESS

Caring for Patients with Diabetic Ketoacidosis (DKA)

Directions: Read the scenario and provide the answers to the following questions.

Scenario: Jason, age 16, is on the school track team, and he was able to maintain a B average in his studies. Jason's mother reports that within the past several months he has lost about 20 pounds, lost interest in his classes at school, and complains of being too tired to study or participate in any sports at school or at home. He began running a fever several days ago with flulike symptoms and now presents to the emergency department with nausea and vomiting. He is listless, flushed, and dehydrated. The emergency department physician makes a medical diagnosis of diabetic ketoacidosis (DKA). ***(929)***

1. What are possible causes of DKA?

   a. ____

   b. ____

   c. ____

   d. ____

2. List at least six physical assessment findings that are likely to be seen with DKA.

   a. ____

   b. ____

   c. ____

   d. ____

   e. ____

   f. ____

3. List four general treatment goals for patients with DKA.

   a. ____

   b. ____

   c. ____

   d. ____

4. Write an expected outcome for the nursing diagnosis: Fluid volume deficit related to hyperosmolar state.

____

____

5. List three nursing interventions (including assessments) that are appropriate to restore fluid balance.

   a. ____

   b. ____

   c. ____

6. List at least two laboratory tests that would be used to evaluate treatment outcomes for a patient in DKA.

   a. ____

   b. ____

7. Which of the following tasks would be appropriate to assign to the nursing assistant?
   a. Assist Jason to don a patient gown.
   b. Take the initial set of vital signs.
   c. Gather emergency equipment.
   d. Inform Jason's mother about wait time.

PRIORITY SETTING

Directions: Read the scenario and prioritize nursing actions.

Scenario: You are working in an extended care facility. You walk into Mr. Jipnak's room and the nursing assistant tells you that Mr. Jipnak refused his breakfast this morning and went out for a brisk walk. He appears pale, diaphoretic, and is too lethargic to swallow. His blood sugar is 30 mg/dL. You have standing orders to treat hypoglycemia with 1 mg Glucagon IM if the patient is unable to swallow. ***(931-932)***

Directions: Prioritize the nursing actions below to assist Mr. Jipnak during this hypoglycemic episode.

______ a. Turn the patient on his side.

______ b. Give a fast-acting source of sugar and a longer-acting source, such as crackers and cheese or a meat sandwich if alert enough to swallow.

______ c. Administer 1 mg of Glucagon by injection after mixing the solution in the bottle until it is clear.

______ d. If the patient does not awaken within 15 minutes, give another dose of Glucagon and inform a physician of the situation immediately.

______ e. Assess ability to swallow after second dose of Glucagon.

______ f. Assess level of consciousness and ability to swallow.

NCLEX-PN® EXAM REVIEW

Directions: Choose the correct answer(s) for the following questions.

1. The patient is a type 1 diabetic who has been admitted for ketoacidosis and influenza. Which assessment findings are most likely to be documented in this patient's record? ***(929)***
   1. Headache, thirst, and anorexia
   2. Weight gain, polyuria, and dizziness
   3. Diaphoresis, headache, and nervousness
   4. Weakness, stomach pain, and sweating

2. When planning nursing care for a patient with ketoacidosis, the nurse would include a primary goal to: ***(929)***
   1. maintain adequate nutrition.
   2. prevent weight loss.
   3. maintain acid-base balance.
   4. prevent swings in blood glucose level.

3. An important safety intervention for type 1 diabetes patients is to: ***(912)***
   1. provide an 1800-calorie ADA diet.
   2. assess for signs of hypoglycemia after insulin is given.
   3. monitor intake and output carefully.
   4. do not allow ambulation without assistance.

4. Evaluation of correct balance of food, exercise, and insulin for a diabetic patient would be to: ***(913)***
   1. assess trends of blood sugar levels.
   2. assess daily weight trends.
   3. determine what the blood pH is now.
   4. determine if electrolytes are in balance.

5. An infection such as influenza can be a cause of ketoacidosis because: ***(929)***
   1. patients continue insulin but do not eat properly.
   2. use of over-the-counter decongestants interferes with insulin.
   3. infection causes an increased metabolic rate and release of extra glucose.
   4. patient does not rest well or sleep because of cough and discomfort.

6. A diagnostic test that monitors the overall progress of a known diabetic is a: ***(925)***
   1. glucose tolerance test.
   2. fasting blood sugar test.
   3. 2-hour postprandial blood sugar test.
   4. glycosylated hemoglobin test.

7. The reason a patient with uncontrolled type 2 diabetes tends to gain weight is because: ***(913)***
   1. he has a big appetite and experiences polyphagia.
   2. of insulin resistance; the food he eats is not fully metabolized.
   3. the excess glucose in his body makes him retain excess water.
   4. he tends to become very sedentary because of little energy.

8. Whenever a type 1 diabetic patient knows that he is going to exercise heavily, he should: ***(914)***
   1. skip his insulin dose both before and after the exercise.
   2. drink a large quantity of water.
   3. eat an extra high-protein snack to prevent hypoglycemia.
   4. take extra insulin to compensate for that used during the exercise.

9. The diabetic patient undergoing surgery experiences considerable stress, which alters his blood sugar levels. For this reason, he is usually given: ***(921)***
   1. an extra allotment of calories before surgery.
   2. intravenous insulin during surgery.
   3. twice as much IV fluid as the usual patient receives.
   4. a large dose of long-acting insulin prior to surgery.

10. One problem that occurs fairly often in elderly type 2 diabetes patients is hyperglycemic hyperosmolar nonketotic syndrome (HHNKS). It occurs most often after: ***(929)***
    1. abdominal surgery and nasogastric suction.
    2. fractures that cause immobility.
    3. multiple diagnostic tests during which patients have been NPO.
    4. a febrile illness or gastrointestinal flu.

11. The treatment for type I diabetes is most likely to include which of the following? ***(910)***
    1. Usually responds to diet and exercise only
    2. Must receive exogenous insulin
    3. Can be managed with oral antihypoglycemics
    4. Islet cell transplantation

12. Patients with type 2 diabetes are typically: ***(910)***
    1. young when first diagnosed.
    2. older and overweight.
    3. noncompliant and prone to ketosis.
    4. active with no history of health problems.

13. The patient has been diagnosed with reactive hypoglycemia. With this disorder, the nurse recognizes the need to watch for signs and symptoms of hypoglycemia that will occur: ***(931-932)***
    1. suddenly several hours after eating carbohydrates.
    2. only after prolonged fasting, (i.e., NPO for procedures).
    3. when he eats breakfast first and then takes insulin.
    4. after excessive exercise or physical therapy.

14. What is the recommended treatment for reactive or spontaneous hypoglycemia? ***(931-932)***
    1. Smaller and more frequent meals
    2. Ingest small amounts of simple sugars
    3. Low protein and low carbohydrate diet
    4. Eat refined sugar and whole grains

15. Which of the following statements by a patient's family member indicates an understanding of the signs and symptoms of hypoglycemia? ***(931-932)***
    1. "He could refuse to eat because he is angry."
    2. "He could be flushed and look dehydrated."
    3. "He could be irritable because his sugar is low."
    4. "He will urinate a lot and be very thirsty."

16. Which viral agent is thought to attack the beta cells of the pancreas causing an onset of insulin-dependent diabetes mellitus (type 1)? ***(911)***
    1. Herpes simplex
    2. *Staphylococcus aureus*
    3. Cytomegalovirus
    4. Coxsackievirus

17. The patient is admitted with a diagnosis of hyperglycemic hyperosmolar nonketotic syndrome. The nurse recognizes that because of the extremely high blood glucose levels associated with this disorder that the priority nursing diagnosis is: ***(929)***
    1. Imbalanced nutrition, more than body requirements, related to alteration in glucose utilization by cells.
    2. Risk for infection related to elevated blood glucose level.
    3. Fluid volume deficit related to hyperosmolar state.
    4. Nausea related to gastrointestinal distress.

18. Which of the following statements by the patient indicates a need for additional teaching on diabetic foot care? ***(927)***
    1. "I should check both feet daily for cracks, blisters, or abrasions."
    2. "I should cut the nails straight across and smooth with an emery board."
    3. "I should elevate my feet whenever possible to improve circulation."
    4. "I should soak my feet in hot water everyday and use mild soap."

19. The nurse is teaching the patient how to manage his diabetes during times of minor illness, such as during mild gastrointestinal upset. Which of the following is appropriate information to tell the patient? ***(927)***
    1. Discontinue your insulin if you are vomiting.
    2. Take at least 1 cup of water or calorie-free, caffeine-free liquid each hour.
    3. Test your blood sugar once or twice a day.
    4. If taking an oral hypoglycemic agent, increase the dose for 2–3 days while ill.

20. The nurse is interviewing a patient to establish a database. The patient has reported being excessively thirsty, but has never been diagnosed with diabetes. Which of the following questions would be appropriate to ask the patient during this initial interview? *(Select all that apply.)* ***(921)***
    1. Have you had any recent weight loss?
    2. Have you become increasingly hungry over the past few months?
    3. Are you having any trouble sticking to your dietary plan?
    4. Do you have to urinate (go to the toilet) more than you used to?
    5. Have you noticed that you are more tired than you were 6 months ago?
    6. Have you made any plans on how to cope with a chronic illness?
    7. Has anyone in your family ever been told he or she has diabetes?

CRITICAL THINKING ACTIVITIES

Scenario: Mrs. Thomas, age 62, has been diagnosed as a type 2 diabetic. She is 50 pounds overweight and leads a very sedentary life. She worked as a secretary until 3 months ago, when she began to feel weak and "tired all the time." Her physician has prescribed diet and exercise and Glucophage for the management of her diabetes. Mrs. Thomas is reluctant about engaging in an exercise program and has many questions about it. How would you answer the following questions? ***(913-914)***

1. What does exercise do for a person with diabetes? ____

   ____

   ____

   ____

2. What kind of exercise do I have to do? ______________________________

3. Do I have to keep a record of exercise, too? ______________________________

4. Will exercising eliminate the need for taking Glucophage or for staying on my diet? If it won't, why not?

____

STEPS TOWARD BETTER COMMUNICATION

VOCABULARY BUILDING GLOSSARY

Term	Pronunciation	Definition
sequelae	se kwe' lee	(plural) unhealthy consequences
brittle	brit' el	easily broken; (referring to diabetes: hard to control, with wide daily variations in glucose level)
postprandial	post' pran' dee al	after a meal
first generation		original in a line of creation or descent: families (e.g., *first-generation* American); objects or inventions (e.g., original is *first generation,* further development is *second generation*)
tight control		control within a narrow range; carefully regulated control
unmask	un mask'	uncover something hidden
basement membrane	bas' ment mem' brane	a delicate membrane in the secreting glands
susceptible	su cep' ti bul	likely or liable to develop; to be affected by

COMPLETION

Directions: Fill in each blank with the appropriate word from the Vocabulary Building Glossary to complete the statement.

1. The child's glucose level was difficult to keep within normal limits because his diabetes mellitus was very ______________________.
2. Diabinese is a ______________________ hypoglycemic agent.
3. The physician was trying to ______________ what was causing the patient's symptoms of extreme shakiness and headaches that occurred periodically.
4. Blindness and renal failure are ______________________ of long-term uncontrolled blood glucose levels.
5. Older adults who are obese seem to be more ______________ to diabetes mellitus.
6. When screening for diabetes mellitus, the physician may order a ______________________ blood sugar level drawn.
7. The best way to avoid complications of diabetes mellitus is to maintain ______________________ of blood glucose.

WORD ATTACK SKILLS

Directions: Sometimes words that you find in daily speech are used in a different way in the hospital or medical setting. Can you give the two meanings for each?

1. Brittle
   a. Medical usage: ______________________
   b. Everyday usage: ______________________
2. Basement
   a. Medical usage: ______________________
   b. Everyday usage: ______________________

PRONUNCIATION SKILLS

melli'tus (mel eye' tus **or** mel ee' tus) (may vary depending on the part of the country where you live)

Somo'gyi (so mo' gee)

Directions: Practice pronouncing the following terms:

HHNK: hyperosmolar hyperglycemic nonketotic

DKA: diabetic ketoacidosis

CULTURAL POINT

Young people in the United States are very sensitive to the opinions of others, especially their peers, about body image, their attractiveness, friends, and capabilities in school and sports. They do not want to appear different. For example, they like to wear the same style of clothing and hair, and eat the same kinds of food. This can make it very difficult for a young person who is diabetic and must eat differently, perform blood sugar checks often, and administer insulin.

You must work with the patient and family to help him or her lead as normal a life as possible. Encouraging sports with guidelines for blood sugar checks, extra snacks, and insulin adjustments promotes safe participation. When the patient wishes to sleep over at a friend's house, appropriate snacks can be sent along and the friend's parents can be made aware of the patient's requirements of blood sugar checks, insulin, and meals. You can teach the patient how to make smart food choices when out with friends at restaurants or fast-food places.

COMMUNICATION EXERCISE

When working with diabetic patients, you must assess for problems with compliance with the treatment prescribed. Trust between you and the patient must be developed before the patient will be open and honest about problems he or she is having sticking to the diet, exercise program, blood glucose monitoring, and medication schedule. There are certain ways of approaching these topics that seem to work better than others.

After each of the following questions nurses often ask diabetic patients, there is an example in italics of a better way to obtain the desired explanation.

"Are you sticking to your meal plan?"

"Tell me about any problems you are having with your meals."

"How much are you exercising now?"

"Are you able to exercise as much as you thought you could?"

"Are you checking your blood sugar before meals?"

"Tell me how your blood sugar checks with the glucometer are going."

"Are you taking your insulin at the times it is scheduled?"

"Are you having any problems giving yourself the insulin at the designated times?"

"Are you checking your feet for problems each day?"

"Tell me when you have managed to work checking your feet into your daily routine."

"Are you remembering to take your oral medication each day?"

"How are things going with taking your oral medication?"

This allows patients, especially teens, to perceive themselves in charge of the situation and avoid what they see as accusatory questions.

CHAPTER 38

Care of Women with Reproductive Disorders

evolve Go to http://evolve.elsevier.com/deWit for additional activities and exercises.

COMPLETION

Health Promotion and Self-Examination

Directions: Fill in the blanks to complete the statements.

1. Lifestyle changes to reduce the incontinence symptoms associated with pelvic relaxation syndrome include increased ______________________ and a ______________ diet to avoid constipation, and maintaining optimum ____________________. ***(958)***

2. A healthy lifestyle that includes exercise and a diet rich in antioxidants and phytoestrogens, such as vegetables, _____________, __________________, and ______________ products may protect against the development of many cancers. ***(948)***

3. Patients at risk for osteoporosis should be advised to stop smoking and to avoid excessive _____________, __________________, ___________, or soft drink intake. ***(947)***

4. ______________________________ is designed to decrease the probability of becoming ill, such as maintaining a health or nutrition history and providing immunizations. ***(948)***

5. Breast self-examination should be done monthly, about ________________ after menstruation begins, or on a specific date each month after menopause. ***(948)***

6. Vulvar self-examination should be performed ___________________. ***(950)***

Medical Examination and Diagnostic Testing

Directions: Fill in the blanks to complete the statements.

1. You should provide ____________________ for the patient undergoing a pelvic examination. ***(952)***

2. The female patient should be advised not to ______________ before a vaginal examination. ***(950)***

3. Regular scheduled mammograms after age __________ are recommended by the American College of Obstetricians and Gynecologists. ***(950)***

4. A _________________________ is to used evaluate abnormal cells and lesions, particularly after a positive Pap smear. ***(950)***

5. A pelvic examination is a visual inspection of the external ________________, ________________, and cervix to obtain specimens such as a Pap smear. ***(950)***

6. Dilation and evacuation can be performed to find the cause of ____________ bleeding; removal of hypertrophied ____________________ lining, retained placenta, or tissue remaining from incomplete ____________________. ***(951)***

7. You should inform the patient who is having an endometrial biopsy that severe ______________ may occur during the procedure. ***(950)***

COMPLETION

Disorders of the Reproductive System

Directions: Fill in the blanks to complete the statements.

1. ______________________________ is a congenital condition in which many cysts develop on one or both ovaries and produce excess estrogen. ***(958)***

2. Uterine bleeding may be considered abnormal if the interval between menstruations is less than __________ days or more than _______ days; the duration of menstrual flow is more than ________ days or the amount of blood loss exceeds ________ mL. ***(959)***

3. ______________________ means absent menstruation. ***(958)***

4. Common symptoms of leiomyoma include backache, a sense of lower ____________ pressure, constipation, urinary ______________ or ______________, and abnormal uterine bleeding. ***(959)***

5. Continuous hormonal contraceptive therapy for endometriosis includes drugs such as ______________________ or ______________________, which suppresses growth of the endometrial tissue. ***(960)***

6. Toxic shock syndrome (TSS) is a rare and potentially fatal disorder caused by strains of ______________________________ that produce toxins that cause shock, coagulation defects, and tissue damage if they enter the bloodstream. ***(961)***

7. For a patient with menorrhagia, the ____________________ and ____________________ should always be assessed to determine seriousness of the blood loss. ***(958)***

8. *Candida albicans* is always present in low levels in the vaginal area; a change in vaginal pH can lead to an overgrowth, resulting in ______________________. ***(960)***

SHORT ANSWER

Nursing Assessment of the Reproductive System

Directions: Read the scenario and answer the following questions about nursing assessment of a patient's gynecologic health status.

Scenario: You are working in a gynecology clinic. Jean Simmons is a new patient who comes in for a routine pelvic examination and her annual Pap smear. You are collecting information that will contribute to identifying problems and educational needs.

1. Why is the female patient's age relevant to a nursing assessment? ***(963)***

___

___

___

2. Why would you be interested in Jean's sexual activities; for example, at what age she became sexually active and how many partners she has had? ***(963)***

___

___

3. List information that would be included in the patient's menstrual history. ***(963)***

a. ___

b. ___

c. ___

d. ___

e. ___

4. List some subjective and objective data that would be useful in assessment of a patient with a gynecologic disorder. ***(953)***

Subjective data:

a. ___

b. ___

c. ___

d. ___

e. ___

Objective data:

a. ______________________________

b. ______________________________

c. ______________________________

d. ______________________________

Hysterectomy

Directions: Read the scenario and answer the questions that follow.

Scenario: Ms. Toliver, age 49, has been divorced from her husband for 5 years. She has been told by her gynecologist that she needs to have a hysterectomy, but she does not want to have this surgery. She is currently dating a man she eventually hopes to marry and is afraid the surgery will make her less attractive to him.

1. List three clinical indications for hysterectomy. ***(957)***

   a. ______________________________

   b. ______________________________

   c. ______________________________

2. List two other factors that should be considered in the decision to have or refuse this type of surgery.

   a. ______________________________

   b. ______________________________

3. Ms. Toliver eventually decided to have the recommended hysterectomy after obtaining a second opinion from another gynecologist. List the kinds of information that should be included in the plan for her discharge after the hysterectomy.

   a. ______________________________

   b. ______________________________

   c. ______________________________

Menopause

Directions: Read the scenario and answer the questions that follow.

Scenario: Mrs. Stahl, age 52, has begun having menstrual irregularity, alternating between a scanty flow and heavy bleeding, and often missing periods. Her gynecologist assures her that she is entering the climacteric and there are no signs of abnormalities of her uterus. Mrs. Stahl is an engineer and she works mostly with men at her office. She asks you for more information.

1. Menopause is described as cessation of menses for a __________-month period due to decreased estrogen production. *(948)*
2. Estrogen production in the female decreases by about ________ % during menopause. *(947)*
3. A physical change that occurs after menopause is that the vaginal lining thins and less _______________ is produced. *(947)*
4. Women may be prescribed vaginal creams containing estrogen to restore _______________ and _________________ to vaginal tissues. *(947)*
5. In addition to menstrual irregularity, list at least seven other psychologic and physiologic symptoms sometimes accompany menopause. *(946-947)*

   a. ______________________________

   b. ______________________________

   c. ______________________________

   d. ______________________________

   e. ______________________________

   f. ______________________________

   g. ______________________________

6. The first sign of osteoporosis is loss of height, back pain, and the development of a _________________ _________________ in which vertebrae fail to support the upper body in an upright position. *(947)*
7. Recent research has offered evidence that hormone replacement therapy can increase the risk of developing ______________________, ______________, and __________________________, and even breast cancer. *(947-948)*
8. Postmenopausal women are at increased risk for coronary heart disease due to changes in ________________ metabolism and a rise in total _______________. *(947)*
9. What are some foods that you could recommend to Mrs. Stahl for nutritional therapy related to menopause? *(948)*

   a. ______________________________

   b. ______________________________

   c. ______________________________

   d. ______________________________

Cancers of the Reproductive System

Directions: Read the scenario and answer the questions that follow.

Scenario: You have been asked to do a community presentation that includes some basic information about gynecologic cancers. You want to share information about the risk factors and signs and symptoms that women should watch for. ***(961-962)***

1. The most common malignant tumor of the female reproductive tract is ____________________ cancer.

2. List six risk factors for cervical cancer.

   a. ____________________

   b. ____________________

   c. ____________________

   d. ____________________

   e. ____________________

   f. ____________________

3. List three risk factors for ovarian cancer.

   a. ____________________

   b. ____________________

   c. ____________________

4. What are the signs and symptoms of vulvar intraepithelial neoplasia (VIN)? ____________________

   ____

5. Explain in your own words why ovarian cancer is known as the "silent cancer." ____________________

   ____

   ____

   ____

6. Regular pelvic examinations and Pap smears may enable early diagnosis of ____________________ and provide opportunity for early and more successful intervention.

7. A newly approved ______________ vaccine given to girls at or before puberty may prevent the type of HPV infection that causes cervical cancer.

PRIORITY SETTING

Directions: Read the scenario and prioritize the steps of assisting with a pelvic exam.

Scenario: Ms. Gian has come in for a pelvic exam and a Pap smear. You are preparing her for examination and will assist the doctor during the procedure.

_____ a. Assemble clean gloves and supplies.

_____ b. Encourage Ms. Gian to void because a full bladder will make the exam more uncomfortable.

_____ c. Stay with Ms. Gian, encourage her, and give information.

_____ d. Orient Ms. Gian to the equipment and the purpose of the exam.

_____ e. Position Ms. Gian appropriately (i.e., lithotomy position).

_____ f. The unit should provide privacy and good lighting.

APPLICATION OF THE NURSING PROCESS

Care of the Patient with Breast Cancer

Directions: Read the scenario and provide the answers to the following questions.

Scenario: Mrs. Donner has been diagnosed with breast cancer and is admitted for a lumpectomy. She has had some preoperative teaching prior to being admitted to the hospital. The RN completed the admission assessment and history.

1. In evaluating preoperative teaching with Ms. Donner, which of the following statements by the patient indicates that she understands what is happening during the procedure of lumpectomy? ***(964)***
   a. The doctor removes only the tumor.
   b. The doctor removes the entire breast and axillary lymph nodes.
   c. The doctor removes the tumor and a portion of the surrounding breast tissue and axillary lymph nodes.
   d. The doctor removes the breast, axillary lymph nodes, and chest wall muscles under the breast.

2. Ms. Donner's maintenance IV is dextrose 5% with normal saline 1000 mL to infuse over 8 hours. What is the pump setting? ____________________

3. What is your first concern for Mrs. Donner when she returns from the operating room? ***(967)***
   a. Risk for depression
   b. Risk for bleeding from the surgical site
   c. Risk for infection
   d. Risk for falls

4. List four specific nursing measures that would be included in the nursing care plan for Ms. Donner immediately after lumpectomy. ***(967-968)***

   a. ____________________

   b. ____________________

   c. ____________________

   d. ____________________

5. Which of the following tasks would be appropriate to assign to the nursing assistant?
   a. Watch Ms. Donner use the spirometer.
   b. Do bilateral pulse checks on the upper extremities.
   c. Inform Ms. Donner that no blood pressures are taken on affected side.
   d. Assist Ms. Donner to ambulate to in the hall.

6. List information that would be helpful to Ms. Donner in planning her discharge after lumpectomy. ***(967-968)***

   a. ______________________________

   b. ______________________________

   c. ______________________________

   d. ______________________________

NCLEX-PN® EXAM REVIEW

Directions: Choose the best answer(s) for the following questions.

1. Which of the following statements by a patient indicates a need for additional teaching about the "morning after pill"? ***(941)***
   1. "It has to be taken 72 hours after unprotected sex."
   2. "It works by preventing ovulation, implantation, or fertilization."
   3. "It may cause nausea and vomiting, so I should take an antiemetic."
   4. "It can be used to terminate a first trimester pregnancy."

2. Which postmenopausal condition is treated with Fosamax? ***(947)***
   1. Hot flashes
   2. Osteoporosis
   3. Fatigue
   4. Elevated lipid levels

3. When should a female start having routine pelvic exams and Pap smears? ***(948)***
   1. As soon as she becomes sexually active or at age 20
   2. At age 16, if she has family history of cervical cancer
   3. When her family doctor or pediatrician directs her to do so
   4. Whenever she starts her menstrual periods

4. The nurse is assessing a patient for risk factors for breast cancer. The nurse asks about which of the following? *(Select all that apply.)* ***(963)***
   1. Family history of relative with breast cancer
   2. Early menarche, late menopause
   3. Late first pregnancy or no children
   4. Abnormal cells in previous breast biopsy
   5. History of being less than ideal body weight

5. When teaching a patient who has premenstrual stress to control her symptoms, the nurse should encourage her to: ***(939)***
   1. eat a high-protein diet.
   2. take vitamin C and iron supplements.
   3. avoid salty and high-sodium foods.
   4. sleep 9–10 hours night.

6. Which of the following contribute to the development of pelvic relaxation syndrome? ***(957)***
   1. Abdominal pain
   2. Vaginal childbirth
   3. Urinary incontinence
   4. A cystocele

7. The nurse is assessing the sexual health of an elderly woman. Which of the following is the most likely physical symptom that an elderly woman would report? ***(937)***
   1. Does not feel attractive any more.
   2. Is always too tired for sex.
   3. Has no sexual desire.
   4. Has decreased vaginal lubrication.

8. The patient is pregnant. Which of the following would the nurse expect to find documented in this patient's chart? ***(958)***
   1. Metrorrhagia
   2. Amenorrhea
   3. Oligomenorrhea
   4. Menorrhagia

9. In an elderly woman, vaginal bleeding is a possible sign of: ***(946)***
   1. hormone imbalance.
   2. cervical or uterine cancer.
   3. breast cancer.
   4. vaginal-rectal fistula.

10. Measures that may decrease the discomfort of dysmenorrhea include: ***(939)***
    1. doing aerobic exercises when the discomfort first starts.
    2. avoiding foods such as asparagus and watermelon.
    3. using a heating pad and doing pelvic rock exercises.
    4. avoiding use of tampons and douching.

11. Motrin, Anaprox, and Advil are examples of drugs used for dysmenorrhea because they inhibit: ***(940)***
    1. the transmission of pain along nerve pathways.
    2. salt and water retention.
    3. smooth muscle spasm in the uterus.
    4. production of prostaglandins.

12. Two measures that have been found to decrease the discomfort of fibrocystic breast changes are: ***(962)***
    1. taking vitamin C and getting sufficient exercise.
    2. decreasing fat and protein in the diet.
    3. controlled weight loss and wearing a support bra.
    4. taking vitamin E and decreasing caffeine intake.

CRITICAL THINKING ACTIVITIES

Scenario: You are talking to several neighbors about sexual activity and the use of birth control among teenagers and young adults. There are various opinions among the parents and you can tell that it is a very controversial topic. Several of the parents want to know your opinion about the how to deal with their sexually active teens and what they should tell them about birth control.

1. What factors are involved in selecting a method of contraception? *(940)* ______________________

____

____

2. What is the only contraceptive method that is 100% effective? *(940)* ______________________

3. What is the advantage of the male condom? *(943)*______________________

____

____

4. What is the female condom? Why is it generally not widely used? *(943)* ______________________

____

____

____

____

STEPS TOWARD BETTER COMMUNICATION

VOCABULARY BUILDING GLOSSARY

Term	Pronunciation	Definition
slough	sluf	(verb) separating and dropping off of dead tissue; shed
period	pir' ee ud	a woman's monthly menstrual flow
"the change of life"		psychological response to menopause

COMPLETION

Directions: Fill in the blank with the correct word from the Vocabulary Building Glossary to complete the sentence.

1. During menstruation, the uterine lining will ____________________.

2. When calculating the due date for pregnancy, the doctor asks the date of the woman's last ______________________________.

3. With family support and an optimistic outlook for the future, a woman can view ______________________________ as a new transitional period.

PRONUNCIATION SKILLS

This exercise gives you practice in speaking and listening for pronunciation of final consonants.

Directions: With a partner, take turns saying the words below. The speaker chooses and pronounces one word in each line, marking the word pronounced. The listener numbers a sheet of paper from 1 to 11 and writes the words heard (or circles the words in the book). Check for listening accuracy. Switch roles and do the exercise again.

1.	birth	burn	bird	
2.	risk	wrist		
3.	weight	weighed	wake	wait
4.	pain	pale	pay	paid
5.	take	tape		
6.	cost	cot		
7.	age	aids		
8.	sigh	sign	sight	side
9.	team	teen	teeth	teach
10.	you	use	used	youth
11.	not	nod		

WORD ATTACK SKILLS

Directions: Using the word elements listed below, give the meaning of each word.

a-	lack, none, not
dys-	bad, difficult
men/o-	month
meta/o-	after, beyond
-rrhea	flow, discharge
-rrage	excessive bleeding
-rrhagia	hemorrhage

1. Menorrhea: ____________________
2. Amenorrhea: ____________________
3. Dysmenorrhea: ____________________
4. Metrorrhagia: ____________________
5. Menorrhagia: ____________________

ABBREVIATIONS

Directions: Write in the meaning for each abbreviation.

1. ART: ______________________________
2. BSE: ______________________________
3. VSE: ______________________________
4. PCOS: ______________________________
5. IUD: ______________________________
6. D&E: ______________________________
7. PMS: ______________________________
8. BBT: ______________________________
9. ORWH: ______________________________
10. HRT: ______________________________

CULTURAL POINTS

Confidentiality

Confidentiality is a nursing responsibility in all patient situations. Because of the personal nature of reproductive problems, it is particularly important to offer the patient reassurance that any information given will remain private. Such information must not be discussed even with other nurses unless they are directly involved in the patient's care.

Culture and Tradition

Culture and tradition play a large part in attitudes and values toward sex and sexuality. Some cultures are very open about sexual matters, while others are very close-mouthed and such issues are not discussed with others. Many cultures have attitudes that lie somewhere in between. In any culture, there are accepted and unacceptable modes of behavior, and there are people who follow the traditions and people who do not. Think about the traditions you grew up with and what you learned about how to feel toward sexual behavior. How is that different from the traditions you see around you today? How do you feel about these differences? How will that affect your behavior as a nurse? Can you be nonjudgmental?

CHAPTER 39

Care of Men with Reproductive Disorders

evolve Go to http://evolve.elsevier.com/deWit for additional activities and exercises.

COMPLETION

Directions: Fill in the blanks to complete the statements.

1. For detection of prostate cancer, the ________________ test should be combined with the ____. ***(978)***
2. Erectile dysfunction has both ________________________ and organic causes. ***(974)***
3. Whenever examining the genital area, ____________________ and providing ______________________________ are essential to prevent embarrassment. ***(978-979)***
4. _______________________ is a persistent abnormal erection that is unrelated to sexual desire. ***(975)***
5. Follow-up care for vasectomy includes a second sperm count that should be done __________________________ later to verify that the vas deferens is not intact. ***(977)***
6. An inflammatory epididymitis may occur after vigorous __________________. ***(986)***
7. Hydrocele causes enlargement of the ______________________ and is usually ____________________________________. ***(979)***
8. Infertility is defined as failure of a couple to achieve a pregnancy after at least ______________________ of frequent, unprotected intercourse. ***(976)***
9. The patient with epididymitis complains of ________________ pain plus ________________________ and pain in the scrotum. ***(986)***
10. Testicular torsion is commonly caused by _______________________ levels in young adult males but can also be the result of ____________________ trauma. ***(980)***
11. _____________________________ is a condition which results in the inability to have a uniform erection of the penis. ***(891)***
12. Cryptorchidism increases the risk of __________________________ cancer. ***(987)***
13. About ______________________ of U.S. males age 40–79 years have some urinary tract problems attributed to BPH. ***(981)***

14. ______________________________ is the gold standard of treatment for benign prostatic hypertrophy (BPH) and is performed under spinal anesthesia. ***(981)***

15. An enlarged prostate may eventually cause ____________________. ***(981)***

16. BPH produces no symptoms until the growth becomes large enough to press against the ____________________. ***(981)***

17. Because hemorrhage always is a danger after prostate surgery, vital signs are taken every __________ hours initially, then every __________ hours. ***(982)***

18. After prostate surgery, a high-fiber diet and stool softeners may be prescribed to prevent straining, which increases ____________________ pressure and can cause further bleeding. ***(982)***

19. If a postprostatectomy patient reports severe pain in the bladder region, you should check for an obstruction in the ______________ or the ______________ before administering an analgesic. ***(982)***

20. Bilateral orchitis is serious and very often causes ____________________. ***(986)***

21. ____________________ usually is given to lessen the severity of Mumps orchitis. ***(986)***

22. Cancer of the penis is rare, occurring mostly in males with ______________________________ infections or males who were not ____________________. ***(987)***

23. As the male ages, testosterone levels slightly ____________________. ***(974)***

24. All males between the ages of ____________________ should practice testicular self-examination regularly on a monthly basis. ***(978)***

25. Men over the age of ______________ should have an annual digital rectal exam and PSA test to help reduce the death rate from ____________________. ***(978)***

26. For postoperative self-care, the physician instructs the patient to drink 12–14 glasses (8 ounces/glass) of water each day. Convert the range of intake/day into mL. ______________________________

APPLICATION OF THE NURSING PROCESS

Care of the Patient with Epididymitis

Directions: Read the scenario and provide the answers to the following questions.

Scenario: You are working at the university student health center. Jack Jones comes in and tells you he would like to see a physician because he thinks he might have an infection. He is reluctant to disclose information to any female nurses or physicians and would "rather talk to a guy."

1. Identify four strategies that you can use to help patients of the opposite gender to feel more comfortable in talking about sexual health. ***(978)***

   a. ____________________

   b. ____________________

   c. ____________________

   d. ____________________

2. List subjective and objective data that should be included in the nursing assessment of a patient with a disorder of the male reproductive system. ***(978-979)***

   Subjective data:

   a. ____________________

   b. ____________________

   c. ____________________

   Objective data:

   a. ____________________

   b. ____________________

   c. ____________________

   d. ____________________

3. The physician tells Mr. Jones that he has epididymitis. What is the treatment for this disorder? ***(986)***

   a. ____________________

   b. ____________________

   c. ____________________

   d. ____________________

   e. ____________________

4. Which of the following nursing diagnoses would be the priority to help Mr. Jones to prevent future problems with reproductive organs and maintain good sexual health? ***(986)***
   a. Knowledge deficit related to self-care and safe sex practices
   b. Risk for sexual dysfunction related to impotence
   c. Anxiety related to health care interview
   d. Risk for infection related to poor hygiene

5. Which of the following statements by Mr. Jones indicates a need for additional patient teaching about the treatment and prevention of epididymitis? ***(986)***
   a. "My sexual partners should be treated for HPV infection."
   b. "My other testicle could become infected."
   c. "Treatment includes antibiotics and analgesics."
   d. "The scrotum is elevated and I can use an ice pack."

SHORT ANSWER

Care of the Patient with Benign Prostatic Hypertrophy

Directions: Read the clinical scenario and answer the questions that follow.

Scenario: Mr. Tillotson is an older man who has always enjoyed good health. He reports some dribbling after urination and also nocturia that has slowly but progressively become more annoying. The physician informs him that he has BPH. ***(981)***

1. Signs and symptoms of BPH include:
   a. ____________________
   b. ____________________
   c. ____________________
   d. ____________________
   e. ____________________

2. What are the drug therapies that are used to treat BPH?
   a. ____________________
   b. ____________________

3. What are some dietary modifications that you could review with Mr. Tillotson?
   a. ____________________
   b. ____________________

CRITICAL THINKING ACTIVITIES

Promoting Men's Reproductive and Sexual Health

Directions: Read the clinical scenario and answer the questions that follow.

Scenario: You are participating in a men's health fair. You have been asked to collect information about various topics regarding men's sexual health and disorders of the reproductive system.

1. What are three ways in which disorders of the male reproductive organs might be prevented? ***(979-981)***

   a. ______________________________

   b. ______________________________

   c. ______________________________

2. Describe when, how, and why a testicular self-examination should be done. ***(987)***

   a. When: ______________________________

   b. How: ______________________________

   c. Why: ______________________________

3. Name four ways that you can be instrumental in the community in promoting male reproductive and sexual health. ***(977)***

   a. ______________________________

   b. ______________________________

   c. ______________________________

   d. ______________________________

PRIORITY SETTING

Directions: Read the scenario and prioritize appropriately.

Scenario: You are working in an emergency department. It is a busy night. Several of the following patients are very uncomfortable and all are anxious to receive care and attention.

1. Which of the following male patients has the condition with the highest priority for attention?
   a. The patient with a testicular torsion
   b. The patient with urinary retention secondary to BPH
   c. The patient with orchitis
   d. The patient with Klinefelter's syndrome

NCLEX-PN® EXAM REVIEW

Directions: Choose the best answer(s) for the following questions.

1. When discussing a prostatectomy with a patient, the nurse reinforces to him that, if the cancer is confined within the capsule of the prostate, then: ***(988)***
   1. radiation is the only other recommended treatment.
   2. hormonal therapy may or may not be recommended.
   3. a bilateral orchiectomy can prevent spread of the tumor.
   4. chemotherapy and biophosphates are recommended.

2. When assessing a patient's history, the nurse looks for risk factors for testicular cancer. She therefore questions him about a: ***(987)***
   1. history of an undescended testicle.
   2. family history of cancer.
   3. history of urinary tract infections
   4. history of exposure to toxic inhalants at work.

3. The patient tells the nurse that he has decided to have a vasectomy. He asks how this will affect his ability to have intercourse. The nurse reinforces to the patient that: ***(977)***
   1. he will be able to achieve an erection, but he will not ejaculate.
   2. there is no sperm production and libido is unaffected.
   3. sexual intercourse may be resumed in about 1–2 months
   4. this surgery has no effect on libido or sexual function.

4. A patient asks the nurse for information about prostate cancer and how it develops. The nurse answers: ***(988)***
   1. "It is a quick-growing cancer and the nodule is small."
   2. "Prostate cancer is a very slow-growing cancer."
   3. "It is a cancer that is related to sexually transmitted viruses."
   4. "This type of cancer is embryonic and continues to grow slowly after birth."

5. When helping a patient with the psychologic preparation for prostate surgery, the nurse encourages the patient to: ***(982)***
   1. discuss his sexual concerns and fears with his wife.
   2. contact his minister or spiritual adviser for support.
   3. visit with family members and friends prior to surgery.
   4. attempt to rid himself of all guilt that he feels from the past.

6. Which of the following diagnostic tests would most likely be performed on an elderly patient who reports nocturia and has a slightly enlarged prostate on physical exam? ***(978)***
   1. Blood sample for prostate-specific antigen
   2. CT scan of the pelvis
   3. Voiding urethrogram
   4. Cystoscopy

7. A patient returns to the physician. He states that for the past month he has been restricting fluids in the late afternoon and evening, but this has not helped to control nocturia. The physician is likely to prescribe a(n): ***(981)***
   1. beta-blocker.
   2. diuretic.
   3. adrenergic blocker.
   4. anti-estrogen agent.

8. Terazosin (Hytrin) is prescribed, and the nurse explains to the patient that it: ***(981)***
   1. lowers testosterone levels.
   2. lowers PSA levels.
   3. decreases the prostate size by 50%.
   4. promotes relaxation of smooth muscle.

9. The nurse teaches a patient that a potential side effect of terazosin (Hytrin) is postural hypotension and that he should: ***(981)***
   1. take his blood pressure each day.
   2. change positions slowly to prevent dizziness.
   3. call the office if he starts having headaches.
   4. rest for half an hour each afternoon.

10. Which of the following would be appropriate to teach a patient about postoperative self-care following a transurethral resection of the prostate (TURP)? *(Select all that apply.)* ***(984)***
    1. Drink 3–4 glasses of water during the day.
    2. Avoid bladder stimulants such as alcohol and spicy foods.
    3. Avoid strenuous exercise for 2–3 weeks after surgery.
    4. Keep follow-up appointments.
    5. Catheterize self as needed to prevent urinary retention.

11. The elderly patient is unable to pass urine. He is diagnosed with BPH and the physician has ordered the insertion of a Foley catheter. Which of the following tasks would be appropriate to assign to the nursing assistant?
    1. Insert the Foley catheter using surgical technique.
    2. Clean the Foley catheter and provide perineal care.
    3. Observe the meatus for skin breakdown during hygienic care.
    4. Evaluate the patient's response to the Foley insertion.

CRITICAL THINKING ACTIVITIES

Scenario: Your neighbor confides that she and her husband have been trying to have a baby for several years without success. They suspect that he may have some infertility problems, because she had a successful and uneventful pregnancy when she was a teenager and ultimately the baby was adopted. Your neighbor tells you that they are having trouble talking about it, because "Jason doesn't think he is unfertile and he is having some trouble with the idea that I was pregnant before. What can I do to get Jason to get checked out? Is there anything that you know that we should or should not be doing?"

1. Would you feel comfortable giving advice to this neighbor? If so, what would you say? ________________

   ____

   ____

   ____

   ____

   ____

2. How is male fertility assessed? ***(976)***

   a. ____

   b. ____

   c. ____

   d. ____

   e. ____

3. What are some of the environmental factors that can affect fertility in males? What are some teaching points that address these factors? *(976)*

   a. ______________________________

   ____

   b. ______________________________

   ____

   c. ______________________________

   ____

STEPS TOWARD BETTER COMMUNICATION

VOCABULARY BUILDING GLOSSARY

Term	Pronunciation	Definition
cessation	ses sa' shun	stopping, ceasing
open-ended questions		questions that cannot be answered by "yes," "no," or a short answer; questions that begin with "What can you tell me about . . ." and do not expect a specific response
gonads	go' nads	sex glands; the testes and ovaries

COMPLETION

Directions: Fill in the blanks with the appropriate words from the Vocabulary Building Glossary to complete the statements.

1. Suppressing secretion of testosterone by the ____________________ is a method of treating prostate cancer.
2. After a TURP, if a clot occludes the urinary catheter, there is a ____________________ of urine drainage.
3. Using ____________________________________ when assessing for sexual dysfunction often elicits the most information.

ABBREVIATIONS

Directions: Write the meaning of each abbreviation. Pronounce each abbreviation.

1. BPH: ______________________________
2. PSA: ______________________________
3. TSE: ______________________________
4. TURP: ______________________________

WORD ATTACK SKILLS

-cele	tumor; hernia

GRAMMAR POINTS

When taking medical histories and performing assessments, use the following phrases to obtain information from the patient.

Occurring currently	**Occurred in the past**	**Continues to occur**
Do you feel	Have you felt	Have you been feeling
Do you have	Have you had	Have you been having
Have you noticed	Have you ever had	What have you been taking
What do you take	What did you take	Have you been using
Do you use	Did you use	
Are you using	Have you used	
Would you describe	Is there a history	
Do you perform		
How much do you drink/eat/sleep		

PRONUNCIATION SKILLS

*Directions: Practice saying these words aloud, giving special attention and emphasis to the syllables with accent marks (') and extra emphasis to the syllables in **boldface**.*

epididymitis (ep' i did' i **mi'** tis)

cryptorchidism (krip **tor'** ki dizm)

suprapubic prostatectomy (su' prah **pu'** bic pro' sta **tek'** to mee)

transure'thral resection of the prostate (trans u **ree'** thral ree sek' shun of the pro state') (TURP)

COMMUNICATION EXERCISE

Practice Assessment

With a male partner, practice performing an assessment by asking the questions in Table 39-1 of the textbook. The partner should listen for clear pronunciation of the questions and should answer clearly. He may ask for an explanation of a question or procedure.

Popular Slang Terminology

There are other terms your patients may use to name sex organs and functions. Proper medical terms are given below in **boldface**. Nonmedical but polite terms are in parentheses ( ). The others are not medical terms and are not polite, but they are words you should understand when you hear them.

genitals, (private parts), privates, down below

penis, dick, cock, dong, shlong, prick

testes, (testicles), gonads, scrotum, balls, nuts

sexual intercourse, (have sex, make love), do it, fuck, screw, make it, bonk, bang

ejaculate, come, have it off, jack, jack-off

CHAPTER 40

Care of Patients with Sexually Transmitted Infections

evolve Go to http://evolve.elsevier.com/deWit for additional activities and exercises.

COMPLETION

Directions: Fill in the blanks to complete the statements.

1. ______________________________ refers to those particular infections spread by intimate physical contact. ***(992)***
2. The largest population groups affected by STIs are ____________________ and ____________________. ***(992)***
3. ______________ and ____________________ associated with STIs increases the risk of developing of human immunodeficiency virus (HIV) infection that can result in AIDS. ***(992)***
4. Although men and women are equally susceptible to STIs, ______________ are diagnosed with STIs at a much higher rate. ***(992)***
5. In men, ________________________ associated with sexual activity may be the first sign of STI. ***(993)***
6. The Centers for Disease Control (CDC) Advisory Committee on Immunization Practices has recommended routine human papillomavirus (HPV) vaccinations for all ________-year-old females. ***(993)***
7. ______________________________ refers to any inflammation in the pelvic cavity. ***(993)***
8. Depending on the organism, STI exposure can lead to a variety of serious problems for the infant, including ________________ and ________________. ***(994)***
9. STIs are primarily passed through intimate contact with ________________. ***(994)***
10. *Condylomata acuminata* in the female, especially on the cervix, is thought to cause ______________________________. ***(995)***
11. Discharge from the skin lesions of a patient with syphilis is contagious in the primary stage until ______________________________. ***(999)***
12. A mother with hepatitis B (HBV) transmits the disease to her fetus via the blood traveling through the ____________________. ***(998)***
13. The treatment for gonorrhea recommended by the CDC is single dose of ____________________ ____________________. ***(997)***

SHORT ANSWER

Care of the Patient with Syphilis

Directions: Read the clinical scenario and answer the questions that follow.

Scenario: You are working in a downtown STI clinic. Mr. Del Rey, a young man, tells you that he had sexual relations several weeks ago and suspects that he may have contracted an STI. The doctor orders a Venereal Disease Research Laboratory (VDRL).

1. List at least four questions that you would ask Mr. Del Rey to collect data regarding his risk for STI. ***(1001)***

   a. ______________________________

   ____

   b. ______________________________

   ____

   c. ______________________________

   ____

   d. ______________________________

   ____

2. What are the symptoms of primary syphilis? ***(999)*** ______________________________

   ____

   ____

   ____

3. What is the treatment for syphilis? ***(999)*** ______________________________

   ____

   ____

4. The doctor orders a STAT dose of benzathine penicillin 1.8 g (2.4 million units) IM. The pharmacy delivers benzathine penicillin 600,000 units/mL. How many mL should you give? ____________ mL

5. What follow-up information related specifically to syphilis would be appropriate for Mr. Del Rey? ***(999)***

   a. ______________________________

   b. ______________________________

   c. ______________________________

   d. ______________________________

PRIORITY SETTING

Directions: Read the scenario and prioritize as appropriate.

Scenario: You are caring for several patients with STIs. Prioritize the order in which you will attend to the needs of these patients.

_____ a. Jill Jones needs information about STIs for a school project.

_____ b. Leandra Rodrieguez needs her first dose of IV antibiotics for acute pelvic inflammatory disease (PID).

_____ c. Joe Kowolski needs reinforcement of follow-up procedure for syphilis.

_____ d. Bill Sakai needs an IM dose of ceftriaxone for gonorrhea.

_____ e. Loki Hantu needs encouragement to identify multiple sexual partners.

APPLICATION OF THE NURSING PROCESS

Care of the Patient with Pelvic Inflammatory Disease

Directions: Read the scenario and provide the answers to the following questions.

Scenario: Ms. Teabo is admitted for acute PID. She is a young woman and she appears to be very ill and suffering with pain. She tells you that she has been treated for an STI in the recent past.

1. What are two possible causes of PID? ***(993)***

   a. ______________________________

   b. ______________________________

2. Which of the following signs and symptoms would you expect to find in the documentation of a patient with acute PID? ***(993)***
   a. Severe abdominal and pelvic pain and fever
   b. Clear, copious, mucuslike vaginal discharge
   c. Multiple open lesions on the labia and vulva
   d. Back pain and heavy menstrual periods

3. Review the procedure for assessing the abdomen and abdominal pain. ______________________________

____

____

____

____

____

____

4. Write a sample outcome for the nursing diagnosis: Abdominal pain related to inflammation.

___

___

Ms. Teabo feels much better after 2 days of IV antibiotics. She tells you that she has had STIs several times, "but I always bounce back from it after the antibiotics."

5. List four or five education points that you could review with Ms. Teabo. ***(1003)***

   a. ___

   b. ___

   c. ___

   d. ___

   e. ___

6. Write a sample evaluation statement for the following nursing diagnosis and patient goal. Knowledge deficit of self-care to prevent recurrence or other STI; Patient will verbalize three ways to prevent recurrence of STIs after patient teaching sessions.

___

___

___

NCLEX-PN® EXAM REVIEW

Directions: Choose the best answer(s) for the following questions.

1. When teaching a patient who is being treated for *Chlamydia trachomatis,* the nurse should stress that: ***(995)***
   1. medication must be taken every day for a month.
   2. partner(s) must be treated concurrently.
   3. swimming or hot tubbing is contraindicated while under treatment.
   4. lesions must be kept clean and dry to prevent secondary infections.

2. The physician or nurse practitioner is most likely to prescribe which drug to treat chlamydial infection? ***(995)***
   1. Clindamycin
   2. Erythromycin
   3. Gentamicin
   4. Doxycycline

3. When the nurse teaches about "safer sex" practices, it should be stated that proper use of condoms includes using:
   1. petroleum jelly as a lubricant.
   2. saliva as a lubricant.
   3. a spermicide containing nonoxynol-9.
   4. lambskin condoms.

4. A patient has come to the clinic after having been notified of exposure to gonorrhea. He states that his exposure occurred 11 days ago. If he is infected, signs and symptoms that would be expected are: ***(997)***
   1. headache, rash, stiff neck, irritability, rash, and joint pain and stiffness.
   2. urinary frequency and burning with purulent discharge from the urethra.
   3. nausea, diarrhea, fever, and urinary frequency and urgency.
   4. burning sensation of the penis and swollen lymph nodes in the groin.

5. Patient information that is appropriate to the new HPV vaccine (Guardasil) includes which of the following? ***(993)***
   1. Only one dose is required.
   2. Should not be used for girls under 12 years old.
   3. Is effective in preventing genital warts.
   4. Is effective in preventing general HPV infections.

6. Which of the following best describes the reporting of STIs as monitored infections? ***(993)***
   1. STIs must be reported to the local Public Health Agency in accordance with state and local statutory requirements.
   2. Individual state authorities establish regulations and provide regular updates and reporting forms to the health care providers.
   3. Syphilis, gonorrhea, chlamydia, hepatitis B, and PID are the most frequently reported diseases in most states.
   4. In some states, HIV infection and AIDS are not reportable diseases because of confidentiality issues.

7. Which of the following are nursing responsibilities related to collecting specimens for diagnosis of STIs? *(Select all that apply.)* ***(994)***
   1. If antimicrobials have been started, note this on the lab slip.
   2. Provide appropriate draping and privacy.
   3. Female patients should douche before vaginal cultures or smears.
   4. Document medication history.
   5. Cultures and smears usually are obtained with a clean swab.
   6. Label specimens and deliver to the lab with the corresponding lab slips.

8. The patient is reluctant to talk about his sexual history. Which of the following statements by the nurse would be the most appropriate to complete the task of obtaining a sexual history, while considering the psychological comfort of the patient? ***(978-979)***
   1. "This will only take a few minutes to complete these questions."
   2. "Let's take a short break; then we can continue."
   3. "Don't be embarrassed. I ask everybody these same questions."
   4. "Let's start with your kidneys. Are you having trouble with urination?"

9. A new nursing assistant expresses fear in caring for patients with HIV/AIDS. Later, the nurse observes this assistant helping a hepatitis B patient with toileting. She is not wearing gloves. Which of the following statements would help the nursing assistant to understand infection control precautions in caring for patients with STIs? ***(120)***
   1. "Use standard precautions for all patients, especially when body fluids are involved."
   2. "Good hand hygiene is adequate when caring for patients with STIs."
   3. "Hepatitis patients and HIV/AIDS patients deserve equal care and attention."
   4. "Hepatitis virus is actually more virulent than HIV/AIDS, so you should be more afraid of hepatitis patients."

10. Which of the following statements made by a patient indicates an understanding of the information and teaching about genital herpes? ***(996)***
    1. "It is highly contagious, but it is only transmitted by sexual contact."
    2. "I am cured once vesicles in the genital area crust over and resolve."
    3. "Numbness and tingling may occur 24 hours before lesions appear."
    4. "If lesions are present, it is best to use a condom and spermicide."

CRITICAL THINKING ACTIVITIES

Scenario: You are talking to a group of young female commercial sex workers at a local community health drop-in center. Most of them report using condoms and they claim awareness of the potential for STIs; however, you decide to take advantage of this teachable moment to reinforce STI information.

1. Explain in your own words why having a treatable STI such as gonorrhea still puts one at higher risk for an untreatable STI such as HIV/AIDS.

____

____

2. Explain in your own words why young women are at an increased risk for STIs. ______________

____

____

____

____

____

____

____

____

3. Explain in your own words the advantage of a single-dose antibiotic treatment for a group such as the commercial sex workers.

____

____

____

____

STEPS TOWARD BETTER COMMUNICATION

VOCABULARY BUILDING GLOSSARY

Term	Pronunciation	Definition
genital	jen'ah tal	pertaining to the reproductive organs
monogamous	mon og' ah mus	a relationship with only one other person
heterosexual	het' ah ro sek' shoo al	prefers sexual relationships with the opposite sex
homosexual	ho' mo sek' shoo al	prefers sexual relationships with the same sex
draping	dra'ping	covering with a sheet or towel to provide privacy and prevent embarrassment
reluctant	re luk' tant	hesitant; not wanting to do something
assurance	ah shur' ans	self-confidence; certainty
nonjudgmental attitude	nonjudgmen'tal at'titude	indicating by words, facial expressions, and body language that you are not having any opinion, good or bad, about what a person has done or what is happening

COMPLETION

Directions: Fill in the blanks with the appropriate words from the Vocabulary Building Glossary to complete the statements.

1. One way to practice "safer sex" is to be ______________________.
2. A person diagnosed with an STI is often ______________ to tell his or her partner.
3. A male-female sexual relationship is called a ____________________ relationship.
4. ______________________ relationships in our society often meet with community condemnation in this country.
5. It takes practice to perform an assessment for sexually transmitted infection with ______________ ______________.
6. You should provide appropriate ____________________ for all examinations and procedures that involve the genital area.
7. You must present a ____________________ when caring for a patient with an STI.

ABBREVIATIONS

Directions: Write out the meaning for the following abbreviations.

1. OC: ____
2. STI: ____

3. HBIG: ______________________________

4. HPV: ______________________________

5. PID: ______________________________

6. HBV: ______________________________

COMMUNICATION EXERCISE

Obtaining a history of sexual activity requires tact, sensitivity, and an objective attitude to make the history-taking easier for you and the patient. Here are some phrases you could use.

"I know this is a sensitive area, but we need to have this information to help you."
"This information is necessary to protect your baby." *(For a pregnant woman or expectant father)*
"Are you willing to give me the names of your former sex partners so they can get the health care they need?"
"I am legally required to ask you about your sex partners for their protection."

Here is some body language you could use.

Introduce yourself and shake hands when you meet.
Smile, but be businesslike rather than overly friendly.
Sit in an alert but relaxed position. Try to seem at ease yourself. Keep a neutral facial expression.
Do not be apologetic; this is necessary business.
Look the person in the eye when you are talking, but not constantly. You may look at your history form some of the time when listening.
Careful, quiet, nonjudgmental listening is helpful.
Maintain an appropriate distance. Getting too close may make the patient uncomfortable; too much distance indicates distaste, formality, or coldness.
A touch on the shoulder or arm at an appropriate time may be reassuring.
Allow sufficient time for the interview so you are not rushed.
Be attentive and quiet; do not fidget.
Offering a tissue to a person who becomes tearful is considerate and shows awareness of the person's feelings.
Using illustrations and models for teaching purposes helps maintain objectivity.
Respect confidentiality and privacy.
Ensure privacy for dressing and undressing; drape the patient for exams.
Knock and pause before entering the room.
Interview in a space where others cannot hear.

CHAPTER 41

The Integumentary System

evolve Go to http://evolve.elsevier.com/deWit for additional activities and exercises.

REVIEW OF ANATOMY AND PHYSIOLOGY

Terminology

Directions: Match the term on the left with the correct definition, function, or statement on the right. ***(1006-1007)***

1. ______ Dermis
2. ______ Epidermis
3. ______ Subcutaneous tissue
4. ______ Stratum corneum
5. ______ Melanocytes
6. ______ Fibroblasts
7. ______ Glands
8. ______ Nails
9. ______ Skin
10. ______ Ultraviolet light
11. ______ Melanin
12. ______ Nerve receptors
13. ______ Hair follicles
14. ______ Sweat glands
15. ______ Change that occurs with aging

a. Act to excrete water and salt
b. Produce new cells to heal skin
c. Skin becomes thinner and more transparent
d. Stratum corium
e. Contain keratin
f. Provides a barrier to bacteria
g. Consists of squamous epithelium
h. Contribute color to skin
i. Attaches skin to underlying structures
j. Transmit feelings of heat, cold, pain, touch, and pressure
k. Absorbs light and protects tissue from ultraviolet light
l. Cells die and slough off
m. Sebaceous, sweat, or ceruminous
n. Skin molecules convert it to vitamin D
o. Produce hair with aging

COMPLETION

Age-related Changes in the Skin

Directions: Fill in the blank with the correct word or phrase.

1. Wrinkling and sagging of skin as we age occurs because the ______________________________ decreases and __________________ tissue diminishes. ***(1007)***

2. The elderly person's skin is more _______________ and slower to heal because there is a loss of __________________________. ***(1007)***

3. Skin of the elderly becomes drier and may itch due to reduced ____ ________________________. ***(1007)***

4. Because of changes in the skin with aging, the elderly are more susceptible to ________________ and ______________________________. ***(1007)***

5. Hair thins as we age because the hair growth rate declines and the number of ________________________ decrease. ***(1007)***

6. Nail characteristics change as we age and this makes the nails more susceptible to ____________________ ________________________. ***(1007)***

7. Melanocyte production changes make the elderly more susceptible to ______________________________ and causes the appearance of ____. ***(1007)***

SHORT ANSWER

Causes and Prevention of Skin Problems

Directions: Write brief statements to answer the questions.

1. List four distinct functions of the skin itself. ***(1005)***

   a. ____

   b. ____

   c. ____

   d. ____

2. What are three ways that a person can help prevent skin problems? ***(1009)***

   a. ____

   b. ____

   c. ____

3. What are four ways to protect yourself against damage caused by ultraviolet rays of the sun? ***(1018)***

   a. ____

   b. ____

   c. ____

   d. ____

4. A factor that should be considered when repositioning a bed-bound patient relevant to the skin is ____. ***(1008)***

5. Skin tears frequently occur in the elderly when they are ____________________ or ____________________ from bed to chair by nursing personnel. ***(1008)***

6. Adequate intake of ________________ and ____________________ is essential for healthy skin. ***(1009)***

7. A standard for preventing pressure ulcers is to ____________________ the patient at least every ______________ hours. ***(1011)***

8. The use of a lifting device, a lift sheet, or a trapeze bar to reposition a patient is beneficial to prevent skin damage from __________________. ***(1011)***

9. Patients with limited mobility need to utilize a ____________________________ device on the bed or in the wheelchair. ***(1011)***

10. Whenever a patient is turned, the ________________________ that were against the bed should be assessed. ***(1011)***

APPLICATION OF THE NURSING PROCESS

1. A ______________________ is used to differentiate benign from malignant skin lesions. ***(1010)***

2. When a rash is considered to be allergic in nature, __________________________ is used to try to identify the responsible allergen. ***(1010)***

3. A skin patch test is considered positive if a ______________ forms. ***(1010)***

SHORT ANSWER

Directions: Provide a brief answer for each of the following questions.

1. A thorough medication history is important in diagnosing skin disorders because __________________ ____. ***(1012)***

2. The two most common complaints patients with skin disorders voice are ________________________ ____. ***(1005)***

3. Seborrheic keratoses in the elderly appear as ____ ____. ***(1012)***

4. Black-skinned people need special hair care because ____ ____. ***(1009)***

5. Skin turgor is determined by: ***(1013)*** ____

____

____

6. The way to tell if a reddened area on the skin is a beginning pressure ulcer is ______________________________ ______________________________. ***(1016)***

7. The characteristics of pressure ulcer stages are: ***(1016)***

Stage	Characteristics
Stage I	
Stage II	
Stage III	
Stage IV	

PRIORITY SETTING

Directions: Your patient has a medicated bath prescribed for a skin problem. Choose the correct actions and place them in order of priority as you would carry them out. Some actions will not be appropriate. ***(1018)***

_____ a. Check the ambient temperature in the tub room or bathroom.

_____ b. Mix the medication into the bathwater evenly.

_____ c. Correctly identify the patient using two identifiers.

_____ d. Check the order for the medicated bath.

_____ e. Pat the patient dry with a towel.

_____ f. Inspect the skin.

_____ g. Gather needed linens for the bath.

_____ h. Draw the bathwater and check the water temperature.

_____ i. Document the bath.

_____ j. Obtain the substance to be used for the medicated bath.

_____ k. Check on the patient every 10 minutes or so.

_____ l. Add warm water as the bathwater cools.

_____ m. Don disposable gloves.

_____ n. Clean up the tub area.

_____ o. Apply topical medication as ordered.

_____ p. Assist patient into the tub.

NCLEX-PN® EXAM REVIEW

Directions: Choose the best answer(s) for the following questions.

1. Removal of the entire skin lesion for cytologic study is called: ***(1010)***
   1. an incision biopsy.
   2. a cytologic smear.
   3. an excision biopsy.
   4. a brush biopsy.

2. A Wood's light is used to assist in the diagnosis of: ***(1011)***
   1. fungal infections of the skin.
   2. malignancies of the skin.
   3. dermatologic viral infections.
   4. parasitic infestations of the skin.

3. Environmental factors that could be responsible for a skin disorder include: *(Select all that apply.)* ***(1009)***
   1. cold weather.
   2. tropical climates.
   3. exposure to chemicals and other irritants.
   4. exposure to malignant lesions.
   5. ultraviolet light exposure.

4. Significant subjective data in the assessment of a patient with a skin disorder includes: ***(1012)***
   1. appearance of skin adjacent to the lesions.
   2. having difficulty falling asleep at night.
   3. localized or generalized edema of the skin.
   4. complaints of itching sensation in the affected area.

5. Health teaching for the prevention of skin disorders should include: ***(1009)***
   1. precautions to avoid gamma radiation.
   2. dietary restrictions to prevent acne.
   3. avoidance of soap when bathing (elderly patients).
   4. proper way to clean the skin and preserve natural oils.

6. When itching is a problem, the physician might ask the nurse to give the patient which type of bath? ***(1018)***
   1. Oatmeal
   2. Oil
   3. Tar
   4. Calamine

7. Your patient is suffering from poison ivy and the physician has prescribed a steroid injection. The order reads: SoluMedrol 35 mg with Decadron 2 mg IM. On hand are SoluMedrol 25 mg/mL and Decadron 4 mg/mL. You will give one combined injection of ____________ mL.

CRITICAL THINKING ACTIVITIES

Scenario A: Mr. Sam Torres is admitted to your unit from the long-term care facility. He is being treated for pneumonia. You discover an area on the right hip that is raw-looking with serous drainage.

1. How would you correctly document this skin problem? ***(1016)***

2. How would you "stage" this ulcer? What stage is it (considering the information above)? ***(1016)***

3. What skin care measures should be instituted? ***(1011)***

Scenario B: Ms. Paula Weiskoff, age 86, is visiting the clinic for a blood pressure check. She has areas of excoriation on her arm and when you ask her about them, she says that her skin itches and the excoriation is from scratching.

1. What would you teach this patient about skin care? ***(1016, 1018)***

2. What would you recommend she do to prevent excoriating the skin? ***(1018)***

STEPS TOWARD BETTER COMMUNICATION

VOCABULARY BUILDING GLOSSARY

Term	Pronunciation	Definition
exasperating	eg zas' pah ray ting	frustrating, psychologically irritating, making one lose patience
trauma	traw' mah	a physical wound or emotional shock

COMPLETION

Directions: Fill in each blank with the correct word from the Vocabulary Building Glossary to complete the statement.

1. A bad burn causes emotional as well as physical ____________________.
2. A skin problem that does not clear up easily can be very ______________________________ for a patient.

WORD ATTACK SKILLS

Word Roots

Root words in English can have several meanings and can be used in many forms. You may need to think about which meaning is being used. It may be a new meaning for you, or it may be a new way to use a word you know. One example from this chapter is the word *compromise* (kom' pro miz). *Compromise* is a verb with two meanings:

1. Take an action that endangers health: *Inadequate fluid replacement may compromise the patient's recovery.*
2. Make a decision by mutual consent where both sides get something they want but neither side gets everything: *The family compromised on the hours they would assist with their father's care.*

Compromise is also a noun meaning "the decision that is made by this method": *The compromise called for fewer hours but less pay for the nurses.*

Compromised is an adjective from the first verb meaning and means "endangered" (it is also the past tense form of the verb): *The patient's health was compromised by the nurse's action.*

PRONUNCIATION SKILLS

wheal (hweel)	itchy, raised, skin area
psori'asis (so ri' ah sis)	skin disorder with patchy areas of silvery scales
es'char (es' kar)	leathery layer of dead tissue resulting from a full-thickness burn or within a pressure ulcer

COMMUNICATION EXERCISE

Write a short dialogue explaining to an aging patient why it is important for him to turn or shift his position in bed and in his chair so that he doesn't develop pressure sores. Make some suggestions to help him to remember. (Turn when the TV commercial comes on, when he turns the page in his magazine, when the old lady across the hall calls out, when he returns from a trip to the bathroom.)

CULTURAL POINT

In some periods and cultures, fair, pale, untanned skin implied wealth and leisure, with no need to be out in the sun working. Today in the United States, it is the opposite. Pale skin to some people indicates the pallor of ill health, or the necessity of working inside. Tanned skin means the person has leisure time and money to be outside at the beach, tennis court, or golf course. A tan is looked upon as more "healthy." Therefore, many people want to look tanned. How can you teach people that tanning can be dangerous to their health?

CHAPTER 42

Care of Patients with Integumentary Disorders and Burns

evolve Go to http://evolve.elsevier.com/deWit for additional activities and exercises.

SHORT ANSWER

Integumentary Disorders

Directions: Supply a brief answer or fill in the blank(s).

1. Infections with herpes simplex virus 1 (HSV-1) most commonly affect the ________________ but can also affect ________________ and ________________. ***(1028)***
2. Herpes virus infection can be spread from one area of the body to another by ________________________________. ***(1027)***
3. Herpes zoster is caused by ________________________ and is ________________________ from one person to another. ***(1027)***
4. Fungal infections of the skin can be prevented by ____. ***(1029)***
5. Scabies mites burrow under the top layers of the skin and cause ________________. ***(1030)***
6. Lice and scabies are eliminated by ________________ and ________________________. ***(1030)***
7. Acne is thought to be due to ________________, ________________, ________________, ________________, and ________________________. ***(1023-1024)***
8. Recommended basic care for teenage facial skin problems includes: ***(1023-1024)*** ________________
____
____
____
____
9. A drug prescribed for cases of inflammatory and cystic acne that do not respond to other forms of treatment is ________________, but it may have serious side effects. ***(1024)***

10. The treatments most often used for persistent psoriasis are: ***(1025)*** ______________________________

____

____

11. The best preventive measure for skin cancer is ______________________________

______________________. ***(1031)***

12. A common skin change in the elderly that can precede cancerous skin lesions is ______________

______________________________. ***(1032)***

13. Nurses have a responsibility to counsel people to stay away from ______________ salons. ***(1031)***

14. Skin tears are usually the result of the forces of ______________________ or

______________________. ***(1035)***

15. Skin tears are very common among the elderly, cause considerable discomfort, are sometimes difficult to heal, and are mostly ____________________. ***(1036)***

MATCHING

Skin Cancers

Directions: Match the type of skin cancer on the left with the characteristics on the right that best describe it. ***(1032)***

1. ______ Basal cell epithelioma
2. ______ Squamous cell epithelioma
3. ______ Malignant melanoma: superficial, spreading
4. ______ Malignant melanoma: nodular
5. ______ Malignant melanoma

a. Arises from a lesion that resembles a large, flat freckle
b. Accounts for 70% of all skin cancers
c. Occurs mainly on head, neck, and hands
d. Horizontal growth can continue for years, vertical growth worsens prognosis
e. Rarely spreads; easily treated
f. Small tumor nodules may ulcerate and bleed
g. Crusted or ulcerated center has a pearly border
h. Itching, oozing, and bleeding may be present
i. Can appear in a variety of colors
j. Has an irregular surface and notched border
k. Is uniformly blackish-grayish color; resembles a blackberry
l. Is somewhat rare
m. Spreads rapidly

COMPLETION

Directions: Fill in the blanks to complete the statements.

1. Is there an age group in which skin cancer is more common? ***(1031-1032)***____________________

2. What is the method of diagnosis for a suspected skin cancer? ***(1031)*** ____________________

   ____

3. What is included in the treatment for melanoma? ***(1032-1033)*** ____________________

   ____

   ____

   ____

TABLE ACTIVITY

Burn Care

Directions: Complete the following table correlating the pathophysiology and clinical management of a major burn.

Pathophysiology	Medical Management	Nursing Interventions
Dilatation of capillaries and small vessels in area; increase in capillary permeability; plasma seeps out; edema ***(1040, 1046-1047)***		
Fluid loss; hemoconcentration; reduced efficiency of circulation ***(1040, 1046, 1047)***		
Fall in blood pressure; hypovolemic shock; cellular dehydration ***(1040, 1046-1049)***		
Sloughing of dead tissue; large open wounds; infection ***(1041, 1046-1047)***		

(Continued)

Pathophysiology	Medical Management	Nursing Interventions
Pulmonary and respiratory changes due to inhalation injury, pulmonary edema, obstructed airway ***(1040-1041, 1046-1047)***		
Pain in response to injury ***(1041, 1046-1047)***		
Emotional shock due to pain, long-term therapy, changed body image; depression, boredom ***(1044, 1046, 1047)***		

LABELING

Directions: For each drawing below showing the appearance of a primary skin lesion, provide the correct label for the lesion and give one or more examples of each. ***(1014)***

1. Name: ______________________________

   Example: ___________________________

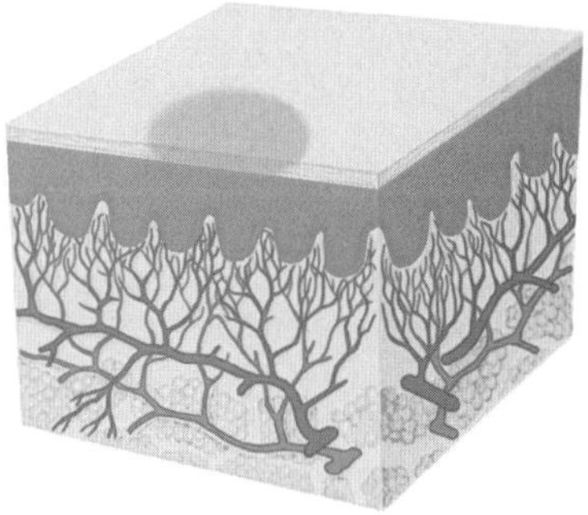

2. Name: ______________________________

   Example: ___________________________

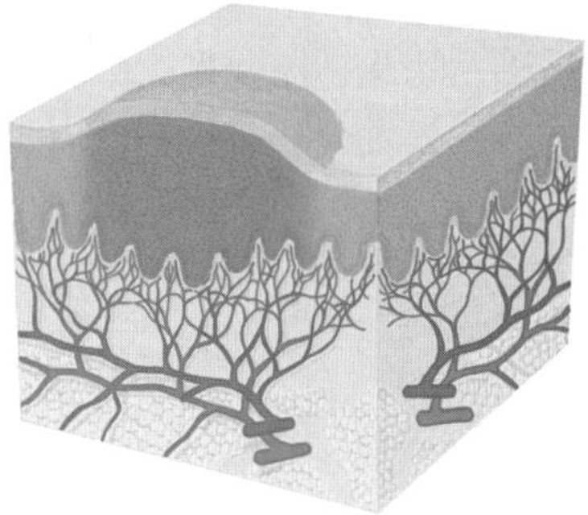

3. Name: ______________________________

   Example: ___________________________

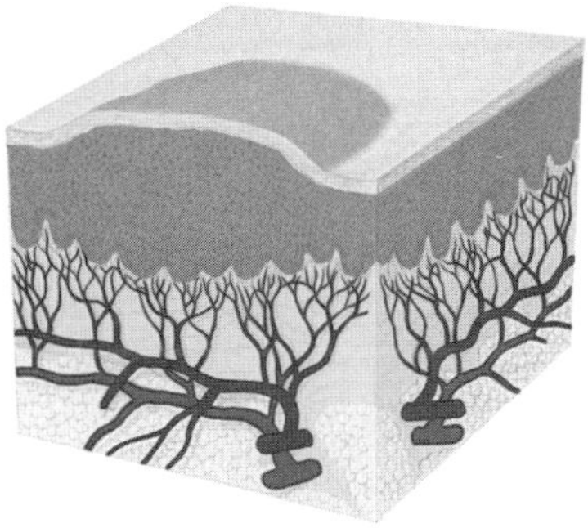

4. Name: ______________________________

   Example: ___________________________

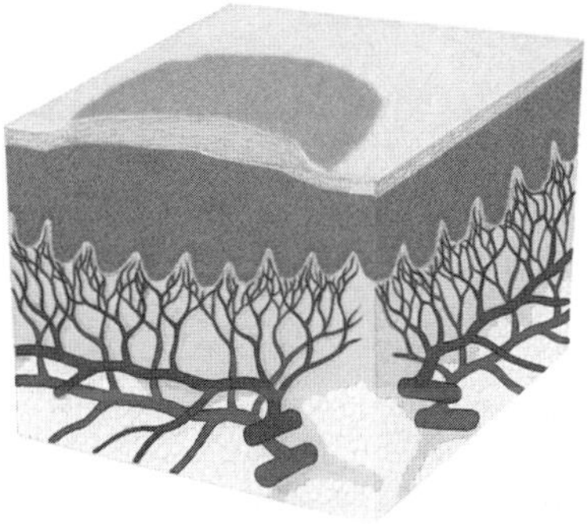

5. Name: ______________________________

   Example: ___________________________

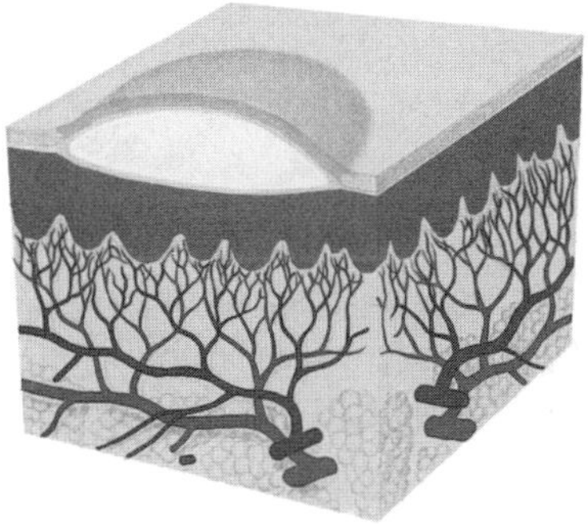

6. Name: ______________________________

   Example: ___________________________

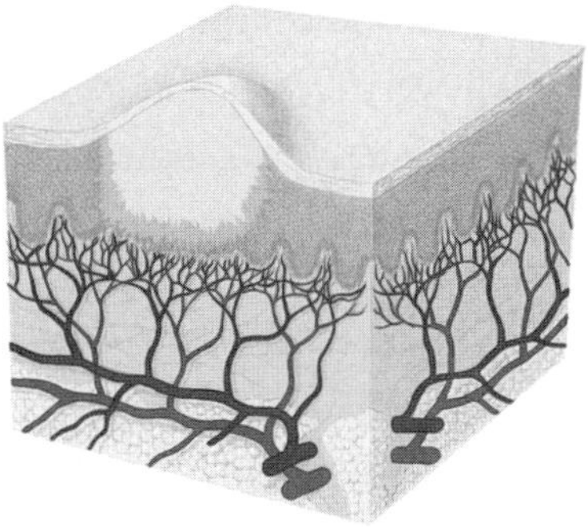

SHORT ANSWER

Directions: Answer the following questions in the spaces provided.

1. An appropriate nursing diagnosis for the patient who has contracted poison ivy on his arms would be: ***(1017)***

   ____

   ____

2. An expected outcome for the above nursing diagnosis for this patient might be: ***(1017)*** ______________

   ____

3. Appropriate nursing measures for the patient who is experiencing poison ivy and considerable itching are: ***(1017)***

   a. ____

   b. ____

   c. ____

   d. ____

   e. ____

4. An expected outcome for the nursing diagnosis of Impaired skin integrity related to presence of a pressure ulcer would be: ***(1017)***

   ____

   ____

5. What evaluation data would you use to evaluate whether the above expected outcome is being met?

   ____

PRIORITY SETTING

You are at a neighborhood barbeque and one of the chef's aprons catches on fire when a large dog knocks over the barbeque. He beats at the apron with his cooking mitt. You rush to help. Place the following actions in the order of priority in which you would perform them. ***(1038-1039)***

______ a. Cover burned areas with a clean or sterile cloth.

______ b. Cool burned areas with cool water continuously for 5 minutes.

______ c. Pull him to the ground and roll him to quench the flames.

______ d. Yell for someone to call 911.

______ e. Tell everyone to stand far back from the fire on the ground.

______ f. Tell someone to get the hose or water and put out the fire.

______ g. Stay with the victim until the paramedics arrive.

NCLEX-PN® EXAM REVIEW

Directions: Choose the best answer(s) for the following questions.

1. Contact dermatitis can be caused by any number of substances. When considering whether a skin problem is contact dermatitis, you would look for the following signs and symptoms indicating that disorder. *(Select all that apply.)* ***(1022)***
   1. Erythema and swelling
   2. Ulcerated lesions
   3. Scaling
   4. Pruritus
   5. Vesicular lesions

2. Stevens-Johnson syndrome may occur around 14 days after beginning drug therapy. The most common drugs causing this allergic syndrome are: ***(1025-1026)***
   1. trimethroprim/sulfamethoxazole, phenytoin, and carbamazepine.
   2. Bactrim, Dilantin, and Cardiazem.
   3. Tegretol, Motrin, and digoxin.
   4. furosemide, Septra, and Cortef.

3. A nursing diagnosis commonly associated with psoriasis is: ***(1025)***
   1. Risk for injury.
   2. Fluid volume excess.
   3. Disturbed body image.
   4. Ineffective thermoregulation.

4. Genital herpes lesions can be from: ***(1026)***
   1. herpes virus type II.
   2. herpes virus type I.
   3. spread by casual contact.
   4. herpes virus type II or type I.

5. Herpes zoster: ***(1027)***
   1. presents as a larger, single lesion.
   2. is manifested by pain, itching, and tenderness.
   3. is usually painless.
   4. is likely to last 1–2 days.

6. Psoriasis in an inflammatory skin condition that: ***(1025)***
   1. is curable with systemic drugs and topical agents.
   2. has scales and underlying inflammation of the dermis.
   3. is an infection caused by *Staphylococcus aureus.*
   4. causes blisters and reddening of the skin.

7. The following statements are true about tinea pedis. It: *(Select all that apply.)* ***(1029)***
   1. is a fungal disease.
   2. displays with cracks between the toes with peeling and itching.
   3. is often contracted in public showers and spas.
   4. is treated by keeping the foot moisturized and covered.
   5. is treated with antibiotic ointments and systemic drugs.
   6. is a bacterial infection.

8. A high-priority intervention for the patient with serious burns is: ***(1040)***
   1. cooling the burn areas every 2 hours with running water.
   2. beginning intravenous fluid administration as soon as possible.
   3. cleansing the burn areas thoroughly as quickly as possible.
   4. administering a tetanus immunization within the first hour of treatment.

9. Which one of the following is the highest priority when caring for the burn patient? ***(1041)***
   1. Preventing contractures from forming.
   2. Grafting to cover open burn areas.
   3. Preventing infection or controlling it.
   4. Providing psychosocial support to the patient.

10. Fluid resuscitation is a high priority during the emergent stage of a serious burn. Your patient weighs 182 lbs. His burn percentage is calculated to be 65% of body surface. You are to infuse Ringer's lactate. Using the formula provided in the chapter, within the first 8 hours after the burn he should receive __________ mL of Ringer's lactate. ***(1040)***

CRITICAL THINKING ACTIVITIES

Scenario A: Mr. Marshall is a 27-year-old truck driver who was burned in a vehicular accident. He has been brought to the emergency department of the community hospital. He has burns over his arms, chest, back, and neck.

1. According to the rule of nines, how would you calculate his burn total percentage? ***(1037)***

2. One of the burns on his chest is a full-thickness burn. What are the characteristics of a full-thickness burn? ***(1038)***

3. What are the two major concerns during the first hour after a burn injury? ***(1040)***

4. How would you assess whether Mr. Marshall has a respiratory injury? ***(1040)***

5. What measures would you expect to be carried out to reduce the risk for infection for Mr. Marshall? ***(1041)***

Scenario B: Mr. Marshall has progressed and débridement and grafting on his chest and arms has been carried out. He is undergoing physical therapy; however, he has become progressively withdrawn and less willing to have visitors.

1. When he expresses concern about the scars that are beginning to form, what would you tell him about scar maturation? ***(1044)***

2. When he resists performing his physical therapy exercises, how would you encourage him to continue them? ***(1044-1045)***

3. What can you do to help him cope with the psychosocial effects of his injuries? ***(1044)***

Scenario C: Mrs. Ruiz, age 78, is being discharged from the long-term care facility following convalescent care and rehabilitation for a fractured hip. She has a healing stage II pressure ulcer on her left buttock.

1. What equipment would you make certain that the patient has at home to help prevent further pressure ulcer development? ***(1033)***

2. What teaching would you provide as to the care of the skin and of the healing pressure ulcer? ***(1033-1034)***

STEPS TOWARD BETTER COMMUNICATION

VOCABULARY BUILDING GLOSSARY

Term	Pronunciation	Definition
proliferation	pro lif' ah ray' shun	rapid increase or multiplication; the reproduction of similar forms, usually meaning cells in medicine
traumatic	traw mat' ik	very emotionally unpleasant

COMPLETION

Directions: Fill in the blanks to complete the statements.

1. Receiving a diagnosis of melanoma would be a ____________________ experience.
2. A squamous cell skin carcinoma is composed of a ________________________ of abnormal cells.

WORD ATTACK SKILLS

Word Elements

auto-	self
allo-	other (same species)
homo-	same, similar
hetero-	different (individual, tissue)
xeno-	foreign, unlike (different species)
epi-	above, on, upon
derm/a-, dermat/o-	skin
-logy	study or science of
-ist	a person who
-graft	to implant or transplant tissue

Using Word Elements

Directions: What word would mean:

1. Study of the skin: ______________________________
2. On the skin: ______________________________
3. A person who studies the skin: ______________________________
4. Transplant tissue from another person: ______________________________
5. Transplant tissue from oneself: ______________________________

PRONUNCIATION SKILLS

débride'ment (da breed' maw)	removal of dead tissues and foreign material from a wound
xen'ograft (zen'o graft)	graft of tissue between animals of different species

COMMUNICATION EXERCISE

a. If you noticed a skin lesion that looked as if it might be a skin cancer on someone you didn't know well, how would you bring it to the person's attention without offending him or her? Americans normally do not like to have attention called to personal matters, especially any deformities that might be considered negative or personal. However, this is such an important matter that you might want to find a way to approach the person. It would be best to catch the person's attention and speak to him or her in a manner that cannot be overheard by others. Write out what you would say to the person.

____

____

____

____

____

b. Describe:

1. The attitude you should take with a patient who has a long-term recovery ahead. ______________________________

   ____

2. The diversional and occupational activities you could suggest. ______________________________

   ____

CHAPTER 43

Care of Patients in Disasters or Bioterrorism Attack

evolve Go to http://evolve.elsevier.com/deWit for additional activities and exercises.

COMPLETION

Directions: Fill in the blanks to complete the statements.

1. A disaster exists when the number of __________________ exceeds the resource capabilities of the area. ***(1051)***
2. The emergency plan is to be tested with drills at least ______________ a year. ***(1054)***
3. A medical command physician will focus on determining the___________, the _____________, and __________________________ of the casualties arriving from the scene of the disaster. ***(1054)***
4. ____________________________ is a top priority when large groups of people are together in a shelter because the incidence of communicable disease is much greater. ***(1056)***
5. Responses of persons coping with a major disaster are similar to those of a person who is overwhelmed with sudden and profound ______________, ______________, or ________________________ of a former way of life. ***(1054)***
6. Triage for a disaster is based on saving those with life-threatening conditions and a likelihood of ______________________________. ***(1056)***
7. Those exposed to toxic chemicals should be ______________________ in the field before transport to a medical facility. ***(1060)***
8. _____________, ___________________, and __________________ are key to the quantity of radiation an individual will receive. ***(1060)***
9. Exposure to high doses of external radiation rays that penetrate the body even for a few minutes may result in acute ______________________________. ***(1063)***
10. Anthrax, primarily a disease of sheep and cows, is caused by the gram-positive bacteria ________________________________ that forms spores. ***(1066)***

SHORT ANSWER

Disaster Management Planning

Directions: Read the clinical scenario and answer the questions that follow.

Scenario: You have been asked to sit on a hospital committee to review and update the hospital's disaster management plan. You have been assigned to investigate the roles and responsibilities of the nursing staff and to develop a list of topics that are relevant to disaster nursing.

1. Identify at least five nursing responsibilities in case of a disaster, according to U.S. Department of Health and Human Services. ***(1056-1057)***

   a. ____________________

   b. ____________________

   c. ____________________

   d. ____________________

   e. ____________________

2. Give four examples of procedures or tasks that you might be expected to perform in the emergency department for patients who may have sustained injury or illness during a disaster. ***(1057-1058)***

   a. ____________________

   b. ____________________

   c. ____________________

   d. ____________________

3. According to the U.S. Department of Health and Human Services, nurses need to be skilled in which three areas if they are providing care during disaster situations? ***(1056)***

   a. ____________________

   b. ____________________

   c. ____________________

4. Which are the six pathogens that are most likely to be used as bioterrorism agents? ***(1065)***

   a. ____________________

   b. ____________________

   c. ____________________

   d. ____________________

   e. ____________________

   f. ____________________

5. What are five categories of chemical agents that might be used in a terrorist attack? ***(1069-1070)***

   a. ______________________________

   b. ______________________________

   c. ______________________________

   d. ______________________________

   e. ______________________________

6. List four general guidelines for your role in bioterrorism preparedness and response? ***(1069)***

   a. ______________________________

   b. ______________________________

   c. ______________________________

   d. ______________________________

TABLE ACTIVITY

Psychological Responses to Disaster

Directions: Fill in the table below by identifying the name of the stage of psychological response and the behaviors associated with each stage. The first block has been done for you. ***(1054-1055)***

Stage	Name of stage	Behaviors and responses of victims
Stage I	Impact stage	Stunned, apathetic, and disorganized; initially may have difficulty following directions; needs strong support and firm guidance.
Stage II	Recoil stage	
Stage III	Post-trauma stage	

APPLICATION OF THE NURSING PROCESS

Caring for a Patient with Botulism

Directions: Read the scenario and provide the answers to the following questions.

Scenario: Ms. Kelso is admitted for botulism. She became sick after eating some home-preserved vegetables. Fortunately, she was the only one to eat the vegetables and her family quickly helped her to seek medical attention.

1. What are the early symptoms of botulism? ***(1066-1067)***

    a. ______________________________

    b. ______________________________

    c. ______________________________

2. What is the classic triad of symptoms for this disorder? ***(1067)***

    a. ______________________________

    b. ______________________________

    c. ______________________________

3. Which of the following is the priority diagnosis for Ms. Kelso? ***(1067)***
    a. Risk for ineffective breathing pattern related to flaccid paralysis
    b. Impaired verbal communication related to muscular weakness
    c. Diarrhea related to food poisoning
    d. Impaired physical activity related to decreased strength

4. List at least four interventions (including assessments) to ensure safety for a patient who is having difficulty swallowing. ***(688)***

    a. ______________________________

    b. ______________________________

    c. ______________________________

    d. ______________________________

5. Which of the following statements by the family indicates an understanding of the treatment plan for Ms. Kelso? ***(1067)***
    a. "The antitoxin will reverse the muscular paralysis."
    b. "She can be treated with gentamycin (Garamycin)."
    c. "Supportive therapy may be needed for several weeks."
    d. "The drug of choice is ciprofloxacin (Cipro)."

PRIORITY SETTING

Disaster Triage

Directions: Read the scenario and correctly tag the disaster victims.

Scenario: You are participating in a disaster drill and have been assigned to assist in the triage area. The drill instructor gives you the following instructions: "An LPN/LVN would not ordinarily be responsible for making initial triage decisions; however, in this scenario, 250 victims have just converged on the hospital and you must do your best to correctly tag patients. You should ask for help in decision-making if you feel that you are unable to accurately assess and appropriately tag the patient. You will have to use your critical thinking skills in each situation." *Correctly tag each patient (RED, YELLOW, GREEN, or BLACK) or refer to RN/MD.* ***(1055)***

______ a. Middle-aged man who is having symptoms of myocardial infarction.
______ b. Child with swollen ankle, decreased ROM, good peripheral pulses.
______ c. Young woman with vomiting, low-grade fever, and mild abdominal pain.
______ d. Young man with dislocated shoulder and decreased peripheral pulses.
______ e. Child with 90% total body burns.
______ f. Teenager with blunt force abdominal trauma, denies distress, but is diaphoretic.
______ g. Elderly man with insect bite, reports tightness in throat, has angioedema.

NCLEX-PN® EXAM REVIEW

Directions: Choose the best answer(s) for the following questions.

1. The nurse is assigned to assist in triage. The purpose and goal of triage is to: ***(1055)***
   1. sort patients by priority of need for treatment.
   2. ensure that all patients receive treatment.
   3. ensure that medical equipment is available.
   4. identify the need for supplies and support.

2. The nurse is advising a community group about what to do in the event of a natural disaster such as an earthquake or flood. Which of the following is appropriate information and advice? ***(1053)***
   1. Evacuate the area and leave immediately.
   2. Take refuge in the basement during a tornado warning.
   3. During an earthquake, drop to the floor and crawl to an exit.
   4. For flood warnings, jam towels in the cracks under the doors.

3. There are multiple victims during a disaster. The majority of these victims will be triaged and identified with which color of tag? ***(1055)***
   1. Red tag
   2. Black tag
   3. Yellow tag
   4. Green tag

4. The patient is being treated for radiation exposure. A chelating agent functions to reduce radiation damage by: ***(1065)***
   1. binding the radioactive material.
   2. blocking specific isotopes.
   3. mobilizing radioactive material.
   4. reducing concentration of radioactive material.

5. What is a simple way to purify water when the supply has been disrupted? ***(1057)***
   1. Rolling boil for 3–5 minutes.
   2. Adding 16 teaspoons of household liquid bleach.
   3. Water that drips from a source into a clean cup.
   4. Boil the water for 20 minutes.

6. Victims who may have residual particulate after radiation or chemical exposure should be decontaminated. Victims should be instructed to: ***(1060)***
   1. remove and burn clothing.
   2. wear protective gear and double gloves.
   3. scrub skin with water and soap and rinse well.
   4. brush off and vacuum residual particulate.

7. A patient is admitted with radiation sickness. Which of the following would the nurse expect to find documented in the patient's chart? ***(1064)***
   1. Cardiac arrhythmias and low blood pressure
   2. Nausea, vomiting, diarrhea, and hair loss
   3. Lethargy, constipation, and blurred vision
   4. Renal failure and electrolyte imbalances

8. The patient is admitted for a diagnosis of anthrax. Which of the following is the physician most likely to order to treat this patient? ***(1067)***
   1. IV fluids and oxygen therapy
   2. Ciprofloxacin (Cipro)
   3. Gentamicin (Garamycin)
   4. Antitoxin type A or B

9. Which of the following tasks related to disaster management would be appropriate to assign to a nursing assistant?
   1. Assisting victims to shower after exposure to toxin.
   2. Debriefing others during a critical incident.
   3. Triaging incoming green-tag victims.
   4. Moving black-tagged victims to designated areas.

10. The nurse is assisting in a temporary housing shelter that has been created for displaced victims of a hurricane. What is the priority diagnosis for this group? ***(1056)***
    1. Anticipatory grieving related to loss of property, friends, family, etc.
    2. Ineffective coping related to sudden catastrophic event
    3. High risk for infection related to crowding, poor hygienic conditions
    4. Fatigue related to unfamiliar surrounding and stress

CRITICAL THINKING ACTIVITIES

Scenario A: Your supervisor asks you to work some extra shifts. There has been an unexpected influx of patients with flulike symptoms. These patients are rapidly progressing into severe respiratory distress. She tells you that your help is really needed; however, you should be aware that relatively healthy young people with no previous health problems are getting sick and the physicians are not exactly sure what is going on with these patients.

1. Discuss how you might feel about being asked to help under these circumstances and/or expose yourself (and your family) to potentially serious communicable disease.

2. When you are comfortable in your first nursing job, what are some things that you could do (or ask) that would prepare you to face a similar scenario?

Scenario B: You are working in a downtown walk-in clinic. Typically the clinic services low-income families and the homeless population and provides routine health services such as immunizations for children, treatment for minor illness or accidents, or prescription service for blood pressure medications, etc.

1. Explain in your own words why you would need to have a working knowledge of bioterrorism for this work setting.

2. List seven signs or events that suggest a bioterrorism incident has occurred. ***(1069)***

   a. ______________________________

   b. ______________________________

   c. ______________________________

   d. ______________________________

   e. ______________________________

   f. ______________________________

   g. ______________________________

Scenario C: You are working in small emergency department in a rural town. There is an explosion in a nearby factory and multiple victims (adult workers) begin to arrive. The physician instructs you to start peripheral IVs (with at least an 18 gauge catheter) on all the patients as they arrive and hang normal saline unless ordered otherwise at 125 mL/hour. The hospital runs out of IV pumps, so you must calculate the flow rate using ordinary IV tubing. Calculate the gtts/min using various tubings.

1. Drop factor 20 gtts/mL ______________________ gtts/min.
2. Drop factor 15 gtts/mL ______________________ gtts/min.
3. Drop factor 10 gtts/mL ______________________ gtts/min.
4. Drop factor 60 gtts/mL ______________________gtts/min.
5. The charge nurse tells you not to use mini-drip (60 gtts/mL) tubing unless there is nothing else available. Why would he say this?

   ____

   ____

   ____

STEPS TOWARD BETTER COMMUNICATION

VOCABULARY BUILDING GLOSSARY

Term	Pronunciation	Definition
catastrophe	ka tas' tro fee	a terrible event, a disaster
disparity	dispar'ity	difference, inequality
duress	duress'	forced hardship or difficulty
improvise	im'provise	to use whatever is available
triage	tree ahzh'	a system for determining priority of need and order or location of treatment

COMPLETION

Directions: Fill in the blanks with the appropriate words from the Vocabulary Building Glossary to complete the statements.

1. The people who had their homes destroyed in the tornado were experiencing considerable ______________________.
2. The man's leg was badly fractured, so the nurse had to ______________ a splint.
3. When Ms. Lyons was admitted, there was evident ________________ between the appearance of one leg and the other.
4. Hurricane Katrina was a major ______________________.
5. The nurse was assigned to ________________ for the victims of the tornado.

WORD ATTACK SKILLS

Word Meanings

Directions: For each word on the left, circle the word or phrase with the same meaning on the right.

1. mitigate: reduce add water delay
2. acuity: distance perception lack of water
3. lethargy: fatal lack of energy skin condition
4. aerosolize: spray with a liquid suspend solid particles in a gas blow dry

ABBREVIATIONS

Directions: Pronounce and give the meaning of each abbreviation.

1. OES: ______________________
2. FEMA: ______________________
3. DMAT: ______________________
4. WMD: ______________________
5. EDTA: ______________________
6. CDC: ______________________
7. CISD (team): ______________________
8. PTSD: ______________________
9. VHF: ______________________
10. EMS: ______________________
11. HEPA (filter mask): ______________________

COMMUNICATION EXERCISE

Idioms

Directions: Explain to a partner what the following idioms mean:

1. Telephone tree: ____

____

____

2. Ground rules: ____

____

____

CHAPTER 44

Care of Patients with Trauma or Shock

evolve Go to http://evolve.elsevier.com/deWit for additional activities and exercises.

TERMINOLOGY

Emergent Conditions

Directions: Match the condition on the left with the symptoms on the right that are most likely to be associated with it.

1. ______	Choking emergency ***(1088)***	a. Rapid, shallow breathing; victim under emotional stress
2. ______	Carbon monoxide poisoning ***(1083)***	b. Hot, dry skin; victim working outside in summer
3. ______	Heatstroke ***(1079)***	c. Ingestion of custards, cream pies, or mayonnaise
4. ______	Hyperventilation ***(54)***	d. Unable to cough or speak, gasping respirations; victim was eating in a restaurant
5. ______	Hypothermia ***(1079)***	e. Vomiting, disorientation, or a deep unnatural sleep in a toddler
6. ______	Food poisoning ***(1082)***	f. Cherry red skin; victim found unconscious in garage
7. ______	Accidental poisoning ***(1081)***	g. Cool, dry skin; impaired mental ability; elderly victim found at home in winter
8. ______	Brown Recluse bite ***(1083)***	h. Severe pain and swelling in the site of injection
9. ______	Venomous snakebite ***(1083)***	i. Tissue sloughs off leaving a deep slow-healing ulcer
10. ______	Anaphylactic shock ***(1092)***	j. Severe hypotension and acute airway emergency

COMPLETION

Directions: Fill in the blanks to complete the statements.

1. Accidents in the home account for about ____________________ of all fatal accidents. ***(1072)***
2. State laws requiring the use of seat belts in automobiles have ____________________ the death rate from auto accidents. ***(1072)***
3. A safety device that has decreased the death rate in automobiles is ________________. ***(1072)***
4. A safety rule that should always be applied to swimming is to never ______________________________ ____________________________. ***(1074)***

5. Before moving an accident victim who may have a spinal injury, the rescuer should stabilize the ____________ and ______________ and move the body and head as a unit. ***(1074, 1077)***

6. An object that has penetrated the body of an accident victim should be ____________________ and ______________________ to prevent movement. ***(1076)***

7. When assisting victims of an accident, the rescuer should also consider factors that might affect ____. ***(1076)***

8. The amount of ______________________ and current involved, the length of __________________, and the condition of the ____________ determine how much damage may have occurred as a result of an electric shock. ***(1084)***

9. The person who sustains a tick bite in a mountainous area may contract _____________ or ____. ***(1084)***

10. If a poison victim is unconscious, the rescuer should never try to ________________________________ ______________________. ***(1081-1082)***

11. The only emergency conditions that have priority over control of hemorrhage are cessation of ____________________ and a ______________________ of the chest. ***(1076)***

12. Blood issuing from an artery is _______________ red and will gush forth in spurts at ___________________________ intervals. ***(1076)***

13. Nonexertional heatstroke occurs more commonly in the very young and very old and those who cannot control their ____________________ or __________________. ***(1079)***

14. The heart is extremely sensitive when cold, and the patient must be handled carefully to prevent _____________________________. ***(1080)***

SHORT ANSWER

Domestic Violence

Directions: Read the clinical scenario and answer the questions that follow.

Scenario: You are working in an outpatient clinic and Ms. Luten comes in for treatment of a broken wrist. She tells you that she slipped and fell. While you are taking her blood pressure you notice bruises on her upper arms and around her neck. Her medical records show that she has been treated for injuries twice within the past year.

1. You suspect that Ms. Luten may be a victim of domestic abuse. What are five questions that you could ask to assess for abuse? ***(1089)***

   a. ______________________________

   b. ______________________________

   c. ______________________________

   d. ______________________________

   e. ______________________________

2. List eight physical signs of battering. ***(1088-1089)***

   a. ______________________________

   b. ______________________________

   c. ______________________________

   d. ______________________________

   e. ______________________________

   f. ______________________________

   g. ______________________________

   h. ______________________________

3. A clue to the need for an assessment for abuse is ________________ in various stages of healing. ***(1089)***

4. What are four potential psychological signs of abuse? ***(1089)***

   a. ______________________________

   b. ______________________________

   c. ______________________________

   d. ______________________________

5. Which of the following tasks would be appropriate to assign to the nursing assistant?
   a. Take photos of Ms. Luten's bruises.
   b. Sit with Ms. Luten to provide support.
   c. Collect evidence such as torn clothes.
   d. Obtain an ice pack for her wrist.

APPLICATION OF THE NURSING PROCESS

Allergic Reaction

Directions: Read the scenario and provide answers to the following questions.

Scenario: You are outside with your children and you hear your neighbor, Ms. Andrews, calling for help. She tells you that she was just stung by a bee and "last time I had a really bad reaction to it." Currently, she is anxious, and you can see the sting mark with some redness on her forearm around the immediate area.

1. What is the first action you should take? ***(1084)***
   a. Call 911 and encourage her to stay calm.
   b. Remove the stinger by gently scraping the skin with a credit card.
   c. Elevate the arm and apply an ice pack.
   d. Assess for hives and general weakness.

2. What are eight signs and symptoms of a systemic reaction to a bee sting? ***(1084)***

   a. ______________________________

   b. ______________________________

   c. ______________________________

   d. ______________________________

   e. ______________________________

   f. ______________________________

   g. ______________________________

   h. ______________________________

You have assessed Ms. Andrews and she does not appear to be having the signs or symptoms of a systemic reaction to the sting; however, she tells her daughter to run into the house and get the anaphylaxis kit so that you can see it "because you are a nurse and I don't really remember anything about what's in the kit, or how to use it."

3. What is the name, the strength, and the dosage of the emergency drug in the anaphylaxis kit? ***(1084)***

   ____

4. What is the name and dose of a typical over-the-counter medication that could be used after the emergency drug is given? ______________________________ ***(1084)***

5. Identify four additional self-care measures for bee stings that Ms. Andrews could do at home. ***(1084)***

   a. ______________________________

   b. ______________________________

   c. ______________________________

   d. ______________________________

6. Ms. Andrews comes over to your house in the evening to thank you for your help. "I really feel silly about making such a fuss and not knowing anything about that kit." You recognize that while she is not really your patient, she does have some health issues that you can assist her with. What is the priority nursing diagnosis at this point?
   a. Impaired skin integrity related to scratching
   b. Knowledge deficit related to bee sting kit
   c. Risk for ineffective breathing related to throat constriction
   d. Anxiety related to future allergic exposures

PRIORITY SETTING

Directions: Read the scenario and prioritize as appropriate.

Scenario: You are at a community swimming pool and there is no lifeguard on duty. Suddenly, one of the women says, "I think my husband is drowning! Please help him! I can't swim!" Prioritize the actions for assisting a drowning victim. ***(1074)***

_______ a. Transport to a medical facility promptly for evaluation and treatment.
_______ b. The rescuer should call for help.
_______ c. Pull the victim slowly to safety.
_______ d. Turn head to one side to prevent aspiration.
_______ e. Try to reach the victim without going in water.
_______ f. Coach the victim to grasp the object.
_______ g. If victim is breathing; place him in the recovery position.
_______ h. Extend an arm, towel, rope, pole, or any long and sturdy object.

NCLEX-PN® EXAM REVIEW

Directions: Choose the best answer(s) for the following questions.

1. Implementation of nursing care for the emergency patient who is admitted with frostbite of the foot includes: ***(1080)***
   1. applying a heating pad to the frostbitten area.
   2. giving the patient hot fluids to drink.
   3. wrapping the foot in warmed blankets.
   4. immersing the foot in warm water.

2. When an accident victim is admitted to the hospital, after assessment of respiration, pulse, and blood pressure, the nurse would next assess for: ***(1075)***
   1. details of the accident.
   2. allergies to medication.
   3. sites of bleeding.
   4. psychologic status.

3. To evaluate the effectiveness of Lasix and morphine for the treatment of pulmonary edema in an emergency patient, the nurse would: ***(470)***
   1. monitor intake and output.
   2. assess respiratory status.
   3. assess for decreased anxiety.
   4. check the strength of peripheral pulses.

4. The priority goal when planning the care of the emergency patient admitted in shock would be to: ***(1089)***
   1. maintain the patient's body warmth to prevent vasodilation.
   2. decrease the patient's pain to lessen vasoconstriction.
   3. restore the patient's circulating blood volume to promote perfusion.
   4. restore the patient's acid-base balance to aid respiration.

5. A high priority in the immediate treatment of burns of the hands is: ***(1085)***
   1. cool burned areas quickly with cool water.
   2. assess ROM to joints and circumferential burns.
   3. cover with blankets or sheets to prevent chilling.
   4. determine the area and degree of the burns.

6. The nurse is at a restaurant and observes a person who appears to be choking. He is conscious and partially able to speak. What is the priority action? ***(1088)***
   1. Have a bystander call 911 and stay with patient.
   2. Encourage him to cough and breathe as deeply as he can.
   3. Get behind him and perform the Heimlich maneuver.
   4. Strike him sharply between the shoulder blades.

7. There is a multi-car motor vehicle accident and several people stop to assist. Under "Good Samaritan" laws, which of the following applies to voluntary rescuers who assist at the scene? ***(1074-1075)***
   1. All rescuers are equally protected against liability.
   2. Rescuers are only protected if they can prove they acted in good faith.
   3. Physicians who stop are held to a higher standard of care than others.
   4. Bad outcomes usually result in liability suits.

8. The patient sustains a venomous snakebite. The current emergency first-aid treatment includes which of the following? ***(1083)***
   1. Wash the wound and elevate the extremity.
   2. Apply suction to the area immediately after the bite.
   3. Make an incision over the wound with a sterile tool.
   4. Place a tourniquet above the wound and check the pulses.

9. The current recommendations for health care provider CPR include which of the following? ***(1086)***
   1. Do 2 minutes of CPR before leaving the victim to call help if the victim has had an airway problem.
   2. Call first, call fast, then begin CPR and maintain compressions and rescue breathing until help arrives.
   3. Ventilation rate of 12–15 breaths per minute; deliver breaths with tidal volume appropriate to age and weight.
   4. Use the AED immediately, regardless of whether the arrest was witnessed or unwitnessed.

10. The nurse is at a community event and a child accidentally sustains a laceration with apparent arterial bleeding. The nurse's immediate action to control the bleeding is to: ***(1076)***
    1. apply pressure directly over the wound with the palm of the hand.
    2. place a sterile or clean dressing over the open wound.
    3. elevate the injured part and immobilize the child and the wound.
    4. periodically remove the original dressing to assess for active bleeding.

11. The patient is a trauma victim who has sustained multiple injuries during a motor vehicle accident. The doctor orders a peritoneal lavage. The purpose of the procedure is to: ***(1078)***
    1. stop the hemorrhage in the peritoneal cavity.
    2. diagnose intra-abdominal bleeding.
    3. wash away debris and clots to prevent infection.
    4. diagnose active or potential peritonitis.

12. The patient is in cardiogenic shock secondary to a myocardial infarction. Which of the following emergency treatments will the physician most likely order for this patient? ***(1090-1091)***
    1. Fluid bolus and volume expanders
    2. Epinephrine and bronchodilators
    3. Isoproterenol, dopamine, or dobutamine
    4. Fluid bolus and corticosteroids

13. An elderly patient is at high risk for septic shock. Which of the following signs and symptoms of shock is more frequently associated with elderly patients compared to younger patients? ***(1095)***
    1. Decreased urinary output
    2. Tachycardia
    3. Hypothermia
    4. Slightly elevated temperature

14. The staff is attempting to de-escalate the behavior of a patient who is becoming increasingly hostile and upset. Which of the following is the best approach? ***(1088)***
    1. Several staff members should surround the patient.
    2. Allow a family member to privately speak to the patient.
    3. Restrain the patient to give a tranquilizing drug.
    4. Explain the purpose of any planned procedures.

15. The nurse has just completed a community presentation about ways to prevent hypothermia during cold weather outings. Which of the following statements from an audience member demonstrates a need for additional teaching? ***(1080)***
    1. "Wearing a hat prevents heat loss through the head."
    2. "I should carry high-energy snacks in case I get lost."
    3. "I should wear or take layers of warm clothing."
    4. "If I get lost I should sit quietly to conserve energy."

CRITICAL THINKING ACTIVITIES

Scenario: You are working in the emergency department. The doctor orders IV fluids for several patients. The RN instructs you to go ahead and hang the fluids and calculate the pump settings.

1. Mrs. Sharon needs a maintenance IV of $D_5$0.45 NS 1000 mL to infuse over 8 hours. What is the pump setting? ______________________

2. Mr. Swan needs a fluid bolus 300 mL of normal saline over 30 minutes. What is the pump setting? ______________________

3. Ms. Phillo needs a fluid bolus 100 mL of 5% dextrose to infuse over 20 minutes. What is the pump setting? ______________________

4. Mr. Damon needs to receive 500 mL before he goes home to infuse at 125 mL/hour. What is the pump setting? ______________________

5. When you are using an IV pump how can you maximize the "volume to be infused" (VTBI) feature to increase the safe delivery of fluids?

____

____

____

____

____

STEPS TOWARD BETTER COMMUNICATION

VOCABULARY BUILDING GLOSSARY

Term	Pronunciation	Definition
aspirate	aspira'te	foreign material becomes lodged in the airway of the respiratory system
battering	bat'tering	hitting often and repeatedly
combative	combat'ive	wanting to fight or argue
corrosive	corro'sive	wearing away by chemical action
extremities	eks trem' ah teez	arms and hands, legs and feet
perfusion	perfu'sion	passage of fluid through the organs or tissues
triage	tree ahzh'	a system for determining priority of need and order or location of treatment

COMPLETION

Directions: Fill in the blanks with the appropriate words from the Vocabulary Building Glossary to complete the statements.

1. The nurse must ______________ patients carefully in order to determine priority and the correct area of treatment.
2. Children frequently ________________________ hot dogs or hard candy.
3. The patient who had sustained a head injury in the accident became ________________________ and started to fight with the nurse.
4. The nurse carefully checked all four _______________ to see if there were any fractures.
5. There were bruises in various stages and cuts on the woman's body indicating that she was a __________________ victim.
6. The child was brought in by the emergency medical team because he had taken a drink of Liquid-Plumr, which is __________________________.

7. A warm feeling to the foot, pinkish color, and the presence of a pedal pulse indicated that ________________________ was occurring in the leg and foot.

SHORT ANSWER

Assessment

Directions: Write a brief answer to each question.

1. What are the ABCDEs of assessment?

   A: ____

   B: ____

   C: ____

   D: ____

   E: ____

2. Describe the head-to-toe assessment. ____

   ____

   ____

   ____

   ____

   ____

   ____

   ____

   ____

   ____

WORD ATTACK SKILLS

Word Meanings

Directions: For each word on the left, circle the word or phrase with the same meaning on the right.

1. cessa'tion: a period of time stopping hard and fast
2. deter'iorate: increase rapidly change into bad condition become smaller

Word Elements

circum-	around
oral	mouth

Directions: Write the meaning of the word.

1. circumoral: ____________________

PRONUNCIATION SKILLS

pto'maine (toh' main)

a'queous epineph'rine (a' kwee us)

CHAPTER 45

Care of Patients with Anxiety, Mood, and Eating Disorders

evolve Go to http://evolve.elsevier.com/deWit for additional activities and exercises.

COMPLETION

Directions: Fill in the blanks to complete the statements.

1. An ____________________ is a recurrent or intrusive thought that the person cannot stop thinking about and these thoughts create anxiety. ***(1102)***
2. Persons diagnosed with post-traumatic stress disorder have experienced ________________________ ______________________ that produce intense horror and recurrent symptoms of anxiety. ***(1102)***
3. Dysthymic individuals feel a sense of ______________________ and ______________ that cannot be alleviated by usual means. ***(1105)***
4. Manic individuals may not ___________ or ___________ for days. ***(1108)***
5. The individual who switches from being extremely depressed to becoming manic has a ______________________ disorder. ***(1105)***
6. The mood of a manic person is often one of ________________________ and general ___________________. ***(1105)***
7. Two hallmarks of mood disorders are the ______________________________ and ___________________. ***(1103-1104)***
8. The depressed patient may have _________________________ retardation. ***(1109)***
9. One way to increase nutritional intake for a manic patient is to provide __________________. ***(1108)***
10. A diagnosis of generalized anxiety disorder can only be made when the anxiety is present for at least _______________ months. ***(1101)***
11. Benzodiazepines are used cautiously for anxiety disorders because they are highly _________________ ______________________________. ***(1103)***
12. The drug of choice to stabilize manic behavior is ___________________________. ***(1105)***
13. The doctor orders 16 mEq of lithium citrate syrup for a patient who has acute manic behavior. The pharmacy delivers a 500 mL bottle of lithium citrate 8 mEq/5 mL. How many mL should be given? ____________________ mL

14. Close observation of the manic patient is essential because a mood of frivolity and joking can quickly escalate to ____________________ and ____. ***(1109)***

15. ______________________________ often mimics depressive symptoms. ***(1109)***

APPLICATION OF THE NURSING PROCESS

Anxiety

Directions: Read the clinical scenario and answer the questions that follow.

Scenario: A bus full of senior citizens is involved in a minor traffic accident in front of the clinic where you work. The emergency medical personnel have asked to use the clinic as a triage area and have also asked the clinic staff to assist by providing emotional support to the passengers until more help can arrive. One passenger appears to have a broken arm but for the others there are no obvious physical injuries; however, many of the passengers are very upset.

1. What are six physical signs of severe anxiety that you might expect to find? ***(1101)***

   a. ____

   b. ____

   c. ____

   d. ____

   e. ____

   f. ____

2. List five feelings of severe anxiety that these passengers could be experiencing. ***(1101)***

   a. ____

   b. ____

   c. ____

   d. ____

   e. ____

3. In the elderly, signs of severe anxiety are often somatic. What three signs might indicate severe anxiety in an elderly person? ***(1104)***

   a. ____

   b. ____

   c. ____

4. What are three medical conditions that should be considered because they can mimic the signs of severe anxiety? ***(1102)***

 a. ______________________________

 b. ______________________________

 c. ______________________________

5. Write a patient goal with outcome criterion for the following nursing diagnosis: Anxiety related to real or perceived threat. ***(1104)***

 ____

 ____

6. List three interventions that could be used to assist a passenger who is experiencing severe anxiety. ***(1104)***

 a. ______________________________

 b. ______________________________

 c. ______________________________

7. Which of the following behaviors indicates that a passenger is responding to intervention for anxiety? ***(1105)***
 a. Passenger cries, but is able to answer questions appropriately.
 b. Passenger cries and repeatedly asks, "What happened to me?"
 c. Passenger is quiet and calm, but will not respond to any questions.
 d. Passenger is wandering around and looking for his "sandwich and milk."

PRIORITY SETTING

Directions: Read the scenario and prioritize as appropriate.

You are caring for several patients in an acute psychiatric admission ward. Mr. Loisi was admitted for major depression and demonstrates marked psychomotor retardation. Ms. Planto has bipolar disorder, and this morning she is very intrusive and loud. Mr. Salest was admitted for a severe episode of generalized anxiety disorder and suicidal ideations. Ms. Tomei has a long history of anorexia nervosa; she denies suicidal thoughts, but she has attempted suicide in the past. Mr. Blanchard was admitted for major depression. Prioritize the order in which the nurse should address the needs of these patients.

______ a. Mr. Loisi had a bowel movement while sitting in the dayroom, but he will not get up and go to the shower.

______ b. Ms. Planto is standing at the nurses' station yelling at the unit secretary.

______ c. Mr. Salest appears secretive as he walks down the hall; he is carrying something large under his shirt.

______ d. Ms. Tomei is doing jumping jacks and jogging around the unit.

______ e. Mr. Blanchard is quiet and appears to be on the verge of crying.

NCLEX-PN® EXAM REVIEW

Directions: Choose the best answer(s) for the following questions.

1. When a patient is showing signs of severe anxiety and it is time for him to bathe and dress, it is best if the nurse: ***(1104)***
   1. leaves the patient alone.
   2. asks the patient why he is feeling so anxious.
   3. explain the rationale for practicing good hygiene.
   4. gives simple directions.

2. Which symptoms are most characteristic of depression? ***(1109)***
   1. Lack of interest, loss of libido, and flight of ideas
   2. Insomnia, poor hygiene, and grandiose ideas
   3. Overeating, hyperactivity, and rapid speech
   4. Insomnia, anorexia, and lack of energy

3. When communicating with a severely depressed patient, the nurse should: ***(1112)***
   1. be quiet while assisting with activities of daily living.
   2. interact and talk with the patient whenever in the room.
   3. make an effort to be cheerful.
   4. speak in simple, direct sentences when necessary.

4. When planning care for a patient with a mood disorder, the highest priority is to: ***(1105)***
   1. encourage the expression of feelings.
   2. engage in therapeutic interaction.
   3. provide a safe environment.
   4. orient the patient to time and place.

5. The nurse is doing discharge teaching for a manic patient. The patient asks, "Will I have to take lithium forever?" The best answer would be: ***(1105)***
   1. "No, only until your symptoms are under control."
   2. "Yes, you will most likely need to take it for your lifetime."
   3. "You will only need to take it for about 4 months."
   4. "No, usually you can do without it after about a year."

6. Which medication is used to treat anxiety? ***(1102-1103)***
   1. Paroxetine (Paxil)
   2. Alprazolam (Xanax)
   3. Phenezine (Nardil)
   4. Amitryptiline (Elavil)

7. In planning care for the depressed patient, the nurse is aware that the risk for self-harm actually increases when the: ***(1107-1108)***
   1. patient is discharged and has to care for himself.
   2. antidepressant medications begin to take effect.
   3. family promises, but fails, to visit him in the hospital.
   4. patient is first admitted and does not trust the staff.

8. An MAO inhibitor such as phenelzine (Nardil) may cause life-threatening: ***(1111)***
   1. respiratory distress.
   2. gastrointestinal bleeding.
   3. cardiac arrhythmias.
   4. hypertensive crisis.

9. The patient is admitted for anorexia nervosa. Which of the following behaviors are associated with this disorder? *(Select all that apply.)* ***(1114)***
   1. Shifts food around the plate.
   2. Collects recipes.
   3. Makes elaborate meals for others.
   4. Has superstitions about food.
   5. Uses laxatives and vomits in secret.
   6. Practices excessive exercise.

10. Which of the following statements by the patient's family indicates the need for more teaching about the treatment of anorexia nervosa? ***(1114)***
    1. "If she'll just eat more, we can take her home and she'll be okay."
    2. "She will have to be hospitalized if she has dehydration or electrolyte imbalance."
    3. "Therapy could take between 1–6 years for this disorder."
    4. "Support groups and family therapy are important aspects of treatment."

11. The patient has bulemia nervosa. Which of the following tasks would be appropriate to assign to the nursing assistant? ***(1114-1115)***
    1. Observe for marks on the knuckles during AM hygiene.
    2. Listen outside the bathroom door for sounds of induced vomiting.
    3. Check the patient's belongings for secret caches of snacks and food.
    4. Escort the patient to group therapy or to occupational therapy.

CRITICAL THINKING ACTIVITIES

Scenario A: Mr. Dell is brought to the clinic by a friend. He has been awake for 2 days and has ridden over 200 miles on a bicycle. Although he appears exhausted, he continues to pace around the waiting room, talking loudly, with rapid pressured speech and wild gestures.

1. Which of the following nursing diagnoses is a priority for Mr. Dell? ***(1108)***
   a. Imbalanced nutrition, less than body requirements, related to shortened attention span while trying to eat
   b. Sleep deprivation related to hyperactivity
   c. Communication, impaired, related to flight of ideas and pressured speech
   d. Risk for injury to self or others related to impulsivity and hyperactivity

2. What are three therapeutic communication interventions that can be used in dealing with a patient in the manic phase? ***(1109)***

   a. ______________________________

   b. ______________________________

   c. ______________________________

3. What are two ways you may be able to prevent further escalation of manic behavior in a patient? ***(1109)***

   a. ______________________________

   b. ______________________________

4. The nurse is teaching the patient about lithium carbonate. Which of the following are appropriate to include in the teaching? *(Select all that apply.)* ***(1108)***
   a. It takes 3–4 days to reach therapeutic levels.
   b. It helps to decrease the manic behavior.
   c. There is a small margin of safety between a therapeutic level and a toxic level.
   d. Maintain salt intake and drink adequate fluids; salt depletion may cause toxicity.
   e. Take the medication on an empty stomach.
   f. Do not become dehydrated.

Scenario B: Dixie Jones is 33 years old. She appears to be slightly overweight and suffers from low self-esteem. After lunch, you and other coworkers can frequently hear her vomiting in the bathroom; however, she says she is okay and becomes embarrassed if anybody shows concern. You suspect that she might be bulimic.

1. Write a brief script that could be used to approach Dixie about your concerns. ***(1115-1116)*** ____________

   ____

   ____

   ____

   ____

   ____

2. What ethical obligations do you have towards a coworker with health problems? ***(1116)*** ____________

   ____

   ____

   ____

   ____

   ____

   ____

STEPS TOWARD BETTER COMMUNICATION

VOCABULARY BUILDING GLOSSARY

Term	Pronunciation	Definition
differentiate	dif er en' shee ate	to see differences
overwhelm'ing	overwhelm'ing	more than a person can cope with
lethargy	leth'argy	extreme tiredness, lack of energy or interest
comprises	kom pri' zez	includes, contains
debilitating	debil'itating	weakening
elation	ee la' shun	extreme happiness
recur	recur'	happen again
somatic	soma'tic	physical, referring to the body
mimic	mim'ic	act like
hypervigilant	hi per vij' ah lant	always watchful
escalate	es'calate	increase, go to higher levels
frivolity	frih vol' ah tee	light-hearted fun, silliness, gaiety
precipitate	pree sip' ah tat	to cause to begin
deprivation	dep rah va' shun	a condition of want and need
conducive	kon du' siv	helping to cause or produce
lethality	lee thal' ah tee	degree of ability to cause death

COMPLETION

Directions: Fill in the blanks with the correct words from the Vocabulary Building Glossary to complete the statements.

1. Martha was experiencing ________________ anxiety after her son was seriously injured and went to surgery.
2. People who are highly anxious may express more ________________ complaints than others.
3. Psychotherapy is ______________________ to resolving moderate depression.
4. During the manic phase, the patient experiences ______________________.
5. The death of her husband seemed to ____________________ a period of depression.
6. The depressed patient usually shows signs of __________________ and is not interested in exercising.
7. Sometimes it is difficult to __________________ between moderate and severe anxiety.
8. Side effects of some of the antidepressant drugs can __________________ signs of a neurologic disorder such as Parkinson's disease.
9. Treatment for depression often ______________________ both psychotherapy and antidepressant medication.
10. Severe anxiety or severe depression can be __________________ to a person's life.
11. Episodes of depression may __________________________.

12. The very anxious person often becomes ____________________, studying everyone in his surroundings.
13. In a person with bipolar disorder, the manic phase can ________________________ quickly.
14. Patients with anxiety disorders may have experienced periods of _____________ as children.
15. The patient who can once again engage in ______________________ is on the way to being well again.
16. When interacting with a patient who has expressed a plan for suicide, you must determine its

    ________________________.

WORD ATTACK SKILLS

Word Elements

The following word elements appear frequently in this chapter:

-thymia	condition of mind, mood
som/a-, somat/o-	body (physical versus mental)

CULTURAL POINT

Attitudes toward suicide vary. Some religions prohibit suicide, while others do not approve of it but feel it is an individual's choice, particularly if one is terminally ill and suffering. There is even an organization called the Hemlock Society that provides information and support for those considering suicide. Their position is that a person has a right to control his or her own life and death. Their concern is "death with dignity." The nurse needs to explore his or her own feelings about suicide. When a patient's views differ from the nurse's, the nurse must try to be nonjudgmental. It is important to recognize the differences in attitudes and beliefs that are found in various people.

COMMUNICATION EXERCISE

The following dialogue is an example of one way to interact with a person who is expressing suicidal thoughts.

Patient: "I just can't live like this anymore. I'm going to escape this world and get out of this pain."

Nurse: "It sounds as if you might be planning to take your life. Is that what I am hearing you say?"

Patient: "Yes, I am thinking about it. I'm just not sure yet."

Nurse: "Do you have a plan in mind?"

Patient: "Pills would probably be the easiest way."

Nurse: "Do you have sufficient pills on hand to accomplish your plan? What do you have?"

Patient: "At the moment, I only have a few pain pills and some antidepressants. I'll have to get some more."

The nurse determines that lethality is not high at the moment.

Nurse: "Have the antidepressants helped you at all?"

Patient: "Not much, and I have been on them for 6 weeks."

Nurse: "How about asking your doctor for a different medication that might work better for you? It might also interact with your pain medication to relieve your pain more."

Patient: "I'll think about it."

CHAPTER 46

Care of Patients with Substance Abuse Disorders

evolve Go to http://evolve.elsevier.com/deWit for additional activities and exercises.

COMPLETION

Directions: Fill in the blanks to complete the statements.

1. Another sign of alcohol intoxication might be ____________________, ____________________, ____________________, or ____________________ speech. ***(1122)***
2. Careful withdrawal from alcohol and certain benzodiazepines is essential because effects can be ____. ***(1122)***
3. It takes the body about __________ hour to metabolize one standard drink. ***(1122)***
4. Among the elderly, alcohol may be used to alleviate ____________________ or ____________________. ***(1122)***
5. Although Wernicke's encephalopathy is reversible, Korsakoff's syndrome is ____________________. ***(1124)***
6. In addition to alcohol, other central nervous system depressants include ____________________ and ____________________. ***(1126)***
7. Withdrawal from opiates is not life-threatening, but causes considerable ____________________. ***(1125)***
8. The greatest danger related to an opiate overdose is ____________________. ***(1125)***
9. For successful rehabilitation of the heroin addict, in addition to long-term treatment, a change in ____________________ is essential. ***(1127)***
10. Treatment for abuse of CNS stimulants is similar to that for ____________________. ***(1127)***
11. When administering medication for a patient who has CNS stimulant abuse, ____________________ or ____________________ can be used for agitation and ____________________ can be used for the depressive symptoms. ***(1127)***
12. Careful monitoring and assessment is essential while a patient is withdrawing from CNS stimulant abuse because ____________________ may occur and cause ____________________. ***(1127)***
13. Chronic methamphetamine users may develop toxic ____________________ and experience ____________________, ____________________, and delusions. ***(1127)***

14. Freebasing cocaine is the most dangerous method and accounts for many ____________________ and ____________________ reactions. *(1127)*

15. Marijuana is thought to be nonaddictive physically, but it may lead to ________________ dependence and a lack of ________________ and ambition. *(1128)*

16. Examples of commonly abused inhalants include glue, ________________, ____________________, ____________________, and other types of solvents. *(1129)*

17. ____________________ are most frequently abused by teens and children because they are inexpensive and easily accessible. *(1129)*

SHORT ANSWER

Caring for a Patient with Cocaine Abuse

Directions: Read the clinical scenario and answer the questions that follow.

Scenario: Carrie Jacks, a 23-year-old secretary, started using cocaine as a recreational drug on weekends "just for fun." Within a very short time, Carrie started using cocaine after work and spending more time with friends who were also using increasingly larger amounts. On several occasions, Carrie's mother has called in sick for Carrie. Carrie's mother brings her to the clinic for vitamins and information about cocaine abuse "for a friend." You should collect data to determine Carrie's baseline knowledge about cocaine and to assess for signs and effects of substance abuse.

1. What are three effects of cocaine that Carrie could be experiencing? *(1125)*

   a. ____

   b. ____

   c. ____

2. You are aware that different methods of using cocaine create different health issues. In what four ways is cocaine used? *(1127)*

   a. ____

   b. ____

   c. ____

   d. ____

3. What are two teaching points to share with Carrie about the risks of using cocaine? *(1125)*

   a. ____

   b. ____

4. What are four common feelings of family members who live with a substance-dependent person? ***(1121)***

   a. ______________________________

   b. ______________________________

   c. ______________________________

   d. ______________________________

5. What two enabling behaviors has Carrie's mother demonstrated? ***(1121)***

   a. ______________________________

   b. ______________________________

APPLICATION OF THE NURSING PROCESS

Caring for a Patient with Chronic Alcohol Abuse

Directions: Read the clinical scenario and answer the questions that follow.

Scenario: Mr. Briganti is a 56-year-old homeless man who frequently comes to the walk-in clinic for health care, and sometimes for food or a place to rest. He admits to chronic alcohol abuse and has expressed some thoughts of quitting, but has never followed up on referrals. Today, he is admitted to the hospital for severe malnutrition and electrolyte imbalances. He admits to drinking heavily just before going to the clinic.

1. The diagnosis of alcohol dependence is based on what criteria? ***(1122)***

   a. ______________________________

   b. ______________________________

   c. ______________________________

   d. ______________________________

   e. ______________________________

2. When assessing Mr. Briganti for a substance use problem, what are three things you should ask about substance abuse during history-taking? ***(1129-1130)***

   a. ______________________________

   b. ______________________________

   c. ______________________________

3. Name three goals of care for a patient with a substance use disorder. ***(1130)***

   a. ______________________________

   b. ______________________________

   c. ______________________________

4. Which of the following is the priority diagnosis for Mr. Briganti? ***(1132)***
   a. Noncompliance related to abstinence from substance
   b. Injury, risk for, related to alcohol withdrawal
   c. Home maintenance management, impaired, related to homelessness
   d. Imbalanced nutrition, less than body requirements, related to excessive alcohol consumption and self-neglect

5. Write a sample outcome statement for Risk for injury related to complications of withdrawal from alcohol. ***(1132)***

   ____

   ____

6. Give three nursing interventions to prevent injuries related to complications of withdrawal from alcohol. ***(1132)***

   a. ____

   b. ____

   c. ____

7. The doctor orders a 500 mL fluid bolus of dextrose 5% with normal saline to infuse over 90 minutes for Mr. Briganti. What is the pump setting? __________ mL

8. Which of the following tasks would be appropriate to assign to the nursing student in providing the care for Mr. Briganti?
   a. IV insertion with your supervision.
   b. Telephoning the doctor to give lab results.
   c. Assessing Mr. Briganti for Risk for injury.
   d. Talking to Mr. Briganti about the alcohol abuse.

PRIORITY SETTING

Prioritizing for a Patient with Alcohol Withdrawal

Directions: Read the clinical scenario and prioritize as appropriate.

Scenario: You are caring for a patient who has a history of chronic alcohol abuse. It has been approximately 8 hours since the patient last had a drink. You are vigilant for the signs of withdrawal. The patient currently has a blood pressure of 160/85, pulse 110. Place the interventions in the order of priority. ***(1122-1134)***

______ a. Orienting the patient to person, place, and time.

______ b. IV fluids are administered to correct dehydration as ordered.

______ c. Encourage a balanced diet high in proteins and multivitamins.

______ d. Give chlordiazepoxide HCl (Librium) as ordered.

______ e. Establish IV access.

NCLEX-PN® EXAM REVIEW

Directions: Choose the best answer(s) for the following questions.

1. What are the two main defense mechanisms used by substance abusers? ***(1121)***
   1. Repression and regression
   2. Sublimation and splitting
   3. Denial and rationalization
   4. Displacement and identification

2. The patient is taking lorazepam (Ativan) for anxiety. The nurse advises him not to drink alcohol while taking this drug for which of the following reasons? ***(1123)***
   1. There is an increase in blood pressure caused by frequent use.
   2. There is an additive effect on the nervous system.
   3. There is a decrease in blood pressure caused by frequent use.
   4. There is increased risk for insomnia and gastrointestinal distress.

3. The nurse is caring for an elderly patient who is prescribed triazolam (Halcion) for insomnia. Benzodiazepines must be used cautiously in the elderly because of which of the following? ***(1125)***
   1. They have a long half-life and are not excreted readily.
   2. They are toxic to the aging liver.
   3. Tolerance causes use of increasing doses.
   4. They may be used along with alcohol.

4. The nurse is caring for a patient with a history of substance abuse. Which of the following is the most important aspect in the initial treatment of the substance-abuse patient? ***(1122)***
   1. Careful detoxification procedures
   2. Empathetic care by all health professionals
   3. Recognition of dependence on the substance
   4. Regular participation in a 12-step program

5. Two serious long-term results of smoking nicotine that may occur are: ***(1128)***
   1. addiction to nicotine and impaired coordination.
   2. low blood pressure and cardiac arrhythmias.
   3. stained teeth and bad breath.
   4. lung cancer and emphysema.

6. During the physical assessment, the nurse notices bruises and needle marks on the patient's antecubital space. Which of the following is the best response? ***(1130)***
   1. "What are these marks? Are you injecting IV drugs?"
   2. "I am going to ask the doctor to look at your arms."
   3. "I see you have some bruises. Can you tell me what happened?"
   4. "Let me clean and bandage your arm to prevent infection."

7. The nurse is talking to the patient's mother about enabling. Which statement by the mother indicates that additional intervention is needed for the enabling behavior? ***(1131)***
   1. "I am going to let her take responsibility for her decisions."
   2. "I'm her mother, I'll always be there for her no matter what."
   3. "We have all been denying the problem for a long time."
   4. "I will support her recovery by attending Al-Anon."

8. Early symptoms of alcohol withdrawal (anxiety, irritability, and agitation) may manifest within: *(1122)*
   1. 1–2 hours after the last drink.
   2. 6–12 hours after the last drink.
   3. 24–48 hours after the last drink.
   4. 2–3 days after the last drink.

9. The doctor has ordered large doses of thiamine for the patient. This treatment is appropriate for which of the following? *(1124)*
   1. Wernicke's encephalopathy
   2. Korsakoff's syndrome
   3. Opiate overdose
   4. Methamphetamine abuse

10. The nurse is assisting the alcohol abuse patient to plan activities that will help him to maintain a healthy lifestyle after he is discharged from the hospital. *(Select all that apply.)* ***(1122-1124)***
    1. Remind the patient that the physical symptoms of withdrawal will not last forever.
    2. Help him to make a list of activities that would distract him from the cravings.
    3. Ask him to contact old drug buddies to tell them that he has stopped using.
    4. Tell him to have a beer with a friend and talk about happier times.
    5. Participate actively and frequently in a 12-step program.

CRITICAL THINKING ACTIVITIES

Scenario: You are asked to help develop a community presentation about smoking cessation. One of your tasks is to collect some accurate information that can be used in the presentation.

1. What are three physical changes that nicotine causes? *(1127-1128)*____________________

   ____

   ____

   ____

2. What are the withdrawal symptoms? *(1128)* ____________________

   ____

   ____

   ____

3. What treatments are available for nicotine addiction? *(1128)* ____________________

   ____

   ____

   ____

STEPS TOWARD BETTER COMMUNICATION

VOCABULARY BUILDING GLOSSARY

Term	Pronunciation	Definition
alleviate	ah lee' vee ate	make easier or less severe
arousal level	ah row' zel lev' el	ease with which a person can be awakened
denial	dee ni' al	a defense mechanism in which a person will not admit unpleasant or painful realities
diminish	dee min' ish	become less, get smaller
eradicate	erad'icate	get rid of; remove
foster	fos'ter	encourage and help
withdrawal	withdraw'al	a group of symptoms that are present when a person stops using a drug
enabling	en ab'ling	making something easier; doing something for an addict that he could do for himself
self-righteous	self ri' chus	very sure that oneself is right and has the correct answers
stigma	stig'ma	a mark of shame

WORD ATTACK SKILLS

Word Meanings

Directions: Underline the correct word in each pair to complete the sentence with the correct meaning.

1. Buying alcohol for an alcoholic spouse who has drunk too much is an example of (self-righteous/enabling) behavior.
2. Extreme jumpiness and nervousness can be a symptom of (denial/withdrawal) from alcohol in the hospitalized patient.
3. Joining a 12-step group such as Alcoholics Anonymous will help (foster/eradicate) a person's decision to stop drinking.

Number Words in Order

Directions: Number these words in order, with the strongest word first.

______ a. alleviate

______ b. diminish

______ c. eradicate

Word Elements

Directions: The following words from Chapter 46 end in the word element -tion. *This ending usually indicates the result of an action. In each word defined below, identify the base word and give its part of speech.*

1. Denomina'tion—a religious group with its own set of beliefs within a larger religion; e.g., a Protestant denomination of Christianity:

   ____

   ____

2. Idea'tion—the formation of ideas or images:

   ____

   ____

3. Predisposi'tion—being more vulnerable or likely to attain something:

   ____

   ____

4. Rationaliza'tion—an unconscious defense mechanism in which a person finds logical reasons for his actions while ignoring the real reasons:

   ____

   ____

5. Valida'tion—showing approval, agreeing to the correctness or appropriateness of an action:

   ____

   ____

PRONUNCIATION SKILLS

Directions: Beneath each "s" in the following words write s *or* z *to show how the letter "s" should be pronounced.*

1. predisposition
2. arousal

COMMUNICATION EXERCISE

With a partner, practice asking and answering the questions in Table 46-7 in the textbook. Ask for clarification if you do not understand the pronunciation or meaning of what your partner is saying.

CHAPTER 47

Care of Patients with Cognitive Disorders

evolve Go to http://evolve.elsevier.com/deWit for additional activities and exercises.

TERMINOLOGY

Directions: Match the term on the right with the meaning on the left.

1. ______	Delirium *(1137)*	a.	Becoming confused and disoriented only at night
2. ______	Cognition *(1137)*	b.	Making up conversation to fill gaps in memory
3. ______	Dementia *(1137)*	c.	Acute confusion
4. ______	Confabulation *(1138)*	d.	Deficit in memory and other cognitive areas
5. ______	Global amnesia *(1148)*	e.	Leaving a place or moving with no plan
6. ______	Poverty of thoughts *(1138)*	f.	Unable to recall events, or remember friends and family
7. ______	Wandering *(1147)*	g.	Thoughts are vague, repetitious, and disconnected
8. ______	Sundowning *(1146)*	h.	Mental processes of perception, memory, judgment, and reasoning

COMPLETION

Delirium and Dementia

Directions: Fill in the blanks to complete the statements.

1. The patient experiencing delirium may demonstrate disorganized and distorted thinking and incoherent ______________________________. *(1137)*

2. One of the first things you should assess in a patient who is exhibiting signs of delirium is what ______________________ the patient is receiving. *(1137)*

3. A difference between delirium and dementia is that dementia occurs over a ______________________ ______________________. *(1138)*

4. Early stages of dementia are marked by loss of ______________________. *(1139)*

5. An assessment of mental status should be done for patients with a cognitive disorder at least ______________________________. *(1137)*

6. When planning nursing care for a patient with a cognitive disorder, ________________ is the number-one priority. *(1140)*

7. When implementing nursing care for the patient with delirium, it is best to ________________ all ________________ in the environment. ***(1150)***

8. Patients with dementia fare better if there is ________________ to their environment and a daily ________________. ***(1140-1141)***

9. For the caregiver who is becoming exhausted because of caring for a family member with dementia, you might explore community possibilities for ________________ or ________________. ***(1150)***

10. The most common degenerative disease of the brain is ________________. ***(1139)***

11. For elders, medications should be given in the ________________ amounts possible and increased when the symptoms indicate. ***(1138)***

SHORT ANSWER

Caring for a Patient with Acute Confusion

Directions: Read the clinical scenario and answer the questions that follow.

Scenario: Mr. James is an elderly man who resides at an assisted living facility. Although he is occasionally forgetful, he is usually alert and cheerful and enjoys telling stories about his family and his career in the military. He is able to function with minimal assistance. The nursing assistant tells you that today Mr. James seems drowsy, disoriented, and extremely irritable.

1. Name four types of medications that could be causing Mr. James' change in behavior. ***(1138)***

   a. ________________

   b. ________________

   c. ________________

   d. ________________

2. What five areas are involved in a quick assessment for delirium and dementia? ***(1145)***

   a. ________________

   b. ________________

   c. ________________

   d. ________________

   e. ________________

3. What are five possible causes of acute confusion? ***(1137)***

 a. ____________________

 b. ____________________

 c. ____________________

 d. ____________________

 e. ____________________

4. List five things you can do to help decrease Mr. James' confusion using reality orientation. ***(1147)***

 a. ____________________

 b. ____________________

 c. ____________________

 d. ____________________

 e. ____________________

APPLICATION OF THE NURSING PROCESS

Caring for a Patient with Alzheimer's Disease

Directions: Provide the answers to the following questions.

Mr. Thompson, age 85, lives with his daughter Jane. He was diagnosed with Alzheimer's disease several years ago. Jane is concerned because her father left the house last week and he was missing for several hours before the neighbor helped him back to the house. Jane also reports that her father has not recognized her on several occasions.

1. The doctor has told Jane that her father may begin to have signs of the middle- to late stage of Alzheimer's. List four of the behaviors associated with the middle- to late stage of Alzheimer's. ***(1139)***

 a. ____________________

 b. ____________________

 c. ____________________

 d. ____________________

2. Jane reports that her father has been losing weight and that she has to remind him to eat and sometimes she even has to feed him. She tells you that, "When Dad was younger, he used to weigh over 250 lbs. and now he is down to about 145 lbs. Convert Mr. Thompson's current weight to kg. __________

3. Which nursing diagnosis would be a priority for Mr. Thompson? ***(1141)***
   a. Confusion, chronic, related to slow progressive memory loss
   b. Thought processes, altered, related to biochemical changes in the brain
   c. Social interaction, impaired, related to inability to recognize friends and family
   d. Injury, risk for, related to faulty judgment
   e. Wandering related to disorientation to time and place
   f. Risk for caregiver role strain related to prolonged 24-hour responsibility to give care

4. List three ways in which you can help Jane to reduce her own stress. ***(1150)***

   a. ______________________________

   b. ______________________________

   c. ______________________________

5. For a patient who is confused or tends to wander, list five teaching points to share with the caregiver to ensure the patient's safety. ***(1144)***

   a. ______________________________

   b. ______________________________

   c. ______________________________

   d. ______________________________

   e. ______________________________

6. Which of the following statements indicates that Jane understands how to manage Mr. Thompson's confusion? ***(1141)***
   a. "If I repeat time, date, and year every morning, he will become oriented to time."
   b. "I'll use several different caregivers; he will be stimulated by other faces."
   c. "I'll provide general orientation to the year by using holiday decorations."
   d. "We'll have big family parties every weekend, just like we used to."

PRIORITY SETTING

Directions: Read the scenario and prioritize as appropriate.

Scenario: You are working in an extended care facility. You have just received shift report on your six patients. Indicate the order in which you would attend to the needs of these patients.

______ a. It is the scheduled time for Mr. Jeandron's AM insulin.

______ b. Mrs. Slipik is more confused today than she usually is.

______ c. Mr. Motton has a complaint about the night-shift nurse.

______ d. Mr. Tize has a low-grade fever.

______ e. Mrs. Palabo has fallen in the bathroom.

______ f. Mr. Newton is asking for his scheduled pain medication.

NCLEX-PN® EXAM REVIEW

Directions: Choose the best answer(s) for the following questions.

1. The nurse is caring for a patient with Alzheimer's. Which of the following are signs and symptoms associated with the early stage of Alzheimer's? *(1139)*
   1. Slow, progressive loss of intellectual ability and difficulty learning new things
   2. Unable to speak or ambulate and profound memory loss
   3. Social withdrawal and decreased in ability to perform usual activities of daily living
   4. Outbursts of anger, hostility, paranoia, and wandering

2. What factors cause elderly patients to be at risk for substance-induced delirium? *(1138)*
   1. Increased metabolism and reduction in cardiac and liver function
   2. Decreased metabolism and reduction in cardiac and respiratory function
   3. Decreased metabolism and reduction in kidney and liver function
   4. Increased metabolism and reduction in neurologic and immune function

3. During data collection, the patient's son tells the nurse that, "Mom can remember her name, but she doesn't seem to know where she is." Based on this information, which question should the nurse ask first? *(1140)*
   1. "How does she like to be addressed?"
   2. "When did you first notice this?"
   3. "What kind of medications does she take?"
   4. "When did she last see the doctor?"

4. The patient is suffering acute delirium related to a systemic infection. During the evening the patient appears to be very frightened by the IV tubing. The nurse recognizes that the patient is experiencing which of the following? *(1138)*
   1. Hallucination
   2. Illusion
   3. Delusion
   4. Confabulation

5. A 25-year-old patient is brought to the emergency department by the police. He is a poor historian, but the police tell the nurse that they were called because he was wandering down the middle of the freeway. He appears confused, disheveled, and malnourished. Which nursing diagnosis on the care plan would be of highest priority for this patient?
   1. Bathing/hygiene/feeding self-care deficit
   2. Wandering related to disorientation to time and place
   3. Injury, risk for, related to faulty judgment
   4. Imbalanced nutrition, less than body requirements

6. The nurse is caring for a patient in the middle- to late stage of Alzheimer's. In planning care, the nurse should anticipate the need for which of the following interventions? *(1139)*
   1. Repeat the date and time frequently.
   2. Restrain the patient to protect from falls and wandering.
   3. Vary routine and provide unstructured environment.
   4. Allot extra time for grooming and toileting.

7. The nurse is working on a busy medical-surgical unit. An elderly patient has fallen out of bed twice, despite repeated verbal instructions to call for assistance. Which of the following are appropriate interventions to ensure safety? *(Select all that apply.)* ***(1149)***
   1. Encourage family members and friends to stay with the patient.
   2. Obtain an order for an anxiolytic medication.
   3. Keep patient close to the nurse's station.
   4. Check on patient frequently to offer nutrition, fluids, pain relief, and toileting.
   5. Place the bed in the lowest position with three side rails up.
   6. Temporarily place restraints and secure knots to the bedrails.

8. The doctor has ordered that the patient be restrained for 24 hours. Which of the following tasks is appropriate to assign to the nursing assistant? ***(1148)***
   1. Selecting the type of restraint.
   2. Checking the circulation in the area distal to the restraint.
   3. Performing 1:1 observation.
   4. Obtaining consent from the patient's family to use restraints.

9. The nursing student is assisting the nurse to apply the restraints to a patient. Which of the following actions by the student indicates that she understands the procedure? ***(1149)***
   1. She checks the circulation and then applies the restraints.
   2. She ties the knot so that it is not readily visible to the patient, family, or staff.
   3. She states that she will check on the patient every 2–4 hours.
   4. She documents the care that was given while the patient was in restraints.

10. The patient is prescribed donepezil (Aricept). Which of the following statements by the patient's wife indicates that she understands the information about the drug? ***(1141)***
    1. "It slows progression of symptoms, but is not a cure."
    2. "If he takes the medication, the symptoms will resolve."
    3. "This medicine may improve memory, but it is experimental."
    4. "The side effects include headaches and blurred vision."

CRITICAL THINKING ACTIVITIES

Scenario: You are working at an extended care facility. In report, you hear that Mr. Kuapoo was restrained during the night for "inappropriate behavior." When you check the chart, you cannot find any order for restraints and the documentation does not include any details about the behavior, the type of restraints, or the care given while the patient was in the restraints.

1. What is your first action?
   a. Call the doctor and obtain an order for restraints.
   b. Call the nurse at home and ask for details.
   c. Report the incident to the nursing supervisor.
   d. Assess the patient and remove the restraints.

2. During the report, what information should be clarified with the nurse before he or she leaves? ***(1148)***

____

____

____

____

3. What are your ethical obligations in this situation? What are the ramifications of following through? *(1148-1149)*

____

____

____

____

____

____

____

STEPS TOWARD BETTER COMMUNICATION

VOCABULARY BUILDING GLOSSARY

Term	Pronunciation	Definition
cognition	kog ni' shun	the mental process of thinking, perceiving, and remembering
confabulation	kon fab u la' shun	inventing or making up untrue or exaggerated stories and answers to questions
abstract	ab strakt'	not concrete, material, or physical; (noun) ideas or theories with no specific application
respite care	res'pit care	short-term care to give relief to the family caregiver for an afternoon or weekend
insight	in' site	ability to see and understand the truth about something
blunted	blun'ted	not sharp or perceptive; plain and flat
remote memory	ree mot' memory	distant in time, long ago
advance directives		instructions about what to do in case of medical emergencies, incapacity, and death; may include power of attorney
confront	kon front	to talk face to face about difficult problems, sometimes argumentative

COMPLETION

Directions: Fill in the blanks with the appropriate words from the Vocabulary Building Glossary to complete the statements.

1. A patient suffering from advanced Alzheimer's disease generally has a ____________________ affect.

2. When dementia is present, the patient has difficulty comprehending ____________________ ideas.

3. When patients begin to have great difficulty with memory, they tend to make things up to fill gaps, this is called ______________________.

4. As dementia worsens, __________________ decreases, although long-term memory may remain intact.

5. The family caregiver of an Alzheimer's patient badly needs occasional ______________________ for the patient.

6. A patient who frequently loses his way does not usually have any ________________ as to why this is happening to him and is frightened.

7. The dementia patient often has difficulty with recent memory but can remember things from childhood which reside in ______________________________.

8. All adults should have ____ in place, in case an accident or illness incapacitates them.

SHORT ANSWER

Memory Examples

Directions: Give two examples each of immediate memory, recent memory, and remote memory.

1. Immediate memory:

   e.g., I just drank a cup of coffee.

   a. ____

   b. ____

2. Recent memory:

   a. ____

   b. ____

3. Remote memory:

   a. ____

   b. ____

WORD ATTACK SKILLS

Word Meanings

Directions: Match the adjectives on the left with their correct meanings on the right.

1. ______	Impaired	a.	Changed from its true nature or shape
2. ______	Fragmented	b.	Damaged
3. ______	Incoherent	c.	Divided in pieces
4. ______	Disturbed	d.	Less, smaller
5. ______	Disoriented	e.	Not certain of time, place, or identity
6. ______	Distorted	f.	Not making sense
7. ______	Disorganized	g.	Upset, worried; not normal
8. ______	Diminished	h.	Without an order or system

PRONUNCIATION SKILLS

Directions: Put the following words in the correct column depending on whether the pronunciation of "-ed" in the word is -id, -d, or -t.

blunted, diminished, disorganized, disoriented, distorted, disturbed, fragmented, impaired

-id	-d	-t

COMMUNICATION EXERCISE

Mr. Jones has become combative while being bathed this morning. The nursing assistant has called you to intervene and help him with this difficult situation. The following is an example of an interaction that could be used in such an instance.

Distraction is the first method to be used, then negotiation.

Nurse: "Mr. Jones, I'm Sandra, the charge nurse on this unit. Did you enjoy your breakfast this morning?"

Mr. Jones: "Well, I guess it was OK."

Nurse: "Would you like to go for a walk outside after you are dressed? It's a beautiful day."

Mr. Jones: "That would be nice, but I don't want to bathe now."

Nurse: "How about watching TV? Your favorite game show is on now."

Mr. Jones: "I don't want to watch TV."

Nurse: "How about rinsing off in the shower rather than bathing at the basin today?"

Mr. Jones: "I always prefer to shower. I don't like people messing with me."

Nurse: "OK. Harold will help you get to the shower room. I'll see you later."

CULTURAL POINT

The elderly often have difficulty with recent memory but like to talk about pleasant memories from the past. Conversation with them might be directed at childhood memories of holidays and special vacations or events. Various foods, smells, and pieces of music may remind them of such times. The nurse's own life can be enriched by such sharing of memories.

CHAPTER 48

Care of Patients with Thought and Personality Disorders

evolve Go to http://evolve.elsevier.com/deWit for additional activities and exercises.

TERMINOLOGY

Thought Disorders

Directions: Match the term on the left with the correct definition or statement on the right.

1. ______	Psychotic features ***(1154)***	a.	Person has an inflated notion of self-importance despite logical reasoning
2. ______	Delusions of grandeur ***(1154)***	b.	Absence or near absence of emotional expression
3. ______	Hallucination ***(1154)***	c.	Misinterpretation of reality
4. ______	Word salad ***(1161)***	d.	Sensory perception without a corresponding stimulus
5. ______	Ideas of reference ***(1160)***	e.	The person feels that objects, events, or people in his environment have an unusual significance only for him
6. ______	Neologisms ***(1160)***	f.	Disorganized mix of words, phrases, and fragments that do not make sense
7. ______	Illusion ***(1155)***	g.	Hallucinations, delusions, and disorganized speech or behavior
8. ______	Flat affect ***(1160)***	h.	Made-up new words for expressing confused thoughts
9. ______	Delusion ***(1154)***	i.	False fixed belief

COMPLETION

Schizophrenia

Directions: Fill in the blanks to complete the sentences.

1. When assessing thought disorders, the interview must be ______________ because it is difficult for the individual to ____________________________ for very long. ***(1158)***

2. Schizophrenia usually develops in ________________ or in the early ____________________. ***(1156)***

3. A schizophrenic's behavior can cause vulnerability to psychosocial problems. These include ________________, ______________, ______________, and __________________. ***(1156)***

4. Examples of atypical antipsychotic medications which are used to treat schizophrenia include ______________________, ________________________, and ____________________________. ***(1158)***

5. Because of the negative symptoms of ____________________________ and ______________________, elderly schizophrenics are not as likely to seek help. ***(1158)***

SHORT ANSWERS

Thought Disorders

Directions: Read the clinical scenario and answer the questions that follow.

Scenario: Ms. Lalani, age 45, was diagnosed with schizophrenia at age 21. She is frequently admitted to the psychiatric unit for relapse. Currently, she is delusional and verbally hostile. Her appearance is disheveled and she wears layers of clothes inside out and backward. She has a flat affect and sits by herself, talking and gesturing to the air. In the past, she has been prescribed the conventional antipsychotic medication, thioridazine (Mellaril). The doctor is trying to give her ziprasidone (Geodon) to see if her symptoms can be controlled by one of the newer medications.

1. List six desirable outcomes for the negative symptoms of schizophrenia. ***(1156)***

   a. ____

   b. ____

   c. ____

   d. ____

   e. ____

   f. ____

2. What are four assessment findings for Ms. Lalani that suggest that she has a thought disorder? ***(1155-1156)***

   a. ____

   b. ____

   c. ____

   d. ____

3. Which nursing diagnoses would be appropriate for Ms. Lalani and are likely to be included in her plan of care? *(Select all that apply.)* ***(1160)***
   a. Thought processes, altered
   b. Sensory perceptions, altered
   c. Activity intolerance
   d. Social interaction, impaired
   e. Bathing/hygiene/feeding self-care deficit
   f. Risk for other-directed or self-directed violence
   g. Dysfunctional grieving

4. What are three nursing interventions for patients with altered thought processes related to delusional thinking? *(1162-1163)*

   a. ______________________________

   b. ______________________________

   c. ______________________________

5. What signs and symptoms should you look for when assessing for extrapyramidal side effects that are associated with antipsychotic medications? *(1156-1157)*

   a. Pseudoparkinsonism: ______________________________

   ____

   b. Dystonic reaction: ______________________________

   ____

   c. Akathisia: ______________________________

   ____

   d. Tardive dyskinesia: ______________________________

   ____

   ____

   ____

6. List six common anticholinergic side effects that are seen with the use of antipsychotic medications. *(1156)*

   a. ______________________________

   b. ______________________________

   c. ______________________________

   d. ______________________________

   e. ______________________________

   f. ______________________________

7. The doctor orders a maximum fluid intake of 2500 mL of free water/24 hours, because Ms. Lalani is known to drink excessive water and this puts her at risk for hyponatremia. Convert 2500 mL into the total number of 8-ounce glasses of water that Ms. Lalani is allowed to drink.
   ____________ glasses

APPLICATION OF THE NURSING PROCESS

Caring for a Patient with Schizophrenia

Directions: Read the scenario and choose the best answer(s) for the following questions.

Scenario: Mr. Hinton is a 25-year-old patient who was recently admitted with the diagnosis of schizophrenia. The police were called to a local restaurant because Mr. Hinton had barricaded himself in the men's room and was yelling about Osama Bin Laden. He is disheveled and appears suspicious and distrustful.

1. In report, the nurse states that Mr. Hinton displays positive symptoms of schizophrenia. Which of the following are positive symptoms? ***(1155)***
   a. Delusions and hallucinations
   b. Self-care deficits and lack of motivation
   c. Blunted affect and poverty of speech
   d. Social withdrawal and manipulative behavior

2. You observe Mr. Hinton. He is standing in a corner by himself and suddenly he puts his hands over his ears and begins to sway back and forth. You hear him say "Shut up, just stop it, shut up!" This behavior suggests which of the following? ***(1155)***
   a. Mr. Hinton is seeking attention.
   b. Mr. Hinton is displaying echolalia.
   c. Mr. Hinton is experiencing a drug side-effect.
   d. Mr. Hinton is having an auditory hallucination.

3. Mr. Hinton insists that Osama Bin Laden once kidnapped him. He is afraid that Bin Laden will return to "finish the job." What is the best response? ***(1161)***
   a. "Tell me more about why you think Bin Laden is after you."
   b. "I can see that you are afraid, but I believe that we are safe here."
   c. "You seem very afraid, but we will protect you from Bin Laden."
   d. "Your story about this kidnapping is frightening, but it's illogical."

4. In the acute phase, which is the priority diagnosis for Mr. Hinton? ***(1162)***
   a. Thought processes, altered, related to a chemical imbalance
   b. Social isolation related to fear and feelings of persecution
   c. Other-directed or self-directed violence, risk for, related to delusional thinking
   d. Self-care deficit related to cognitive impairment

5. Mr. Hinton loudly argues with the medication nurse and refuses to take his morning medications. "She is with Bin Laden and is trying to poison all the patients!" What is your first action? ***(1166)***
   a. Point out to Mr. Hinton that other patients are taking the medicines without ill effects.
   b. Call the physician and ask for a temporary emergency order to administer medications.
   c. Support the authority of the medication nurse by gathering 4 or 5 other staff members.
   d. Distract Mr. Hinton and then later see if he will accept the medication from another nurse.

6. Which activity would be most appropriate for Mr. Hinton in the early acute phase of hospitalization? ***(1161)***
   a. Attending a music therapy class.
   b. Walking in an enclosed patio garden.
   c. Playing cards or checkers in the day room.
   d. Sleeping in his room undisturbed.

COMPLETION

Personality Disorders

Directions: Fill in the blanks to complete the sentences.

1. Personality disorders are enduring patterns of behavior with no loss of ____________________ or impaired cognition. ***(1165)***
2. Patients with borderline personality disorder fear real or ____________________. ***(1165)***
3. Two behaviors often seen in patients with borderline personality disorder are ____________________ and ____________________. ***(1165)***
4. To be effective with a patient with borderline personality disorder, you need to maintain ____________________ without being controlling, rigid, or ____________________. ***(1168)***

SHORT ANSWER

Borderline Personality Disorder

Directions: Read the clinical scenario and answer the questions that follow.

Scenario: You are working on a medical-surgical unit. You hear in report that all of the nurses are having trouble dealing with Ms. Aunders, who was admitted several days ago. One of the RNs suggests a psychiatric consult be obtained, because the patient is manipulative, demanding, and "unlikely to follow the treatment plan." Old medical records show that Ms. Aunders has been previously diagnosed with a borderline personality disorder.

1. What are the four characteristics of personality disorders? ***(1166)***
   a. ____________________
   b. ____________________
   c. ____________________
   d. ____________________
2. What are four things to assess for in a patient whom you think might have a personality disorder? ***(1167)***
   a. ____________________
   b. ____________________
   c. ____________________
   d. ____________________
3. Write an outcome for the nursing diagnosis: Self-esteem, chronic low, related to past failures and negative responses from significant others. ***(1171)***

____

____

____

4. What are two nursing interventions used to deal with manipulative behavior of patients who have personality disorders? *(1166)*

   a. ______________________________

   b. ______________________________

PRIORITY SETTING AND ASSIGNMENT

Directions: Read the scenario and prioritize as appropriate.

Scenario: You are caring for Mr. Radcheck. He has been rocking and fidgeting and refuses to interact with the staff or other patients. You have observed him talking to himself and you suspect that he may be having command hallucinations.

1. Which of the following is the priority nursing diagnosis? ***(1166)***
   a. Thought processes, disturbed (delusions)
   b. Sensory perceptions, disturbed (hallucinations)
   c. Social interaction, impaired
   d. Risk for other-directed or self-directed violence

Mr. Radcheck is now pacing. He yells at one of the other patients and then comes to you and says, "That blearsoning boop is rounding, rounding! Get her down! Stick her with a knife and glass and dead her head!"

2. What is the priority intervention? ***(1166)***
   a. Try to figure out what he is saying and empathize.
   b. Firmly instruct him to calm down and go sit down.
   c. Gently tell him his behavior is inappropriate.
   d. Redirect him to a quiet and isolated area.

3. Mr. Radcheck is unable to follow your verbal instructions. His pacing increases and he begins to wildly gesture. What is the priority action? ***(1166)***
   a. Remove the other patients and allow him to pace.
   b. Gather several staff members to stand behind you.
   c. Call the doctor for an order for chemical restraints.
   d. Repeat your verbal instructions and state the consequences.

4. The nursing assistant is available to help you with Mr. Radcheck. What task would be appropriate to assign to the assistant? ***(1168)***
   a. Ask the assistant to try to calm him down.
   b. Ask the assistant to go call the doctor.
   c. Have the assistant do 1:1 as ordered by the doctor.
   d. Assign the assistant to put the patient in four-point restraint.

5. The next day, Mr. Radcheck is calm and quiet. Which of the following tasks would be appropriate to assign to the nursing assistant? ***(1168)***
   a. Sit with Mr. Radcheck and ask him how he is feeling.
   b. Encourage Mr. Radcheck to take a shower.
   c. Talk with Mr. Radcheck about his future plans.
   d. Observe Mr. Radcheck for any agitated behavior.

NCLEX-PN® EXAM REVIEW

Directions: Choose the best answer(s) for the following questions.

1. A nurse is caring for a patient with paranoid schizophrenia. Which of following behaviors indicates that the patient is having delusions of persecution? ***(1152)***
   1. Tilts head and appears to be listening.
   2. Paces around the dayroom with arms folded.
   3. Refuses to eat food unless it is packaged.
   4. Strikes out at a curtain that is waving in the breeze.

2. The patient is taking an antipsychotic medication, fluphanzine (Prolixin). Which of following side effects, if noted, should the nurse identify as most significant, requiring immediate intervention? ***(1156)***
   1. A fixed upward gaze
   2. A shuffling gait
   3. Tapping of the foot
   4. Irritability

3. The patient was admitted yesterday following an episode of violence at a library. He is currently quiet, but displays psychotic behaviors. When planning care for the patient, the nurse plans to avoid which of the following? *(Select all that apply.)* ***(1166)***
   1. Address the patient by name and establish rapport.
   2. Use therapeutic touch to communicate caring.
   3. Control environmental stimuli such as loud music.
   4. Allow the patient to move about in an enclosed area.

4. The patient tells the nurse that there are a several men in dark coats that are watching her and planning to steal her belongings. The best response from the nurse is: ***(1161)***
   1. "There are no men watching you."
   2. "Tell me more about these men."
   3. " I did not see any men."
   4. " They won't hurt you."

5. The nurse is working in an acute admission ward in a psychiatric facility. Which of the following safety precautions should the nurse take when caring for these acutely ill patients? *(Select all that apply.)* ***(1160)***
   1. Avoid wearing flashing or dangling jewelry.
   2. Avoid wearing a white coat or white uniform.
   3. Avoid wearing a stethoscope, scarf, or tie around the neck.
   4. Avoid casual touching without asking permission.
   5. Avoid doorways and exits.
   6. Avoid any patients who appear sullen or depressed.

6. The patient is taking olanzapine (Zyprexa) as prescribed. Which patient comment suggests that the medication is successfully treating the patient's positive symptoms? ***(1158)***
   1. "I can leave the hospital whenever I want to."
   2. "Nurse, I am ready to go home. Would you call my mother?"
   3. "I can still hear the voices, but they are very distant."
   4. "The angel stopped talking; now she just sits and waves."

7. The patient is ready to be discharged. The nurse teaches him about his antipsychotic medication and he asks, "What will happen if I stop taking my medication when I go home?" Which is the best reply? ***(1161)***
   1. "You should never stop taking your medication."
   2. "Someday you may be able to do without the medication."
   3. "If you can get organized and reduce stress, perhaps you can get along without it."
   4. "If you stop taking your medication, the symptoms will probably return."

8. The patient will be discharged within a day or two. Which statement by the patient's family indicates a need for further discussion about the diagnosis of schizophrenia? ***(1158)***
   1. "A stable home environment will help to prevent relapse."
   2. "He might always hear voices, but the medications will help."
   3. "Medication will eliminate his blunted affect and social isolation."
   4. "If he fails to take his medication, it will probably lead to readmission."

9. A patient is admitted to the unit with a diagnosis of borderline personality disorder. Which characteristic is associated with this disorder? ***(1165)***
   1. Indecisive
   2. Submissive
   3. Impulsive
   4. Aggressive

10. The nurse is talking with a patient who has a borderline personality disorder. The patient says, "I'll tell you a secret, because you are the best nurse here." Which of following comments should the nurse identify as most significant, requiring notification of the registered nurse? ***(1165)***
    1. "I lied to get in here, because I was sick of living with my mother."
    2. "The charge nurse is a lesbian. I've seen her in the lesbo clubs."
    3. "I am going to give myself a little superficial cut, so that the doctor will see me."
    4. "I stole some money from my father and he might hurt me when I get out."

11. The nursing diagnosis for a patient is Chronic low self-esteem. The nurse instructs the patient to do which of the following to promote self-esteem? *(Select all that apply.)* ***(1161)***
    1. Make a list of things that she is good at.
    2. Give and receive positive feedback.
    3. Set small, realistic goals.
    4. Describe personal failures in detail to a friend.
    5. Critique personal performance for errors.
    6. Keep a journal of success stories.

CRITICAL THINKING ACTIVITIES

Scenario: You have talked to Christy Smith and feel that rapport has been established. Ms. Smith has shared personal information with you. She states, "I really like talking to you." You leave Ms. Smith to admit a new patient. Later, when you return, Ms. Smith hits you and tries to run out the door.

1. What are your initial thoughts about this scenario? ____________________

____

____

____

____

2. What factors may have triggered Ms. Smith's aggressive behavior? ***(1166)*** ______________________

____

____

____

____

____

3. What types of things should you do to protect yourself, patients, and others? ***(1166)***______________

____

____

____

____

STEP TOWARD BETTER COMMUNICATION

VOCABULARY BUILDING GLOSSARY

Term	Pronunciation	Definition
trigger	trig'ger	start a reaction, cause to begin
de-escalation	dee esk ah la' shun	process of coming back down, as in the calming of a nervous, hyperactive patient
extrapyramidal	eks' trah pir ram' ah dal	symptoms outside the pyramidal tracts of the nervous system
erratic	ah rat'ik	inconsistent, not performing normally; irregular
odd	awd	something or someone different, strange, unusual, or surprising
eccentric	ek sen' trik	showing unusual behavior; unconventional, peculiar
impulsive	im pul' sive	acting on sudden urges or desires without thinking of the consequences
boundaries	bown'dreez	limits to behavior or movement
recur	ree ker'	happen again
rationale	rah shun al'	the reason for doing something; the thoughts about why to do something
acting out		expressing feelings through nonverbal behavior
borderline	bor' der line	on the edge or boundary
"get under the skin"		causing a reaction, such as irritation or attraction
traits		characteristic actions or behaviors
subsequent	sub' see kwent	later, following

CHOOSING THE CORRECT WORD

Directions: Underline the word in parentheses that correctly completes the thought.

1. The patient would often take things from stores; this is an example of (eccentric/impulsive) behavior.
2. The patient was removing her clothes in the dayroom after her husband came to visit; this is an example of (subsequent/acting out) behavior.
3. The patient demonstrated (erratic/odd) behavior by weaving pieces of styrofoam and old milk cartons into her hair.
4. The nurse was firm with the borderline personality disorder patient, setting (boundaries/rationale) for acceptable behavior.
5. The family did not know what would (trigger/recur) manic behavior in the patient.
6. Lying and manipulative behaviors are characteristic (traits/de-escalation) of people with borderline personality disorders.

ABBREVIATIONS

Directions: Write out the meaning for the following abbreviations.

DSM-IV: ______________________________

NOS: ______________________________

APA: ______________________________

COMMUNICATION

The following is a sample dialogue showing how a nurse can intervene when a patient is becoming agitated. The patient, Anna, is speaking in a loud voice and waving her hands in her daughter's face.

Anna: "You must accept Jesus as your savior or you won't go to heaven. Why haven't you been going to church? You'll be damned forever. I'm saved. Why can't you save yourself?"

Nurse (to patient): "Anna, I see your daughter is here to visit. I like the dress you have on, Anna. You have on your new shoes too!"

Nurse (to daughter): "Did you know that Anna managed to dress herself today?"

Daughter: "No, I didn't know that."

Nurse: "Yes, she is all ready to have lunch with you in the garden room. Anna, are you hungry? Shall we go down to lunch?"

The nurse has used distraction to de-escalate Anna's behavior. At the same time, the attention to Anna and the sincere compliments help increase Anna's self-esteem and establish that the nurse is caring and empathetic.

DESCRIPTIVE TERMS

Directions: Place the characteristic behaviors listed below with the correct type of disorder in Cluster A, B, or C as listed in Table 48-6 in the textbook.

clinging
attention-seeking
distrustful
lacks empathy
grandiosity
lability of emotions
impulsive
submissiveness
need for admiration
odd
disregards rights of others
perfectionist
suspicious
fears rejection
need for control
extremely emotional
socially inhibited
eccentric
distorted thinking
feels inadequate
needy
distorted feelings

Cluster A (Odd/Eccentric)	Cluster B (Dramatic/Erratic)	Cluster C (Anxious/Fearful)
1.	1.	1.
2.	2.	2.
3.	3.	3.
4.	4.	4.
5.	5.	5.
6.	6.	6.
	7.	7.
	8.	8.